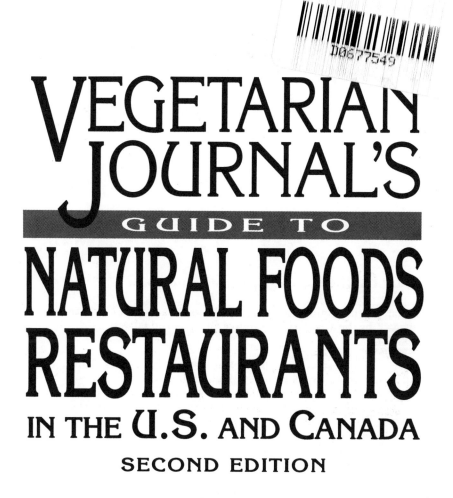

Vegetarian Journal's

GUIDE TO

NATURAL FOODS RESTAURANTS

IN THE U.S. AND CANADA

SECOND EDITION

THE VEGETARIAN RESOURCE GROUP

FOREWORD BY LINDSAY WAGNER

Avery Publishing Group

Garden City Park, New York

Information compiled by: Sally Clinton and Debra Wasserman
Cover Design: Ann Vestal and Rudy Shur
In-House Editor: Linda Comac
Typesetter: Bonnie Fried

Library of Congress Cataloging-in-Publication Data

Vegetarian journal's guide to natural foods restaurants in the U.S. and
  Canada / by the Vegetarian Resource Group.—2nd ed.
    p. cm.
  ISBN 0-89529-654-3 (pbk.)
    1. Vegetarian restaurants—United States—Guidebooks.   2. Natural
  food restaurants—United States—Guidebooks.   3. Vegetarian
  restaurants—Canada—Guidebooks.   4. Natural foods restaurants-
  -Canada—Guidebooks.   I. Vegetarian Resource Group.   II. Vegetarian
  journal.   III. Title: Guide to natural foods restaurants in the U.S.
  and Canada.
  TX907.2.V44   1995
  647.9573—dc20   93-33255
                                                         CIP

Second printing contains updated material

Printed in the United States of America

10   9   8   7   6   5   4   3   2

CONTENTS

Natural Foods Restaurants in Canada

Acknowledgments

As you can imagine, putting together a natural foods restaurant guide of this proportion is a tremendous task. Sally Clinton's huge job would have been impossible without the help of many individuals. A very grateful "thank you" to these members of The Vegetarian Resource Group and readers of *Vegetarian Journal* who recommended restaurants for inclusion in this guide:

Michael Zarky, E.S. Wilson, Libby Williams, Ann and Wes Weaver, Mr. and Ms. Wayman, Gail Watson, Salli Vogler, Karla Verbeck, the Vaupels, Dennie Van Tassel, Lauren Turner, Carol Tracy, Rocky Totino, Judy Terry, Joe Taksel, Christine Szcepanski, Ziona and Tom Swigart, Patricia Swanson, Diane Stathe, Maxine and Stuart Stahler, Sharon Smithline, Wayne Smeltz, Geri Singer, John Lowell Simcox, Eve Sicurella, Keith Seifert, Brad Scott, Susan Havrilla Schneider, David Schneider, Socorro Sargent, Marianne Sanford, Judith Ruiz, Wendy Rozov, John Rouse, Denise Rosen, Mark Rolloson, Max Robinowitz, S. Reilly, Jennifer Raymond, Susan Pritchard, James Pirretti, Sheila Pierson, Melinda Kjarum Peterson, Marcia Pearson, Patti Park, Dan Nussbaum, Sally Nelson, Valerie Mortensen, Margaret Moran, Becky Moody, Lila Moffitt, Judith Miner, Thomas Mills, Lynn Tschantre-Mills, Dorothy Millard, M. McMahon, Marianne Matte, Reed Mangels, Marlene Mannella, Helen Mader, Eric Lynn, Barbara Lovitts, Atsuko Livernois, Susan Lincke, Phoebe Liebig, Ellen Levy, Pat LeBlanc, Kate Lawrence, the Landens, Kathryn Lance, T. Kramer, Stacey Koltonow, Celeste Knofczynski, Robert and Roberta Kalechofsky, Sharon Jonas, Jolene Johnson, Elizabeth Jennings, Matthew Jaquith, J.D. Jackson (*Bunny Huggers' Gazette*), Charlene Inglis, Nancy Howerter, Marilyn Havill, Juliana Harrison, Alison Harlow, Kimberly Hardy, Carole Hamlin, Shari Greenfield, Gigi Green, the Gouldings, Janet Gotlieb, Chris Goss, Shari Goodman, Sheree Gonzalez, Sharlene Goldberg, Amy Gilliland, Peter Gilder, The Fund For Animals, Inc., South Central Regional Office, Powell Foster, Barbara Fontaine, Dan Flaherty,

Mary Faith, Alice Espey, Cate Eisenberg, Pat Ehlinger, Stuart F. Eckman, M. Drummond, David R. Crooks, Matt and Jean Craig, Carmen Corbeil, S. Conroy, Brenda Collins, Suzanne L. Cole, Naomi Cohen, Bill and Ginger Clinton, Mary Clifford, Joan Chowdhury, Bob Chorush (Animal-Free Trade), Elizabeth Caro, Mary Beth Burgmeier, Patti Breitman, Parris Boyd, Darlene Boord, Marilyn Berry, Dr. Richard Berman, Andrea Bennington, Robert Beaumont III, R. Baumgarten, Marcia Anderson, Arnie Alper, Aleithia's Kennels.

Special thanks to Brad Scott, Jennifer Raymond, Jon and Kathleen Shoemaker, Ann Truelove, and Ziona Swigart who helped us meet the deadline of this book. Our appreciation to Rudy Shur of Avery Publishing Group for having a personal interest in this project and to Linda Comac of Avery for editing the final manuscript.

Debra Wasserman
Charles Stahler
Editors of *Vegetarian Journal*,
Coordinators of The Vegetarian
Resource Group

FOREWORD

I am so excited to be writing a foreword for an entire book of restaurants in the United States that cater to vegetarians. I may seem easily pleased. However, I've been a performer struggling to maintain a vegetarian lifestyle for almost twenty years. Here's what a good number of those years on the road looked like . . .

Limousine drives up to the Ritz-Carlton. Chauffeur opens the door. Doorman approaches. "Welcome, Ms. Wagner, glad to have you with us." The Bellman leads the way to the luxurious suite. "Where shall I put the bags?" I reply, "Those three go in the bedroom. THAT BAG stays here." After lifting THAT BAG off the trolley, the bellman is clearly relieved it isn't going very far. And there I am, on location for a film and in one of the finest hotels in the country unpacking THAT BAG. Out comes my two-burner hot plate, two stainless steel pans, brown rice, adzuki beans, tamari sauce, Bragg's amino acid, whole-wheat tortillas and, of course, the ever-present cayenne pepper.

Life was rough in the '70s and '80s for vegetarians on the road. Eventually I learned to inquire (first thing) about the ethnic restaurants in town. (Most other countries around the world seem to understand nutrition without such a heavy carnivorous bent.) That made life much easier and resulted in setting off far fewer smoke alarms.

I now can take my *Guide to Natural Foods Restaurants* with me (in a much smaller bag) and know that my children and I will have a much easier time traveling and working in a healthy, sated way.

God bless the *Guide to Natural Foods Restaurants*!

Lindsay Wagner

INTRODUCTION

One of the aspects of traveling I most treasure is stumbling upon the many wonderful vegetarian or natural foods restaurants in the most unexpected places. Wherever the restaurant happens to be, it seems like an oasis, and the food tastes better than any food you've ever had. Not too long ago, the search for good vegetarian food while traveling did seem comparable to seeking a lake in a desert—an oasis of healthy foods amidst the desolate menus of mainstream eateries. While the United States had been a culinary desert for vegetarians in the past, today it is being reclaimed by health food delis, juice bars, and vegetarian and natural foods restaurants. These eateries are springing up like puddles, and are being joined by numerous mainstream restaurants that are expanding their menus to include options for vegetarians.

A survey conducted by Gallup for the National Restaurant Association in 1991 indicated that when eating out, 20 percent of American adults are likely or very likely to look for a restaurant that serves vegetarian items. This same study revealed that 30 percent or more are likely to order specific vegetarian items. Almost any vegetarian, by personal experience alone, can tell you that these trends are reflected in what is offered at restaurants today, and that the acceptability and availability of vegetarian foods is greater than ever before. Numerous restaurants have "heart-healthy or "light" menu items and still others are willing to accommodate special diets. With all of these factors combined, it seems that now vegetarians often have several options, and no longer have to subsist on steamed vegetables and bread. Now, we more frequently have the opportunity to explore the vast array of creative and delicious tastes, textures, and flavors that are prevalent in the world of healthy, vegetarian cuisine.

In compiling this restaurant guide, we've tried to map out as many vegetarian-oriented treasures as we could find, as well as list the long-established vegetarian oases that have been both welcoming to and appreciated by health-conscious individuals for decades. The information is very usable, listed alphabetically by state, then city, then restaurant. At the beginning of the description of each restaurant, an italicized phrase indicates the type of restaurant (eg., *Italian* or *health-food-store deli*); this is followed by whatever detailed information we can provide. Each listing concludes with a quick reference section in bold that provides some of the basic information you may need. This includes hours or days the restaurants are open; type of service (full, limited, or cafeteria style); availability, if known, of vegan (dairyless) or macrobiotic options; beverages including freshly squeezed juices, espresso/cappuccino, non-alcoholic beer and wine, and wine, beer, and alcohol; provision for take-out; accepted credit cards; and the price range, which is explained in the key box on page 5 and on the bottom of various pages throughout the restaurant listing.

We have tried to make this guide as thorough as possible, but in many cases the information listed is limited by what was provided to us. We wrote to every restaurant requesting that our survey be completed and returned with a copy of the restaurant's menu. Sometimes, however, we did not receive a copy of the menu or the survey was incomplete; consequently, there are some gaps in the information provided. So if "vegan options" or credit card information isn't provided in this publication, you should call the restaurant with your questions. In general, it is wise to check first, especially if you are traveling a good distance to visit a restaurant. Restaurant hours and menus change frequently so there is no guarantee the information listed will remain the same.

We were also limited in our ability to ascertain which menu items are vegan. A listing of "vegan options" may only indicate that our review of the menu led us to the conclusion that vegan options are available. Once again, you might want to double-check to be sure.

While the availability of vegetarian foods certainly has increased significantly, there are still some places where you'll feel as though you're in a desert. In these areas, the selections we have listed may not make your taste buds jump for joy, but there will be options that let you get by. If there aren't any listings for your locality, check out any ethnic restaurants you can find. You can almost always find something to eat at Asian, Indian, Italian, Ethiopian, Mexican, and Middle Eastern eateries. You can also try calling a local health food store, if there is one, and asking for the recommendation of a place to dine. If you are really having trouble, we have listed some local contacts (see page 279) and resources that might be able to help you. We have also included a "vegetarian vacation guide" that lists camps, resorts, spas, bed-and-breakfasts, and tour services that cater to vegetarians.

Finally, if you do find a place we've missed, please let us know!! We never would have been able to compile this guide without the help of vegetarian groups and health-conscious eaters around the country, and we'd love your help in keeping the listing current. For your convenience, a form is included in the back of the book for your replies.

Thank you for thinking and caring about what you eat. I hope this guide makes your travels more enjoyable. And I hope you always find yourself in an oasis of delicious vegetarian foods!

Sally Clinton
The Vegetarian Resource Group,
publisher of *Vegetarian Journal*

Natural Foods Restaurants

Below are the symbols and primary abbreviations that will provide you with important information about each entry.

  ❧ Reviewers' choice
  • Vegetarian restaurant
  •• Vegan restaurant
  $ less than $6
  $$ $6–$12
  $$$ more than $12
  AMX–American Express accepted
  MC–MasterCard accepted
  DISC–Discover Card accepted
  DC–Diner's Club accepted
  VISA–Visa Card accepted
  Non-alc.–Non-alcoholic
  Fresh juices–freshly squeezed in
    the restaurant, e.g., carrot juice

An abbreviated version of the above codes can be found on the bottom of various pages throughout the guide.

In addition, at the beginning of a number of the larger city entries, there appears a listing of towns, suburbs, and/or localities that are in close proximity to the respective city. The names within these listings can be used to locate additional restaurants in these neighboring areas.

ALABAMA

• Golden Temple Natural Grocery & Cafe
1901 11th Ave. S., Birmingham, AL 35205   **(205) 933-6333**

Vegetarian. Sandwiches, salads, drinks, and daily specials are offered at this quick-service vegetarian cafe. Low-salt, low-fat meals are also available. **Open Monday through Saturday. Limited service, vegan options, fresh juices, take-out, VISA/MC, $**

Caribbean House Restaurant
2612B Jordan Lane, Huntsville, AL 35816   **(205) 837-1231**
or (800) 764-7684

Caribbean. A separate vegetarian menu includes oven fried tofu, calypso salad, and veggie burgers. Specials vary day to day, and include barbecued tofu, cornmeal casserole, gluten pepper steak, and Caribbean house pasta and sauce. Try carob chip cookies or tofu cheesecake for dessert. **Open Sunday through Thursday for lunch and dinner, Friday and Saturday lunch only, closed Monday. Limited service, vegan options, catering, take-out, $–$$**

ALASKA

The Marx Brothers Cafe
627 W. 3rd Ave., Anchorage, AK 99501   **(907) 278-2133**

Regional. Some vegetarian options are offered at Marx Brothers, which is also willing to prepare special meals for vegetarians. Herbs, spices, lettuce, and edible flowers are grown on the premises in the summer. **Open for dinner Monday through Saturday. Full service, wine/beer, VISA/MC, $$$**

Cafe de Paris
801 Pioneer Rd., Fairbanks, AK 99701   **(907) 456-1669**

International. Located in a sixty-year-old Victorian house with a beautiful redwood deck, Cafe de Paris serves a wide variety of foods using only the freshest ingredients available. Lettuce and most fresh vegetables are grown for the restaurant by a local gardener. A large variety of European desserts and pastries is served. **Lunch only. Closed Sunday. Full service, cappuccino/espresso, take-out, VISA/MC/AMX/DC, $$**

Gambardella's Pasta Bella
706 2nd Ave., Fairbanks, AK 99701   **(907) 456-3417**

Italian. The Gambardellas pride themselves on generations of fabulous Italian food. Vegetarian entrees are conveniently indicated on the menu. Examples include Pasta Marinara, Fettucini Alfredo, Eggplant Parmesan, Pesto Pasta, and Gourmet Pizza. **Open Monday through Saturday and on Sundays in summer. Full service, cappuc- cino/espresso, wine/beer, take-out, VISA/MC, $—lunch, $$—dinner**

JUNEAU

Fiddlehead Restaurant & Bakery
429 W. Willoughby Ave., Juneau, AK 99801 (907) 586-3150

Natural foods. Fiddlehead offers full gourmet natural foods. Breakfast, lunch, and dinner menus include salads, omelettes, sandwiches, soups, bean burgers, and entrees. Local artwork is displayed, and there is live piano music evenings with a weekend jazz club. The upstairs dining room offers a view of Mt. Juneau. No smoking. **Open daily. Full service, vegan options, fresh juices, wine/beer/alco- hol, take-out, VISA/MC/AMX, $$**

PETERSBURG

Helse Restaurant
#17 Sing Lee Alley, Petersburg, AK 99833 (907) 772-3444

Natural foods. Helse's reputation is based on its soup and homemade bread special offered every day except Monday. Helse offers three vegetarian sandwiches (two of which are vegan), tofu salad, and a garden salad in addition to various seafood and meat sandwiches. A natural foods store is located adjacent to the restaurant. **Open every day except Sunday. Full service, vegan options, cappuccino/espresso, take-out, $$**

ARIZONA

FLAGSTAFF

Cafe Espress
16 N. San Francisco, Flagstaff, AZ 86001 (602) 774-0541

Natural foods. A cafe, bakery, and gallery all in one, with a menu that's actually a little newspaper with ads and interesting info, Cafe Espress can feed your body and mind a variety of vegetarian foods and facts about the area. Options include salads, soups, sandwiches, chili, and hot entrees plus a salad bar. Fresh baked breads, pastries, and desserts. **Open for three meals daily. Full service, vegan options, fresh juices, wine/beer, take-out, VISA, $**

Dara Thai Restaurant
1612 E. Santa Fe Ave., Flagstaff, AZ 86001 (602) 774-0047

Thai. Dara Thai serves delicious vegetarian food from either its regular menu or a separate sheet of additional dishes that includes Veggie Rolls and several tofu specials. The restaurant is also willing to make a vegetarian version of any meat dish. **Open daily except Mondays in winter. Full service, vegan options, alcohol, take-out, VISA/MC, $$**

PHOENIX

Indian Delhi Palace
5050 E. McDowell Rd., Phoenix, AZ 85008   **(602) 244-8181**
Indian. Indian Delhi Palace offers many vegetarian dishes including Roasted Eggplant, Garbanzo Beans with Ginger; Fresh Okra with Onions, Cauliflower and Potatoes; samosas; and fresh breads. **Open for lunch and dinner daily. Full service, beer/wine/alcohol, take-out, VISA/MC/AMX/DISC/DC, $$**

•• Supreme Master Ching Hai Vegetarian House
4812 N. 7th Ave., Phoenix, AZ 85013   **(602) 264-3480**
Vegan/Chinese. Enjoy a wide range of vegan Chinese dishes including Tofu with Vegetables in Brown Sauce, Spring Rolls, Sizzling Rice Soup, and Broccoli with Chinese Mushrooms. **Open Monday through Saturday. Closed Sunday. Full service, vegan only, take-out, MC, $–$$**

Yusef's
15236 N. Cave Creek Rd., Phoenix, AZ 85032   **(602) 867-2957**
Middle Eastern. This combination grocery, restaurant, and deli serves vegetarian dishes including falafel, vegetarian grape leaves, and tabouleh salad. **Open Monday through Saturday for lunch and dinner. Full service, vegan options, take-out, VISA/MC/AMX/DC, $**

PRESCOTT

•• Super Carrot Natural Food Market & Cafe
236 S. Montezuma, Prescott, AZ 86303   **(520) 776-0365**
Vegan. Daily specials instead of a set menu are offered at the Super Carrot. **Open Monday through Friday. Very casual, vegan options, limited service, fresh juices, $**

SCOTTSDALE

Jewel of the Crown
4141 N. Scottsdale Rd., Suite 110, Scottsdale, AZ 85251   **(602) 840-2412**
Indian. Jewel of the Crown offers a wide variety of vegetarian entrees including a curry dish, a lentil dish, and various vegetable dishes. Fresh baked Indian breads are served. **Open daily for lunch and dinner. Full service, non-alc. beer/wine, wine/beer/alcohol, vegan options, catering, take-out, VISA/MC/AMX/DISC/DC, $$**

Marche Gourmet
4121 N. Marshall Way, Scottsdale, AZ 85251   **(602) 994-4568**
Natural foods. Breakfast, lunch, and dinner menus include vegetarian items. Pasta, salads, couscous, and five tofu dishes are offered. **Open daily but closed Sunday evenings. Breakfast offered until 2 P.M. Full service, vegan options, take-out, $$**

SEDONA

La Mediterranee
Atop the Quality Inn, 771 Hwy. 179, Sedona, AZ 86339   (602) 282-7006
Lebanese. Vegetarian selections include Falafel, Stuffed Grape Leaves, Hummus, a vegetarian combination plate, Stuffed Zucchini, homemade bread, plus much more. **Open daily for lunch and dinner. Full service, fresh juices, wine/beer/alcohol, VISA/MC/DISC, $$**

Lotus Garden
Bashas' Shopping Center
164-H Coffee Pot Dr., Sedona, AZ 86336   (602) 282-3118
Chinese. Lotus Garden offers more than fifteen vegetarian dishes, including Mushrooms and Chinese Greens, Eggplant with Garlic Sauce, Tofu in Brown Sauce, and Braised String Beans. **Open daily for lunch and dinner. Full service, vegan options, take-out, $$**

Oaxaca Restaurant & Cantina
231 N. Hwy. 89A, Sedona, AZ 86336   (602) 282-4179
Mexican. Oaxaca offers regional and Southwestern entrees, featuring blue-corn and whole-wheat tortillas. Heart-healthy dishes and vegetarian meals are planned by a registered dietitian. All food is prepared fresh daily without additives or animal fat. **Open every day. Full service, cappuccino/espresso, wine/beer/alcohol, take-out, VISA/MC/DISC, $$**

Sedona Salad Co.
2370 W. Hwy. 89A, Sedona, AZ 86336   (602) 282-0299
American. The Sedona Salad Co. boasts a salad bar with over sixty items, some of which are organic. Sandwiches and potato bar, soup bar, and regular menu. **Limited service, take-out, $**

Thai Spices
2986 W. Hwy. 89A, Sedona, AZ 86336   (602) 282-0599
Thai. Vegetarians can dine on Pad Thai (a rice noodle, vegetable, and tofu dish), Thai Fried Rice, Vegetable Curry, Organic Brown Rice, and other dishes at Thai Spices. **Open Monday through Saturday for lunch and dinner. Open Sunday for dinner only. Full service, vegan options, take-out, VISA/MC, $$**

TEMPE

Gentle Strength Deli
234 W. University, Tempe, AZ 85282   (602) 968-4831

ﺕ Reviewer's choice   ● Vegetarian restaurant   ●● Vegan restaurant
$ less than $6 $$ $6–$12 $$$ more than $12
VISA/AMX/MC/DISC/DC—credit cards accepted
Non-alc.–Non-alcoholic   Fresh juices—freshly squeezed

Natural foods. The Gentle Strength Deli is located within a cooperatively owned natural food store. The deli strives to provide vegetarian, vegan, and macrobiotic choices in a healthy, pleasing atmosphere. Featured are award-winning muffins, noteworthy soups, fresh sandwiches, daily specials, and desserts. **Open daily. Sunday brunch only. Limited service, vegan/macrobiotic options, take-out, VISA/MC, $**

Healthy Heart
6340 S. Rural Rd., Tempe, AZ 85283   **(602) 831-6464**

Natural foods. Healthy Heart restaurant offers low-fat, low-cholesterol food. Meat is offered on the menu, but there is a good selection of vegetarian fare. No nitrates, citrates, or MSG is used. **Closed on Sunday. Self-service, vegan options, take-out, no credit cards, $**

TUCSON

El Adobe Mexican Restaurant
40 W. Broadway, Tucson, AZ 85701   **(602) 791-7458**

Mexican. Located in the historic Charles O. Brown House, one of Tucson's oldest structures, El Adobe features Sonoran style "heart-healthy Mexican food." Butter, lard, MSG, and sulfites are never used. All of the traditional Mexican dishes include beans or vegetable fillings as options. **Full service, vegan options, iced cappuccino, non-alc. beer, wine/beer/alcohol, take-out, VISA/MC/AMX/ DISC/DC, $$**

Good Earth Restaurant & Bakery
6366 E. Broadway, Tucson, AZ 85710   **(602) 745-6600**

American. The restaurant features an extensive menu offering pasta and vegetarian entrees as well as soups, salads, sandwiches, entrees, and desserts. Breads, pastries, and desserts are baked on the premises. Premium wine and beer are served by the glass. **Open daily for breakfast, lunch, and dinner. Full service, fresh juices, espresso/cappuccino, wine/beer, take-out, no credit cards, $$**

• Govinda's
711 E. Blacklidge Dr., Tucson, AZ 85719   **(602) 792-0630**

Vegetarian. Govinda's offers a natural foods buffet featuring international dishes, fresh juice, and a sandwich bar. Most of the dishes are vegan and include items such as Veggie Croquettes in Spinach Sauce, Mock Fish Fillet with Almond Tartar Sauce, Vegetarian Lasagna, etc. **Open Wednesday through Saturday for lunch and dinner. Cafeteria style, vegan options, take-out, VISA/MC, $$**

La Indita
622 N. 4th Ave., Tucson, AZ 85705   **(602) 792-0523**

8578 E. Broadway, Tucson, AZ 85701   **(602) 886-9191**

Mexican. "La Indita," an affectionate term for a little female Indian in Spanish, features the unique recipes of its own "little Indian woman," Maria Garcia, a Tarascan Indian from Michoacan, Mexico. The restaurant offers a mixture of traditional Mexican food, popular Indian fry breads, and Maria Garcia's own family recipes. No lard is used and vegetarian items are indicated on the menu.

Outdoor patio at 4th Ave. location. **Open daily. Full service, vegan options, fresh juices, wine/beer, take-out, $**

Selamat Makan Restaurant
3502 E. Grant Rd., Tucson, AZ 85716   **(602) 325-6755**
Malaysian. Vegetarian dishes are available. **Full service, wine/beer, take-out, VISA/MC/AMX/DISC, $$**

ARKANSAS

EUREKA SPRINGS

Dairy Hollow House
515 Spring St., Eureka Springs, AR 72632   **(501) 253-7444**
Natural foods. This is an award-winning country inn and restaurant. Seven nights a week from April 1 through December 31 and on weekends during February and March, dinner is served at one seating, 7 P.M. The vegetarian owners make sure the soups are vegetarian, and there is always at least one vegetarian selection for the main course. They are willing to accommodate vegans with notice. **Reservations required. Formal, full service, VISA/MC/AMX/DISC/DC/Carte Blanche, $$$**

LITTLE ROCK

Beans, Grains, & Things
300 S. Rodney Parham Rd., Little Rock, AR 72205   **(501) 221-2331**
Natural foods deli. This deli is located in a health food store. **Open daily. Self-service, VISA/MC, $**

CALIFORNIA

ANAHEIM

Alisan Restaurant
115 W. Katella Ave., Anaheim, CA 92802   **(714) 772-4160**
Mandarin/Taiwanese. Specializing in unique and interesting vegetarian dishes, Alisan has a menu that lists more than twenty-five vegetarian items on the back page. Included are many tofu dishes, mushroom creations, and noodle entrees. No MSG or eggs are used. Alisan Restaurant is within walking distance of both Disneyland and the Anaheim Convention Center. **Open daily. Dinner served only on Sundays. Full service, vegan options, wine/beer, take-out, $$**

Ashoka
2021 S. Harbor Blvd., Anaheim, CA 92801   **(714) 663-8501**
Indian. Ashoka offers a wide range of vegetarian Indian dishes including Masala Dosas, vegetable pakoras, samosas, Baked Eggplant, and an okra dish. The restau-

rant is located near the Anaheim Convention Center as well as Disneyland. **Open daily for three meals. Full service, take-out, VISA/MC, $–$$**

Sitar Indian Restaurant
2632 W. La Palma Ave., Anaheim, CA 92801   **(714) 821-8333**

Indian. More than ten vegetarian entrees are offered. **Open daily for lunch and dinner. Full service, vegan options, wine/beer/alcohol, take-out, VISA/MC/ AMX, $$**

ARCATA

Daybreak Cafe
768 18th St., Arcata, CA 95521   **(707) 826-7543**

Natural foods. Ginger wok veggies almondine, vegan Florentine, and vegan daybreak potatoes are a few of the specials at this primarily vegetarian cafe. **Open daily for breakfast and lunch. Limited service, vegan options, smoothies, $**

Spoons Take-Out Kitchen
Arcata Co-op, 811 I St., Arcata, CA 95521   **(707) 822-5947**

Natural foods deli. Spoons is a deli-style kitchen in a natural foods co-op supermarket. Ethnic foods, salads, and entrees are offered, most of which are meatless. Locally grown organic foods are used whenever possible. **Deli style, vegan options, fresh juices, wine/beer in store, take-out, $**

• The Tofu Shop
100 Erickson Ct. #150, Arcata, CA 95521   **(707) 822-7401**

Vegetarian. Arcata's Tofu Shop is modeled after the traditional neighborhood tofu shops in Japan. Fresh tofu is made daily, and a wide variety of tofu entrees, salads, and desserts are offered on the menu. Organic and locally produced ingredients are used when possible. **Open daily. Closed on major holidays. Cafeteria style, vegan options, take-out, $**

• Wildflower Cafe and Bakery
1604 G St., Arcata, CA 95521   **(707) 822-0360**

Macrobiotic/vegetarian. Wildflower features gourmet vegetarian and macrobiotic foods, using local organic fruits and vegetables when possible. Feast on the nut loaf sandwich, West Indian curry, mushroom stroganoff, or one of the many other vegetarian selections. The fresh baked breads and sweets are excellent. Families are welcome. **Open Monday through Saturday for breakfast, lunch, and dinner; Sundays from 10 A.M. to 2 P.M. Full service, vegan/macrobiotic options, fresh juice, catering, no credit cards, $**

ARTESIA

Ashoka
18614 S. Pioneer Blvd., Artesia, CA 90701   **(310) 809-4229**

Indian. See description under Anaheim.

AUBURN

Latitudes
130 Maple St. #11, Auburn, CA 95603 **(916) 885-9535**
Natural foods. Offering multicultural cuisine with an excellent vegetarian selection, Latitudes has a tropical decor with indoor and outdoor dining. It features an extensive micro-brewery and California wine selection. Families are welcome. **Lunch Monday through Friday, dinner Monday and Thursday through Saturday, brunch Sunday. Full service, vegan options, fresh juice, catering, take-out, VISA/MC/AMX, lunch/brunch—$$, dinner—$$$**

BERKELEY

Blue Nile
2525 Telegraph Ave., Berkeley, CA 94704 **(510) 540-6777**
Ethiopian. The Blue Nile of Berkeley serves authentic Ethiopian cuisine in a warm and inviting environment. Vegetarian dishes are clearly indicated and described. **Open daily. Full service, vegan options, wine/beer, take-out, VISA/MC, $–$$**

Brick Hut
3222 Adeline, Berkeley, CA 94703 **(510) 658-5555**
Natural foods. Waffles, omelettes, tofu burgers, chili, and salads are featured. **Open daily for breakfast and lunch. Full service, take-out, $$**

Cafe Intermezzo
2442 Telegraph Ave., Berkeley, CA 94704 **(510) 849-4592**
Natural foods. This restaurant serves mostly vegetarian food. Soups, salads, and sandwiches are featured. **Open daily. Full service, fresh juices, wine/beer, take-out, $**

Elmwood Natural Foods
2944 College Ave., Berkeley, CA 94705 **(510) 841-3871**
Natural foods deli. This organic grocery offers soup, sandwiches, and take-out macrobiotic meals. Non-dairy, whole-grain desserts and baked goods made without refined sugar are also available. **Open daily. Counter service, macrobiotic, take-out, VISA/MC, $**

• Govinda's
2334 Stuart St., Berkeley, CA 94705 **(510) 644-2777**
Vegetarian. Govinda's offers a vegetarian all-you-can-eat buffet. **Closed Sunday and Monday. $**

Long Life Vegi House
2129 University Ave., Berkeley, CA 94704 **(510) 845-6072**
Chinese. The Vegi House menu has more than forty vegetarian entrees including mock chicken, beef and pork, tofu and vegetarian soups, and appetizers such as Pot Stickers or Fresh Garlic Seaweed Salad. Even the pickiest eaters should find something they like here! Upon request, no MSG is used. **Open daily. Full service, vegan options, wine/beer, catering, take-out, VISA/MC, $$**

Maharani
1025 University Ave., Berkeley, CA 94710   (510) 848-7777
Indian. This Indian restaurant has an extensive vegetarian menu. **Open daily. Full service, vegan options, wine/beer, take-out, VISA/MC/AMX/DISC, $$**

Petrouchka
2930 College Ave., Berkeley, CA 94705   (510) 848-7860
Russian. Vegetarian options are available. **Full service, wine/beer, take-out, VISA/MC, $$$**

• Smokey Joe's Cafe
1620 Shattuck, Berkeley, CA 94709   (510) 548-4616
Vegetarian. Vegetarian fast food includes Falafel and Hash Browns. **Open daily. $**

• Vegi Food, Inc.
2083 Vine St., Berkeley, CA 94709   (510) 548-5244
Vegetarian. **Open daily, Mondays for dinner only. Full service, $**

Whole Foods Market
3000 Telegraph Ave., Berkeley, CA 94705   (510) 649-1333
Natural foods deli. **Cafeteria style, fresh juice, take-out, VISA/MC, $–$$**

BEVERLY HILLS

• Akasha's Vegetarian Cuisine
221 N Robertson Blvd., Suite C1, Beverly Hills, CA 90210   (310) 201-0429
Vegetarian catering. This vegetarian delivery service uses only fresh ingredients. Foods are delivered to home or office for individuals, private parties, or conventions. **Monday, Wednesday, Friday delivery. Delivery only, vegan options, $$**

BRENTWOOD

A Votre Santé
13016 San Vicente, Brentwood, CA 90049   (310) 451-1813
Natural foods. Salads, pasta, and Mediterranean cuisine are featured. **Full service, vegan options, fresh juices, wine/beer, take-out, VISA/MC/AMX, $$**

BURLINGAME

•• Osho's Health Express
1207 Capuchino Ave., Burlingame, CA 94010   (415) 348-8015
Vegan. You can dine on pasta, soups, salads, veggie burgers, burritos, and more. **Closed Saturday. Counter service, vegan, fresh juices, take-out, $**

ᘏ Reviewer's choice   • Vegetarian restaurant   •• Vegan restaurant
$ less than $6 $$ $6–$12 $$$ more than $12
VISA/AMX/MC/DISC/DC–credit cards accepted
Non-alc.–Non-alcoholic   Fresh juices–freshly squeezed

Bread of Life
1690 S. Bascom Ave., Campbell, CA 95008 **(408) 371-5000**
Health-food-store deli. Bread of Life offers a salad bar with more than forty items including sushi, quiche, and cakes. Also available are more than thirty salads, twenty desserts, and twenty sandwiches. **Limited service, fresh juices, take-out, VISA/MC/DISC, $**

Royal Taj India Cuisine
1350 Camden Ave., Campbell, CA 95008 **(408) 559-6801**
Indian. Thirteen vegetarian specialties are available at this restaurant offering authentic Indian cuisine at five locations. Pakora, samosa, Dahl Soup, salads, and many Indian breads are also on the menu. **Open daily for lunch and dinner. Full service, vegan options, wine/beer, take-out, VISA/MC/AMX/DISC, $**

Bombay Gate
20252 Saticoy St., Canoga Park, CA 91306 **(818) 998-2727**
Indian. Choose from several traditional vegetarian Indian dishes like samosas, breads, dals, and several entrees. **Open Wednesday-Monday for lunch and dinner. Closed Tuesday. Full service, vegan options, VISA/MC/AMX/DISC, $$**

• Follow Your Heart Natural Foods and Cafe ❧
21825 Sherman Way, Canoga Park, CA 91303 **(818) 348-3240**
Vegetarian. This classic vegetarian restaurant offers an excellent selection of natural foods—salads, sandwiches, entrees with vegetarian (rennet-free) cheese, tofu dishes, and other vegetarian favorites. The beverages consist of juices, teas, raw milk, and shakes. The full breakfast menu, weekend brunch, and all dishes are vegetarian without eggs, sugar, or harmful additives. Heart-healthy items are indicated on the menu. **Open for three meals daily. Full service, vegan options, fresh juices, organic coffee, BYOB, take-out, VISA/MC, $$**

Book Cafe
1475 41st Ave., Capitola, CA 95010 **(408) 462-4415**
Natural foods. The Book Cafe features Lasagna, soups, deli salads, and pastries. **Closed Sunday. Counter service, $**

• Dharma's Restaurant
4250 Capitola Rd., Capitola, CA 95010 **(408) 462-1742**
Vegetarian. A smiling cow wearing dark sunglasses graces the front of Dharma's menu. This is followed by statistics on the number of rainforest acres and cows saved by eating Dharma's vegetarian burgers. No bull! A serious mission with a sense of humor and excellent food is a combination worth exploring. Dharma's offers a wide range of international vegetarian dishes including Mexican, Italian, Chinese, Japanese, and Thai in addition to the old American stand-bys, great muffins, and desserts. The

majority of the foods are organic. **Open for three meals daily. Cafeteria style, limited service, many vegan options, fresh juices, espresso, wine/beer, take-out, $**

CARMEL
Royal Taj India Cuisine
230 Crossroads Blvd., Carmel, CA 93923   **(408) 624-9110**
Indian. See entry under Campbell, CA.

CARMICHAEL
• Mima's Homestyle All Vegetarian Kitchen
7630 Fair Oaks Blvd., Carmichael, CA 95608   **(916) 944-7000**
Vegetarian. Located inside Carmichael Natural Food Market, this restaurant offers soups, salads, sandwiches, veggie burgers, Mexican dishes, and more. Many of the meals meet Dr. McDougal's guidelines for a low-fat diet. There's also a salad bar. **Open for lunch Monday through Friday. Closed Saturday and Sunday. Limited service, vegan options, take-out, $**

CERRITOS
• Madhu's Dasaprakash
11321 E. 183rd St., Cerritos, CA 90701   **(310) 924-0879**
Vegetarian/Indian. South Indian vegetarian cuisine is featured at this all-vegetarian restaurant. The usual vegetarian Indian dishes are available, such as samosas, pakodas, and poories, and there are many more unique dishes featuring crêpes and stuffed patties. **Closed on Monday. Full service, vegan options, wine/beer, take-out, VISA/MC, $**

CHICO
• Cafe Sandino
817 Main St., Chico, CA 95928   **(916) 894-6515**
Vegetarian. Home of "Today's Tomales," Cafe Sandino is a vegetarian restaurant that strives to use organically grown ingredients, and uses unrefined canola and olive oils. **Lunch Monday through Saturday, dinner Wednesday through Saturday. Full service, vegan options, organic juice, organic coffee, wine/beer, take-out, $–$$**

CORONA DEL MAR
Mayur
2931 E. Coast Hwy., Corona del Mar, CA 92625   **(714) 675-6622**
Indian. Mayur offers several vegetarian entrees including Vegetable Jalfrezi, Dal, Roasted Eggplant, and Creamed Spinach with Cheese. **Open daily for lunch and dinner. Full service, vegan options, take-out, VISA/MC/AMX, $$**

CORONADO

Stretch's Coronado Cafe
943 Orange Ave., Coronado, CA 92118 **(619) 435-8886**
Natural foods. Stretch's takes pride in the quality of the food and the variety offered to both vegetarians and non-vegetarians. All food is prepared fresh daily. **Self-serve, fresh juices, wine, take-out, $**

Tiffiny's Deli-Juice Bar
1120 Adella Ave., Coronado, CA 92118 **(619) 437-1368**
Natural foods. Amidst old-fashioned decor, this deli-juice bar offers sandwiches and smoothies. Open daily for breakfast, lunch, and dinner. **Counter service, vegan options, beer/wine, catering, take-out, VISA/MC, $**

Viva Nova
1138 Orange Ave., Coronado, CA 92118 **(619) 435-2124**
Health-food-store deli. Enjoy fresh juices, hot veggie pocket sandwiches, quiche, baked potatoes, Vegetarian Chili, burritos, enchiladas, and soup at Viva Nova. **Limited service, fresh juices, vegan options, take-out, $**

COSTA MESA

Forty Carrots
South Coast Plaza Mall, Bristol at 405
Costa Mesa, CA 92626 **(714) 556-9700**
Natural foods. Forty Carrots serves pasta, Mexican foods, soups, and salad. **Open daily. Full service, wine/beer, VISA/MC/AMX, $$**

Mother's Market & Kitchen
225 E. 17th St., Costa Mesa, CA 92627 **(714) 631-4741**
Natural foods. Mother's has a vegetarian menu except for tuna. Centrally located within the natural foods store, the restaurant offers a wide assortment of delicious appetizers, salads, entrees, pastas, sandwiches, and ethnic and side dishes. A children's menu is available. **Full service, fresh juices, non-alc. wine/beer, take-out, $**

CULVER CITY

• Chandri Vegetarian Cuisine of India
3808 Bagley Ave., Culver City, CA 90232 **(310) 839-0482**
Vegetarian. This vegetarian Indian restaurant offers a wide range of appetizers, soups, breads, and entrees. **Open daily for lunch and dinner. Full service, vegan options, take-out, $–$$**

CUPERTINO

Bread of Life
10983 N. Wolfe Rd., Cupertino, CA 95014 **(408) 257-7000**
Health-food-store deli. See entry under Campbell, CA.

The Good Earth
20807 Stevens Creek Blvd., Cupertino, CA 95014   (408) 252-3555
Natural foods. Enjoy wok dishes, Vegetarian Scramble, Tofu Scramble, Vegetarian Burger, burritos, tostadas, Eggplant Sandwich, salads, Pasta Primavera, Walnut Mushroom Au Gratin, Guatamalan Rice and Tofu. **Open daily. Full service, wine/beer, VISA/MC/AMX, $$**

Hobee's Restaurant
21267 Stevens Creek Blvd., Cupertino, CA 95014   (408) 255-6010
Restaurant chain. Mexican favorites, Veggie Patty, Black Bean Chili, and a salad bar make up the vegetarian options at Hobee's. **Open daily. Full service, fresh juices, wine/beer, take-out, VISA/MC, $$**

DAVIS

• The Blue Mango
330 G St., Davis, CA 95616   (916) 756-2616
Vegetarian. A cooperatively run restaurant, Blue Mango features burritos, tostadas, sandwiches, salads, and Indian entrees. Enjoy indoor and outdoor seating, and live entertainment. **Full service, vegan options, $**

DEL MAR

•• Garden Taste
1555 Camino Del Mar #101A
Del Mar Plaza, Del Mar, CA 92014   (619) 793-1500
Vegan. All organic, this restaurant offers raw soups, sprouted salads, non-wheat, non-dairy pizza, and sprouted veggie burgers. No oil, sugar, or salt is used. **Open daily, full service, completely vegan, fresh juices, take-out, $**

Souplantation/Sweet Tomatoes
Corporate offices in Del Mar, CA 92014   (619) 792-0713
Restaurant chain. An extensive salad bar includes fresh bakery items, a vegetarian soup option, fresh fruits, and desserts. There are twenty-six locations in Northern California. **Closed Sunday. Buffet style, take-out, $–$$**

DUNCAN MILLS

The Blue Heron
1 Steelhead Blvd., Duncan Mills, CA 95430   (707) 865-2269
Ethnic foods. Ethnic dishes, salads, and pasta dishes are featured. **Open daily in summer. Hours vary in winter. Wine/beer/alcohol, take-out, VISA/MC, $$$**

---

๕ Reviewers' choice   • Vegetarian restaurant   •• Vegan restaurant
$ less than $6 $$ $6–$12 $$$ more than $12
VISA/AMX/MC/DISC/DC—credit cards accepted
Non-alc.—Non-alcoholic   Fresh juices—freshly squeezed

EMERYVILLE

Hobee's Restaurant
5765 Christie Ave., Emeryville, CA 95608   **(415) 652-5944**
Restaurant chain. See entry under Cupertino, CA.

ENCINITAS

• Casady's Cafe and Deli
745 1st St., Encinitas, CA 92024   **(619) 633-3663**
Vegetarian. Striving to provide organic, unrefined foods is a goal at Casady's. Try the cornucopia cakes—egg and dairy-free pancakes—for breakfast, or have one of the vegetarian sandwiches or specials. Dine in the cafe, or on the front porch in good weather. An entire menu of fresh-made juices is also available. **Open daily for lunch and dinner. Limited service, vegan options, fresh juices, take-out, VISA/MC/AMX/DISC/DC, $**

• Fountain of Juice
1163 First St., Encinitas, CA 92024   **(619) 944-0612**
Vegetarian. This vegetarian restaurant offers an organic salad bar and a wide variety of entrees including Curried Vegetables, Black Bean Burritos, and mock meat dishes. Open daily. **Counter service, vegan options, organic juices, smoothies, catering, take-out, $**

• Roxy Restaurant and Ice Cream
517 First St., Encinitas, CA 92024   **(619) 436-5001**
Vegetarian. International dishes are featured. **Open daily. Full service, take-out, fresh juices, wine/beer/alcohol, VISA/MC/AMX/DISC, $$**

EUREKA

• East West Center
1122 M St., Eureka, CA 95501   **(707) 445-2290**
Vegetarian. On Thursday nights only, Meredith McCarty, author of *Fresh*, presents a wonderful four- to six-course feast including fresh market produce, organic grains and beans, and great desserts. Reservations are required by Wednesday; call Tuesday through Friday from 9 A.M. to 4 P.M. **Open for dinner Thursday. Reservations required. Limited service, macrobiotic options, $$**

Tomaso's Tomato Pies
216 E St., Eureka, CA 95501   **(707) 445-0100**
Italian. Tomaso's, an institution in Old Town, Eureka, for many years, serves spinach pies, spinzones, vegetarian soups, salads, whole-wheat pizza, and various vegetarian entrees. **Full service, wine/beer, take-out, VISA/MC/AMX/DISC, $$**

Tomo Japanese Restaurant
2120 4th St., Eureka, CA 95501   **(707) 444-3318**
Japanese. Tomo serves Japanese country-style whole food, and traditional and non-fish sushi. Most entrees are available without meat. **Full service, wine/beer, macrobiotic, VISA/MC/DISC, $$**

FAIR OAKS

Eat Your Vegetables
11755 Fair Oaks Blvd., Fair Oaks, CA 95628   **(916) 863-7050**
Natural foods. A mega salad bar includes soup, salad, baked potato, pasta, breads, and desserts. Vegan and wheat-free options featured daily. **Open daily. Cafeteria style, VISA/MC, $$**

• Sunflower Natural Foods Drive In
10344 Fair Oaks Blvd., Fair Oaks, CA 95628   **(916) 967-4331**
Vegetarian. Vegetarian fast food—including burgers, burritos, Chili, and sandwiches—is made primarily on the premises with an emphasis on raw foods. Sunflower is adjacent to a park. **Open daily. Limited service, take-out, VISA/MC/ DISC, $**

FOSTER CITY

Joy Restaurant
1495 Beach Park Blvd., Foster City, CA 94404   **(415) 345-1762**
Mandarin/Szechuan. Several statements on Joy's menu assure vegetarians they are welcome and encouraged to request any special vegetarian dish they would like. Any type of meatless "chicken" is available, and cooking without meat and eggs is not a problem here. Vegetarian appetizers, soup, and entrees are offered. **Open daily. Full service, vegan options, wine/beer, take-out, VISA/MC/AMX, $$**

FREMONT

Hobee's Restaurant
39222 Fremont Blvd., Fremont, CA 94538   **(510) 797-1244**
Restaurant chain. See entry under Cupertino, CA.

• Manju Farsan House
Freemont Shopping Center
40645 Fremont Blvd., Fremont, CA 94538   **(510) 656-2336**
Vegetarian/Indian. Indian vegetarian fast-food items are offered including samosas and many entrees. **Open daily for lunch and dinner. Full service, vegan options, catering, take-out, $**

FULLERTON

Chin Ting
1939 Sunnycrest Dr., Fullerton, CA 92635   **(714) 738-1978**
Chinese. Choose from several vegetarian dishes. **Open Sunday through Friday dinner only. Open Saturday for lunch and dinner. Full service, vegan options, take-out, VISA/MC/AMX/DISC/DC, $$**

Rutabegorz

211 N. Pomona, Fullerton, CA 92632 **(714) 871-1632**

International. Specializing in homemade food, this bohemian-style coffeehouse has an extensive coffee menu as well as Veggie Burritos, pastas, Spinach Lasagna, Stuffed Mushrooms, etc. **Closed Sunday. Full service, vegan options, fresh juices, wine/beer/alcohol, $$**

GARBERVILLE

Woodrose Cafe

911 Redwood Dr., Garberville, CA 95440 **(707) 923-3191**

Natural foods. The many vegetarian options contain a lot of cheese and eggs. Organic and local ingredients are used. **Open for breakfast daily; open for lunch Monday through Friday. Full service, vegan options, fresh juices, non-alc. beer, wine/beer, take-out, $**

GARDEN GROVE

New Moon II Healthfood Store & Lunch Bar

12536 Valley View St., Garden Grove, CA 92645 **(714) 893-0301**

Health-food-store deli. New Moon II offers soups, sandwiches, and non-dairy frozen desserts. Open for lunch daily. **Limited service, vegan options, take-out, VISA/ MC, $**

Yogurt and More

12892 Main St., Garden Grove, CA 92640 **(714) 530-9505**

Natural foods. Dine on yogurt, vegetarian lasagna, burritos, avocado sandwiches, and a wide variety of salads. **Open Monday through Saturday for lunch and early dinner. Limited service, take-out, $**

GLENDALE

• Glendale Adventist Medical Center

1509 Wilson Terrace, Glendale, CA 91206 **(818) 409-8090**

Vegetarian. **Open for three meals daily. Cafeteria style, take-out, $**

GOLETA

Good Earth

5955 Calle Real, Goleta, CA 93117 **(805) 683-6101**

Natural foods. This restaurant offers soups and salads, casseroles, stir-fries, and Mexican specialties. **Open daily for three meals. Full service, wine/beer, catering, take-out, VISA/MC/AMX/DISC, $$**

ﱠ Reviewers' choice   • Vegetarian restaurant   •• Vegan restaurant
$ less than $6 $$ $6–$12 $$$ more than $12
VISA/AMX/MC/DISC/DC–credit cards accepted
Non-alc.–Non-alcoholic   Fresh juices–freshly squeezed

• Healing Moon Health Foods
523 Main St., Half Moon Bay, CA 94019   **(415) 726-7881**
Health-food-store deli. Entrees include soups, brown rice dishes, pasta, tofu, Veggie Burgers, and salads. All foods are organic, and soy cheese is used. **Open daily. Counter service, vegan options, take-out, $**

Siam Clift Cuisine of Thailand
1605 W. Pacific Coast Hwy. #106, Harbor City, CA 90710   **(310) 325-0844**
Thai. Enjoy Thai curry, stir-fried entrees, and various specials in a beautiful dining room. **Closed Sunday. Full service, wine/beer, catering, take-out, VISA/MC/AMX, $**

• The Spot Natural Food Restaurant
110 Second St., Hermosa Beach, CA 90254   **(310) 376-2355**
Vegetarian. This friendly, "local" beach restaurant offers only vegetarian fare with many vegan items. Specialties include burritos, Veggie Burgers, and steamed vegetable plates ("Steamers") with tasty sauces. **Open daily. Full service, vegan options, fresh juices, wine/beer, take-out, $$**

Flowering Tree
8253 Santa Monica Blvd., W. Hollywood, CA 90046   **(213) 654-4332**
Natural foods. Flowering Tree features Veggie Burgers, Baked Sesame Tofu, and other delicious entrees. **Open late daily. Counter service, vegan options, non-alc. beer, take-out, $**

Gengis Cohen
740 N. Fairfax Ave., Hollywood, CA 90046   **(213) 653-0640**
Chinese. No MSG is used, but be sure to request no chicken broth. An acoustic music showroom is featured. **Open for lunch Monday through Friday, dinner daily. Full service, vegan options, wine/beer/alcohol, take-out, VISA/MC/AMX/DC, $$**

• Parus Indian Vegetarian Restaurant
5140 Sunset Blvd., Hollywood, CA 90027   **(213) 661-7600**
Vegetarian/Indian. Most of the main dishes are non-dairy, corn oil is used for cooking, and exotic Indian beverages are available. A brunch special is offered on Saturday and Sunday. Patio service is available. **Full service, wine/beer, take-out, VISA/MC, $$**

The Source Restaurant & Sidewalk Cafe
8301 Sunset Blvd., W. Hollywood, CA 90069   **(213) 656-6388**
Natural foods. This is "the place to see and be seen" says *The Source.* The natural foods menu includes some gourmet vegetarian dishes such as Whole-Wheat Lasagna, Mother's Eggplant, and Cheese and Walnut Loaf. There is only one vegan

entree on the menu, however. Sandwiches, appetizers, and salads make up the rest of the menu. Outdoor patio. **Breakfast served every day. Full service, fresh juices, espresso/cappuccino, take-out, VISA/MC/AMX/DC, $$**

• Eight Immortals of Tao
8841 Adams Ave., Huntington Beach, CA 92646　　　　　　**(714) 965-8894**
Vegetarian. Enjoy creative, unusual, and tasty vegetarian dishes including tofu, vegetables, and mock meat plus six appetizers and seven soups. **Open daily for lunch and dinner. Full service, vegan options, take-out, $–$$**

Mother's Market & Kitchen
19770 Beach Blvd., Huntington Beach, CA 92648　　　　　　**(714) 963-6667**
Natural foods. See entry under Costa Mesa, California.

The Wok Chinese Restaurant
7572 Edinger Ave., Huntington Beach, CA 92648　　　　　　**(714) 842-5698**
Mandarin/Szechuan Chinese. The Wok serves natural and fresh Chinese food without MSG. Vegetarian dishes are available. **Open daily. Full service, vegan options, wine/beer, take-out, VISA/MC, $**

Clay Oven
15435 Jeffrey Rd., Irvine, CA 92714　　　　　　**(714) 552-2851**
Indian. Clay Oven, which takes a healthy approach to Indian cooking, offers nine vegetable entrees. **Full service, vegan options, wine/beer, VISA/MC/AMX/DISC, $$**

• Juice Club
17595 Harvard Ave., Suite F, Irvine, CA 92714　　　　　　**(714) 250-3348**
Vegetarian juice bar. Enjoy a wide variety of fresh juices at this juice bar. **Open daily. Counter service, vegan options, take-out, $**

• Ché Café
UCSD, 9500 Gilman Dr., Student Ctr., 0323-C
La Jolla, CA 92093　　　　　　**(619) 534-2311**
Vegetarian. This is a not-for-profit vegetarian collective on the UCSD campus. Ché Café serves mostly vegan foods. Live music shows are held most weekends. **Always open Wednesday; call for other times and information. Limited service, take-out, $**

Star of India Restaurant
1025 Prospect St. #100, La Jolla, CA 92037　　　　　　**(619) 459-3355**
Indian. See entry under Encinitas, CA.

• Cafe Zinc

350 Ocean Ave., Laguna Beach, CA 92651   **(714) 494-6302**

Vegetarian. Cafe Zinc offers salads, soups, mini- and full-sized pizzas. Indoor and outdoor seatings are available. **Hours vary. Call for information. Counter service, wine/beer, take-out, $**

•• The Downtown Stand

347 Mermaid St., Laguna Beach, CA 92651   **(714) 494-9499**

Vegan. See The Stand below.

• Gauranga's

285 Legion St., Laguna Beach, CA 92651   **(714) 494-7029**

Vegetarian. If you're hungry, Gauranga's all-you-can-eat vegetarian buffet might be just what you need. The steam table includes two soups, brown and basmati rice, steamed veggies, pasta and sauce, mixed Indian-style veggies, and entrees that vary daily. Tuesday and Thursday entrees are vegan. No eggs are used. **Closed Sunday. Cafeteria style, vegan options, take-out, VISA/MC, $**

•• The Stand Natural Foods Restaurant

238 Thalia St., Laguna Beach, CA 92651   **(714) 494-8101**

Vegan. If you're looking for a restaurant with a commitment to quality and excellent vegan food, then The Stand is for you. In business for more than twenty-one years, The Stand offers a wide selection of international salads, sandwiches, side orders, burritos, tamales, main dishes, and treats. All foods are vegan and made without refined sugar, salt, or artificial ingredients. **Open daily. Limited service, completely vegan, fresh juices, take-out, $**

•• Garden of Eatin' Cafe

474 Magnolia Ave., Larkspur, CA 94939   **(415) 927-7611**

Vegan. Eden may be a ways from Larkspur, California, but the Garden of Eatin' does offer a bit of heaven for vegans and others who want healthful, high-quality fast food in a charming environment. Located in a historic building in downtown Larkspur, the Garden offers sandwiches, veggie hot dogs, burgers, oil-free fries, salads, and rolls with some ethnic options. Customers can eat inside or outside on the patio in the herb and flower garden. No sugar, white flour, preservatives, or artificial ingredients are used; honey is used in some items. Organic goods are used when possible. **Open Monday through Saturday. Deli counter, vegan options, fresh juices, organic coffee, catering, take-out, $**

ʔ₳ Reviewers' choice   • Vegetarian restaurant   •• Vegan restaurant
$ less than $6 $$ $6–$12 $$$ more than $12
VISA/AMX/MC/DISC/DC—credit cards accepted
Non-alc.—Non-alcoholic   Fresh juices—freshly squeezed

LEUCADIA

Papa Gus Restaurant
698 Hwy. 101, Leucadia, CA 92024 **(619) 944-9168**
Caribbean/Mexican. This cafe offers many vegetarian options including Fruit Pancakes, Tamales with Soy Cheese, Caribbean Veggie Pizza, burritos, quesadillas, non-dairy smoothies, plus much more. **Open daily. Limited service, vegan options, smoothies, fresh juices, take-out, $**

LOMA LINDA

• Loma Linda University Medical Center Cafeteria
Anderson and Barton Rds., Loma Linda, CA 92354 **(714) 824-4365**
Vegetarian. The cafeteria offers soups, salads, casseroles, and mock meat dishes. **Open daily. Cafeteria service, vegan options, take-out, $**

LOS ANGELES

(For restaurant listings in the surrounding areas, see Anaheim, Beverly Hills, Brentwood, Canoga Park, Costa Mesa, Fullerton, Garden Grove, Glendale, Harbor City, Hermosa Beach, Hollywood, Huntington Beach, Irvine, Laguna Beach, Monterey Park, Newport Beach, Northridge, Norwalk, Orange, Pasadena, Riverside, Rosemead, Santa Ana, Santa Monica, Sherman Oaks, South Pasadena, Studio City, Tarzana, Topanga Canyon, Tustin, Venice, Ventura, and Westlake Village.)

A Votre Santé
345 N. LaBrea, Los Angeles, CA 90036 **(213) 857-0412**
Natural foods. See entry under Brentwood, CA.

•• Beverly Hills Juice Club
8382 Beverly Blvd., Los Angeles, CA 90048 **(213) 655-8300**
Juice bar. Enjoy fresh juices and some foods prepared from local organic produce. Shakes and wheatgrass are made to order. Tahini, Sauerkraut, Hummusushi, Applesauce, Dairy-free Ice Cream, and other treats are prepared on the premises. **Open Monday through Saturday. Fresh juices, take-out only, $**

• The Bodhi Garden Vegetarian Restaurant
1498 Sunset Blvd. #2, Los Angeles, CA 90026 **(213) 250-9023**
Vegetarian/Chinese. Many appetizers, lunch specials, soups, and entrees are offered. **Closed Tuesday. Full service, vegan options, take-out, $**

• Country Life Vegetarian Buffet
888 S. Figueroa St., Los Angeles, CA 90017 **(213) 489-4118**
Vegetarian. International vegetarian cuisine is offered in a contemporary setting with a pleasant atmosphere. The buffet is composed of creative entrees that rotate daily, including Nutty Tofu Croquettes and Vegetable Pocket Quiches. There are also desserts and home-baked goods such as Tofu Cheesecake, and a full salad and

fruit bar. **Open for lunch Monday through Friday. Buffet, vegan options, fresh juices, catering, take-out, $**

Don's Fountain of Health
3606 W. 6th St., Los Angeles, CA 90020   **(213) 387-6621**
Natural foods. Sample the Veggie Burgers, Chili, freshly squeezed juices, and cakes and cookies made on the premises. **Open daily. Full service, fresh juices, catering, take-out, $**

Eat a Pita
465 N. Fairfax Ave., Los Angeles, CA 90036   **(213) 651-0188**
Mediterranean. Eat a Pita offers many vegetarian selections including Tabouli, Hummus, Baba Ghanouj, and Falafel. Seating is outdoors in a casual, friendly environment. **Open daily for lunch and dinner. Counter service, vegan options, take-out, $**

Erewhon Foods Deli
7660 Beverly Blvd., Los Angeles, CA 90048   **(213) 937-0777**
Health-food-store deli. The menu features Stir-Fried Veggies, Steamed Veggies, Millet Loaf, lentil dishes, and Spinach Lasagna. **Open daily. Counter service, VISA/MC, $$**

• Fragrant Vegetable 🍃
11859 Wilshire Blvd., Los Angeles, CA 90025   **(310) 312-1442**
Vegetarian/Chinese. Mock meat, mock poultry, and mock fish dishes made with tofu and wheat gluten are featured. **Open daily. Full service, reservations recommended, vegan options, wine/beer, take-out, VISA/MC/AMX, $$**

• Govinda's
3764 Watseko Ave., Los Angeles, CA 90034   **(310) 836-1269**
Vegetarian. Govinda's specializes in natural foods, featuring a variety of ethnic cuisines. Dairy products are used, but no eggs. **Closed on Sunday. Full service, catering, take-out, VISA/MC, $**

Inaka Natural Foods Restaurant
131 S. La Brea Ave., Los Angeles, CA 90036   **(213) 936-9353**
Macrobiotic/natural foods. No eggs or dairy products are used, and foods are vegetarian except for some fish plates. Brown rice and different beans are featured with vegetables. **Closed Sunday; open for dinner Monday through Saturday and for lunch Monday through Friday. Full service, vegan options, take-out, VISA/MC, $$**

India's Tandoori
5947 W. Pico Blvd., Los Angeles, CA 90035   **(213) 936-2050**
Indian. Fresh clay-oven-baked breads are the specialty here. India's Tandoori has a vegetarian section on the menu plus vegetarian appetizers such as samosas and Onion Balls. **Open daily. Full service, vegan options, wine/beer, take-out, VISA/ MC, $**

Kukatonor African Restaurant
4212 W. Pico Blvd., Los Angeles, CA 90019   **(213) 937-2208**

African/American. At Kukatonor (meaning "We are one"), African masks, plants, and the echoing drums of African music provide an authentic atmosphere in which to sample African cuisine. Kukatonor offers a good range of unique, tasty, and filling vegetarian foods that are traditional Liberian dishes. A local member recommends the "Fufu," a dumpling-like staple, with Palava Sauce or Groundnut Stew. **Open daily. Full service, vegan options, fresh juices, wine/beer, take-out, VISA/MC, $$**

La Salsa

Corporate office   **(213) 857- 1275 or (800) La Salsa**

Restaurant chain. This Mexican food restaurant chain has many locations throughout California and gladly accommodates vegetarian requests. Call for locations. **Open daily. Full service, take-out, $**

La Toque

8171 Sunset Blvd., Los Angeles, CA 90046   **(213) 656-7515**

French. Fine dining at this French restaurant always includes vegetarian options. The menu changes daily, and reservations are required. **Full service, fresh juices, non-alc. beverages, wine/beer/alcohol, VISA/MC/AMX, $$$**

• Mani's Bakery

519 S. Fairfax Ave., Los Angeles, CA 90036   **(213) 938-8800**

Vegetarian bakery/coffeehouse. Try Mani's Bakery for after-dinner treats such as turnovers, deep dish pies, and truffles. **Open late daily. Counter service, take-out, VISA/MC/AMX/DISC, $**

Mother Earth Restaurant

11277 National Blvd., Los Angeles, CA 90064   **(213) 477-0555**

Natural foods. Over ten vegetarian entrees are listed on Mother Earth's menu. The vegan options include Fried Tofu, Stuffed Acorn Squash, and Stuffed Cabbage Rolls with Vegetables. No preservatives, added sugar, or salt is used. **Open for lunch and dinner every day except Sunday. Full service, vegan options, fresh juices, wine/beer/alcohol, take-out, VISA/MC, $–$$**

• Naturally Fast

11661 Santa Monica Blvd., Los Angeles, CA 90025   **(310) 444-7886**

Vegetarian. This natural fast-food restaurant features inexpensive soups, salads, baked potatoes, sandwiches, burgers, hot entrees, daily vegan specials, and desserts without eggs or sugar. **Open daily. Full service, vegan options, take-out, $**

• Nature Club Cafe 🍴

7174 Melrose Ave., Los Angeles, CA 90046   **(213) 931-8994**

🍴 Reviewers' choice   • Vegetarian restaurant   •• Vegan restaurant
$ less than $6 $$ $6–$12 $$$ more than $12
VISA/AMX/MC/DISC/DC—credit cards accepted
Non-alc.—Non-alcoholic   Fresh juices—freshly squeezed

Vegetarian. This relatively new vegetarian restaurant offers a wide variety of dishes including salads, sandwiches, veggie burgers, pasta primavera, Szechuan potstickers, vegetable samosas, and more. **Open for lunch and dinner Monday through Saturday. Full service, fresh juices, vegan options, espresso/cappuccino, catering, take-out, VISA/MC/AMC, $–$$**

Nowhere Cafe ᶻᵃ

8009 Beverly Blvd., Los Angeles, CA 90048   **(213) 655-8895**

Gourmet natural foods. With its gourmet natural cuisine, Nowhere will take your taste buds where they've never been before. Next door to the Nowhere natural foods market, the cafe takes extra measures to utilize fresh, organic produce in its dishes, which are often free from fats, oils, preservatives, sugar, and dairy products. Nowhere caters to special diets. **Open daily. Full service, vegan options, fresh juices, espresso/cappuccino, wine/beer, catering, take-out, VISA/MC/AMX/DISC, $$**

Osteria Romana Orsini

9575 W. Pico Blvd., Los Angeles, CA 90035   **(310) 277-6050**

Italian. Osteria features a large selection of meatless items. Open Monday through Saturday for lunch and dinner. **Closed Sunday. Full service, wine/beer/ alcohol, take-out, VISA/MC/AMX, $$–$$$**

Shekarchi Restaurant

1712 Westwood Blvd., Los Angeles, CA 90024   **(310) 474-6911**

Persian. Several vegetarian plates are featured. **Open daily. Full service, catering, take-out, VISA/MC/AMX, $$**

White Memorial Medical Center Cafeteria

1720 Brooklyn Ave., Los Angeles, CA 90025   **(213) 268-5000 x 1318**

Hospital cafeteria. This cafeteria is in a Seventh-day Adventist hospital. **Open daily. Cafeteria style, take-out, $$**

LOS GATOS

• Richard's Natural Foods

111 E. Main St., Los Gatos, CA 95032   **(408) 354-0588**

Vegetarian health-food-store deli. Enjoy soups, an organic salad bar, and dairyless cakes and pies. **Open daily. Counter service, take-out, VISA/MC, $**

Rooh's Cafe Salsa

New Town Center, 15515 Los Gatos Blvd.
Los Gatos, CA 95032   **(408) 358-ROOH**

Mexican/restaurant chain. Entrees include Enchilada de Rooh's featuring lentils, and pancake pizzas. Rooh's does not use lard, sugar, preservatives, or MSG. Nutritional fact sheets about the food are available. **Open daily. Limited service, take-out, VISA/MC, $**

MENLO PARK

Flea Street Cafe
3607 Alameda de la Pulgas, Menlo Park, CA 94025   **(415) 854-1226**
Natural foods. The chef at this very fancy and formal restaurant will improvise to accommodate vegans. Organic produce is used. **Open daily for lunch and dinner, weekends for brunch. Full service, vegan options, wine/beer, take-out, VISA/MC, $$$**

Fresh Choice
600 Santa Cruz Cove, Menlo Park, CA 94025   **(415) 323-4061**
American. The salad selection is extensive and there is always one vegetarian soup and usually at least one vegetarian pasta. Fixed price includes everything including bread and dessert. **Open daily. Cafeteria style, wine/beer, VISA/ MC, $$**

Late for the Train
150 Middlefield Rd., Menlo Park, CA 94025   **(415) 321-6124**
Natural foods. This country-style restaurant prepares food to order, and serves meals in the "wholest form possible." Produce is organic when available. Chemicals, preservatives, and artificial coloring are not added. Most of the vegetarian dishes include dairy. There's a full breakfast menu. **Open daily but hours vary. Full service, espresso/cappuccino, wine/beer, take-out, VISA/MC, $$**

MISSION VIEJO

The Healthy Gourmet
23162 Los Alisos Blvd., Mission Viejo, CA 92690   **(714) 855-0552**
Natural foods. Vegetarian and "California Lite" cuisines characterize the creative cooking. Low-fat items are offered. Smoking is not allowed. **Open for three meals daily. Full service, vegan options, fresh juices, take-out, VISA/MC/DISC, $$**

MONTEREY

Amarin Thai Cuisine
807 Cannery Row, Monterey, CA 93942   **(408) 373-8811**
Thai. Enjoy authentic Thai cuisine in an informal Thai atmosphere. Tofu can be substituted for the meat in any dish. **Open daily for lunch and dinner. Full service, wine/beer, take-out, VISA/MC/AMX/DISC, $$**

MONTEREY PARK

• Merit Grove Vegetarian Restaurant
206 S. Garfield Ave., Monterey Park, CA 91754   **(818) 280-7430**
Vegetarian/Chinese. Don't be fooled by the meat dishes listed on the menu. It's all soy protein. More than eighty main dishes are offered; a few list oyster sauce. **Open daily. Limited service, vegan options, take-out, VISA/MC/DISC, $$**

MORENO VALLEY

Dragon House Restaurant
22456 Alessandro Blvd., Moreno Valley, CA 92507   (714) 653-1442
Chinese. Dragon House features a complete vegetarian menu including "vegetarian meats" made from soybean protein so don't be surprised when you see chicken, beef, and scallop dishes on the vegetarian menu. **Open daily for lunch and dinner. Full service, vegan options, wine/beer/alcohol, take-out, VISA/MC/AMX, $$**

MOUNTAIN VIEW

Country Gourmet
2098 El Camino Real, Mountain View, CA 94040   (415) 962-0239
Natural foods. Enjoy Veggie Burritos, Taco Salad, and pasta dishes. **Open daily. Counter service, wine/beer, take-out, VISA/MC/DISC, $$**

•• Garden Fresh Vegetarian Restaurant
1245 W. El Camino Real, Mountain View, CA 94040   (415) 961-7795
Vegan/Chinese. At this smoke-free establishment, you'll enjoy vegan dishes including Spring Rolls, Scallion Pancakes, Steamed Dumplings, Vegetarian Sushi, several soups, Stir-Fried Brown Rice with Mixed Vegetables, Stuffed Chinese Cabbage, Tofu Delight, plus much more. **Open daily for lunch and dinner. Full service, vegan options, take-out, VISA/MC, $$**

Hobee's Restaurant
2312 Central Expressway, Mountain View, CA 94043   (415) 968-6050
Restaurant chain. See entry under Cupertino, CA.

Rooh's Cafe Salsa
650 Castro St., Mountain View, CA 94041   (415) 969-6393
Mexican/restaurant chain. See entry under Los Gatos, CA.

NEEDLES

Irene's Drive Inn
703 Broadway, Needles, CA 92363   (619) 326-2342
Fast food. This is a typical fast-food hamburger place that has window service. From a distance, there is no indication of the wonderful, large vegetarian tacos and burritos that are also available on the menu. Vegetarian food is available because, historically, there has been a Seventh-day Adventist community in the area. This is certainly an oasis in the desert! You can buy food to eat in your car or at the picnic table outside. **Open daily. Window service, fresh juices, take-out, $**

🐾 Reviewers' choice   • Vegetarian restaurant   •• Vegan restaurant
$ less than $6 $$ $6–$12 $$$ more than $12
VISA/AMX/MC/DISC/DC—credit cards accepted
Non-alc.—Non-alcoholic   Fresh juices—freshly squeezed

NEVADA CITY

• Earth Song Market & Cafe

727 Zion St., Nevada City, CA 95959   **(916) 265-8025**

Vegetarian. Located adjacent to a natural foods market in the Sierra Nevada foothills, this vegetarian restaurant offers salads, Veggie Burgers, sandwiches, and entrees using fresh organic vegetables and grains when available. Several soups and specials are prepared each day. **Open daily. Full service, vegan/macrobiotic options, fresh juices, take-out, VISA/MC, $**

NEWPORT BEACH

Far Pavillions

1520 West Coast Hwy., Newport Beach, CA 92663   **(714) 548-7167**

Indian. This restaurant is located along the Pacific coast. The menu has a vegetable section that features twelve vegetarian dishes plus traditional appetizers such as samosas and pakoras. **Full service, vegan options, $$**

Royal Thai Cuisine

4001 W. Pacific Coast Hwy., Newport Beach, CA 92663   **(714) 650-3322**

Thai. Royal Thai offers nine vegetarian entrees plus appetizers, soups, and salads. **Open Monday through Friday for lunch, Saturday and Sunday for dinner. Sunday Brunch. Full service, wine/beer/alcohol, VISA/MC/AMX/DISC, $$**

NORTH HOLLYWOOD

• Leonor's

11402 Victory Blvd., North Hollywood, CA 91606   **(818) 980-9011**

Vegetarian. Leonor's is a vegetarian Mexican restaurant. It offers tostadas, tacos, enchiladas, quesadillas, and burritos using soy cheese and soy "meats." It also serves pizza, sandwiches, and salads. **Open for lunch and dinner daily. Full service, fresh juices, vegan options, take-out, $–$$**

NORTHRIDGE

Canopy of the Sky

9351 Reseda Blvd., Northridge, CA 91325   **(818) 885-1875**

Gourmet natural foods. Recommended by a member, this small restaurant has a wonderful hand-painted decor. Each meal is prepared individually so be prepared for leisurely dining. Delicious nut-vegetable and vegetable soups. **Open daily. Reservations recommended. Full service, vegan options, wine/beer, take-out, VISA/MC/AMX/DISC, $$–$$$**

• Paru's

9545 Reseda Blvd., #16, Northridge, CA 91324   **(818) 349-3546**

Indian/vegetarian. Paru's features South Indian cuisine without preservatives or additives and mostly non-dairy. This is a tiny restaurant with delightful service and delicious food. **Closed Monday. Full service, vegan options, take-out, VISA/MC, $$**

• Our Daily Bread Bakery
12201 Firestone Blvd., Norwalk, CA 90650   **(310) 863-6897**

Vegetarian/deli. The entree menu rotates every twenty-one days, and there are twelve different soups, breads, cookies, Macaroni and Cheese, Stuffed Peppers, enchiladas, and quiche. **Open Monday through Thursday late morning and afternoon, and Friday morning. Counter service, vegan options, $**

Granny Feels Great
5020 Woodminster Lane, Oakland, CA 94602   **(510) 530-6723**

Natural foods. Granny's primarily offers sandwiches. Vegetarian options using cheese or dairy are available. The menu also lists a salad plate, Potato Salad, and Carrot-Raisin Salad. **Closed Sunday. Deli style, fresh juices, take-out, $**

Holyland Kosher Foods
677 Rand Ave., Oakland, CA 94610   **(510) 272-0535**

Kosher. Enjoy salads and Hummus, Tabouleh, Falafel, and Stuffed Grape Leaves. Indoor and outdoor seating. **Open Sunday through Thursday afternoon and evening; open Friday until noon. Closed Saturday. Full service, fresh juices, wine/beer, catering, take-out, $**

• Macrobiotic Grocery/Organic Cafe
1050 40th St., Oakland, CA 94608   **(510) 653-6510**

Vegetarian/macrobiotic. Gourmet macrobiotic food is prepared with organic ingredients by a team of internationally trained macrobiotic cooks. Every meal is unique. Desserts are made without refined sugars, honey, eggs, or dairy products. **Open for three meals daily. Full service, vegan/macrobiotic options, catering, take-out, $$**

Nan Yang Rockridge
6048 College Ave., Oakland,CA 94618   **(510) 655-3298**

Burmese. The wide variety of vegetarian dishes includes Fried Tropical Squash, Hot and Sour Soup, Stir-fried Brussels Sprouts and Baby Corn, Stir-fried Jicama, Burmese Cold Noodles, and more. Savor curry, black, coconut, or chili rice. **Open Tuesday through Sunday. Full service, vegan options, wine/beer, take-out, VISA/MC, $$**

Tandoor Cuisine of India
1132 E. Katella Ave., Orange, CA 92667   **(714) 538-2234**

Indian. Minutes from Disneyland and the Anaheim Convention Center, Tandoor has a good selection of vegetarian Indian specialties including appetizers, salad, rice dishes, and entrees that taste excellent! **Open daily. Full service, vegan options, take-out, $$**

OROVILLE
Vega Macrobiotic Center
1511 Robinson St., Oroville, CA 95965 (916) 533-7702
Macrobiotic. Vega offers a variety of macrobiotic meals ranging from simple to international gourmet, depending on which cooking course is in progress on the day you eat there. **Open Monday through Friday. Reservations required. Limited service, take-out, VISA/MC/AMX, $$–$$$**

PACIFIC GROVE
Tillie Gort's Cafe & Restaurant
111 Central, Pacific Grove, CA 93950 (408) 373-0335
Natural foods. Tillie Gort's restaurant/coffeehouse and impromptu art gallery has been a fixture on Central Ave. in Pacific Grove for twenty-three years. Tillie's serves a wide variety of foods including some that qualify as "health food" and organic. Many vegetarian options are offered, including the No Meat Loaf, Veggie Pasta, and Eggplant Parmesan. **Open for three meals daily. Full service, vegan options, fresh juices, espresso/cappuccino, wine/beer, take-out, VISA/MC, $$**

PALM SPRINGS
• Nature's Express
555 S. Sunrise Way #301, Palm Springs, CA 92264 (619) 323-9487
Vegetarian. Enjoy Granola with Soymilk, Deluxe Belgian Waffles, nut butter sandwiches, Mock Egg Salad, beans and rice, veggie burgers, Tamale Plate, burritos, and Vegetarian Sushi at Nature's Express. **Open daily for three meals. Limited service, vegan options, take-out, $**

PALO ALTO
Country Sun Natural Foods Deli
440 California Ave., Palo Alto, CA 94306 (415) 328-4120
Health-food-store deli. The Country Sun deli offers breakfast and lunch every day with a variety of vegetarian options. Organically grown grains, beans, fruits and vegetables are used whenever possible. The menu features homemade vegetarian pizza, a wide variety of salads, hot entrees, vegetarian burgers, and sandwiches. **Open daily. Deli style, vegan/macrobiotic options, fresh juices, limited seating, take-out, $**

Fresh Choice
Stanford Shopping Center, Palo Alto, CA 94304 (415) 322-6995
American. See entry under Menlo Park.

Gaylord India Restaurant
317 Stanford Shopping Center, Palo Alto, CA 94304   (415) 326-8761
Indian. "Vegetarian selections as extensive as the delicate spices which are added to taste. When we say vegetarian menu, we mean more than steamed broccoli." Eleven vegetarian entrees are offered. **Open daily. Reservations accepted. Formal, full service, vegan options, wine/beer/alcohol, take-out, VISA/MC/AMX/ DC/Carte Blanche, $$–$$$**

The Good Earth
185 University Ave., Palo Alto, CA 94301   (415) 321-9449
Natural foods. Enjoy wok dishes, Vegetarian Scramble, Tofu Scramble, vegetarian burger, burritos, tostadas, Eggplant Sandwich, salads, Pasta Primavera, Walnut Mushroom Au Gratin, Guatamalan Rice and Tofu. **Open daily. Full service, wine/beer, VISA/MC/AMX, $$**

Hobee's Restaurant
4224 El Camino Real, Palo Alto, CA 94306   (415) 856-6124

67 Town & Country Village, Palo Alto, CA 94301   (415) 327-4111
Restaurant chain. A seven-vegetable sauté, tofu, veggie patties, Black Bean Chili, and a salad bar are among the vegetarian options at Hobee's. **Open every day. Full service, fresh juices, wine/beer, take-out, VISA/MC/AMX/DISC, $$**

• Juice Club
69 Town and Country Village, Palo Alto, CA 94301   (415) 325-2582
Vegetarian juice bar. See description under Irvine.

Nataraja Indian Cuisine
117 University Ave., Palo Alto, CA 94301   (415) 321-6161
Indian. "Walk in and get the feeling of being transported into another culture far, far away with ambience, aroma, and gracious hospitality"; so reads the front of Nataraja's menu. There are several vegetarian entrees and vegetarian appetizers such as samosas and pakoras in addition to eleven "country-style side orders." Fresh vegetables are used in all veggie entrees. **Closed Sunday. Full service, wine/beer/alcohol, catering, take-out, VISA/MC/AMX, $$**

Tokyo
448 University Ave., Palo Alto, CA 94301   (415) 325-1605
Ethnic. Enjoy tempura tofu dishes and mock (gluten) meats. **Open daily. Full service, beer/wine, VISA/MC, $$**

Whole Foods Market & Deli
774 Emerson St., Palo Alto, CA 94301   (415) 326-8676
Natural foods deli. This gourmet natural foods deli offers thirty-five all natural and organic salads. Specialty items include homemade vegetable knishes, pizzas, and vegetable sushi. There are also hot food selections including vegan entrees, vegetable lasagna, and two daily soups. Breakfast is served and box lunches to go are available. **Open daily. Deli style, vegan options, fresh juices, wine/beer, catering, take-out, VISA/MC, $**

PALOMAR MOUNTAIN

• Mother's Kitchen
Junction of S6 and S7, Palomar Mountain, CA 92060   (619) 742-4233
Vegetarian/juice bar. Any visitor to San Diego who drives up the mountain to see the famous Mt. Palomar telescope will drive right past Mother's. It's the only eatery on the mountain. In this rustic mountaintop cabin, you'll find soups, salads, sandwiches, nutburgers, and fruit smoothies. **Closed Tuesday and Wednesday. Full service, fresh juices, wine/beer, take-out, $$**

PARADISE

• Feather River Hospital Cafeteria
5974 Pentz Rd., Paradise, CA 95969   (916) 877-9361
Vegetarian. Sample the Spinach Tortellini or Spaghetti, Mushroom Loaf, Zucchini Quiche, Enchilada, Garbanzo Casserole, salad bar, pizza bar, and veggie burger bar. **Open daily for lunch and dinner. Cafeteria style, take-out, $**

PASADENA

Clearwater Cafe
168 Colorado Blvd., Pasadena, CA 91105   (818) 356-0959
Natural foods. This smoke-free cafe offers many vegetarian dishes such as Organic Brown Rice Risotto with Lemon and Herbs, Chinese Long Beans with Black Bean-Ginger Sauce, Mixed Grill of Vegetables with Creamy Polenta, Tempura Vegetables with Organic Ventura Bananas and Ponzu Sauce, several salads, plus more. Menu changes daily. **Open daily for lunch and dinner. Brunch served on weekends. Full service, vegan options, take-out, VISA/MC/AMX, $$$**

The Good Earth
257 N. Rosemead Blvd., Pasadena, CA 91107   (818) 351-5488
Natural foods. Good Earth offers Walnut Mushroom Casserole, Eggplant Parmesan, soups, salads, etc. **Open daily. Full service, fresh juices, wine/beer, take-out, VISA/MC/AMX, $$**

PETALUMA

Markey's Cafe
316 Western Ave., Petaluma, CA 94952   (707) 763-2429
Natural foods cafe/bakery. The majority of the menu items are vegetarian and include sandwiches, tempeh burgers, soups, salads, entrees, smoothies, and desserts. **Open daily. Cafeteria style, vegan options, cappuccino/espresso, wine/beer, VISA/MC, $**

REDWOOD CITY

Joy Meadow
701 El Camino Real, Redwood City, CA 94063   (415) 365-3550
Natural foods. In the relaxing atmosphere of Joy Meadow, you can enjoy a variety of unique vegetarian dishes such as Nepal Loaf, Golden Chalice (stuffed eggplant), and Enchanted Forest (tofu marinated in plum sauce with broccoli). They have an extensive vegetarian menu section plus a Light and Tasty section that includes

many vegetarian and vegan options. Next door to the restaurant is the Harmony Bookshop, part of Joy Meadow Inc., featuring New Age books and related items. **Open daily for lunch and dinner. Reservations accepted. Full service, vegan options, espresso/cappuccino, wine/beer, take-out, VISA/MC/AMX/DISC, $$**

RIVERSIDE
Dragon House Restaurant
10466 Magnolia Ave., Riverside, CA 92505   **(714) 354-2080**
Chinese. See entry under Moreno Valley, CA.

ROSEMEAD
Chameli
8752 Valley Blvd., Rosemead, CA 91770   **(818) 280-1947**
Ethnic. You'll eat ethnic foods while listening to classical Indian sitar. **Closed Tuesday. Full service, wine/beer, catering, take-out, VISA/MC/AMX, $$**

SACRAMENTO
Eat Your Vegetables
1841 Howe Ave., Sacramento, CA 95825   **(916) 922-8454**
Natural foods. See entry under Fair Oaks, CA.

Good Earth
2024 Arden Way, Sacramento, CA 95616   **(916) 920-5544**
Natural foods. Food is prepared without artificial ingredients or preservatives. Wok dishes, Mexican cuisine, and casseroles are among the offerings. **Open daily for three meals. Full service, vegan options, fresh juices, non-alc. beer, wine/ beer, VISA/MC, $$**

Juliana's Kitchen
1401 G St., Sacramento, CA 95814   **(916) 444-0966**
Middle Eastern/natural foods. Juliana's Kitchen specializes in a variety of vegetarian pita bread sandwiches from the Middle East along with a daily Middle Eastern special. Salads, desserts, and organic juice sections are also on the menu. **Limited service, vegan options, wine/beer, take-out, $**

•• Marline's Vegetable Patch
1119 8th St., Sacramento, CA 95814   **(916) 448-3327**
Vegan. Marline's completely vegan menu features Mexican dishes with soy cream; vegan sandwiches such as the Tomacado Nut Burger and the "So-Cal" Sub served on whole-wheat buns, bread or pita; and several side orders. Delicious fruit smoothies and fresh fruit juices are also available. **Open for lunch Monday through Friday. Limited service, vegan, fresh juices, take-out, VISA/MC/AMX/ DISC, $**

• Mums
2968 Freeport Blvd., Sacramento, CA 95818   **(916) 444-3015**
Vegetarian. Mums has a cozy dining room, and outside seating in the summertime. Eggs are used only in omelettes. Dishes that can be prepared without eggs or wheat are clearly indicated on the menu, which includes salads, appetizers, and children's dinner, lunch and brunch sections. **Closed Monday; only brunch is served Sunday. Full service, vegan options, fresh juices, wine/beer, limited catering, take-out, VISA/MC/AMX, $$**

Sacramento Natural Foods Co-op
1900 Alkambra Blvd., Sacramento, CA 95818   **(916) 455-COOP**
Deli/juice bar. This co-op features grilled items, soups, salads, sandwiches, and baked goods. **Open daily. Vegan options, $**

Taj Mahal
2355 Arden Way, Sacramento, CA 95825   **(916) 924-8378**
Indian. Vegetarian curry and tandoori dishes are featured at Taj Mahal. **Open daily for lunch and dinner. Full service, wine/beer, VISA/MC/AMX/DC, $$**

SAINT HELENA

• St. Helena Health Center Dining Room
650 Sanitarium Rd., St. Helena, CA 94576   **(707) 963-6214**
Vegetarian. The food service is for participants at the health center, but non-participants can be accommodated with reservations. **Open daily for three meals. Reservations required. Cafeteria style.**

SAN BRUNO

Hobee's Restaurant
#12 Bayhill Shopping Center, San Bruno Ave.
San Bruno, CA 94066   **(415) 588-9662**
Restaurant chain. See entry under Cupertino, CA.

SAN DIEGO

(For more restaurant listings in the surrounding areas, see Coronado, Del Mar, El Cajon, Encinitas, La Jolla, Palomar Mountain—on the way from L.A.—and Solana Beach.)

Ashoka
9474 Black Mountain Rd., San Diego, CA 92126   **(619) 695-9749**
Indian. See description under Anaheim.

ℛ Reviewers' choice   • Vegetarian restaurant   •• Vegan restaurant
$ less than $6 $$ $6–$12 $$$ more than $12
VISA/AMX/MC/DISC/DC—credit cards accepted
Non-alc.–Non-alcoholic   Fresh juices—freshly squeezed

Cafe Greentree
3560 Mt. Acadia Blvd., San Diego, CA 92111   **(619) 560-1975**
Natural foods. Cafe Greentree has an extensive vegetarian menu. **Open daily. Full service, VISA/MC, $**

Casa De Pico
2754 Calhoun St., San Diego, CA 92110   **(619) 296-3267**
Mexican. Located in the heart of Bazaar Del Mundo Shopping Complex in old-town San Diego's historic state park, Casa De Pico offers many vegetarian options. A special menu for the health-conscious offers foods low in salt, fat, and cholesterol. Enjoy live mariachi music nightly on an open air patio. **Open daily. Full service, wine/beer/alcohol, take-out, VISA/MC/AMX/DISC, $-$$**

• Faque Burgers
6109 University Ave., San Diego, CA 92115   **(619) 583-9520**
Vegetarian. Faque Burgers is a fast-food joint for vegetarians, complete with drive-thru window and homemade fries. Vegan burgers and dairy-free shakes can be enjoyed on an outdoor patio. **Open Sunday through Thursday 10 A.M. until 1 A.M., Friday until 4 P.M. only, Saturday 8:30 P.M. to 2 A.M. Limited service, vegan options, take-out, $**

• Gelato Vero Cafe
3753 India St., San Diego, CA 92103   **(619) 295-9269**
Vegetarian. The menu is limited at this coffeehouse cafe—soup, salad, and fresh bread. **Open every evening. Counter service, fresh juices, take-out, AMX, $**

• Govinda's
1030 Grand Ave., San Diego, CA 92109   **(619) 483-5266**
Vegetarian. Govinda's is located three blocks from the beach and offers both indoor and outdoor seating. Enjoy international dishes at the all-you-can-eat buffet. **Closed Sunday and Monday. Open Tuesday through Saturday for lunch and dinner. Cafeteria style, vegan/macrobiotic options, take-out, $**

• Great Harvest Bread Company
1808 Garnet Ave., San Diego, CA 92109   **(619) 272-3521**
Vegetarian bakery. This bakery prepares mostly vegan breads but there are some vegetarian breads that contain cheese. Great Harvest uses stone-ground Montana wheat to make flour for the baked goods. **Open daily. Take-out only, vegan options, $**

Greentree Grocers
3560 Mt. Acadia, San Diego, CA 92111   **(619) 560-1975**
Natural foods deli. Vegetarian options available at this full-service health-food-store deli include twenty different salads and fresh baked goods. **Full service, take-out, $**

• Jimbo's Vegetarian Restaurant
3918 30th St., San Diego, CA 92104   **(619) 294-8055**

12853 El Camino Real, San Diego, CA 92130   **(619) 793-7755**

Vegetarian/health-food-store deli. The back of Jimbo's menu states, "By supporting organic agricultural techniques, we hope to have a positive impact on the environment, our own health, and the health of others," which of itself is an excellent reason to patronize this restaurant. Jimbo's takes extra measures to create healthy dishes using only organic whole-wheat flour, filtered water, and sea salt. Jimbo's features primarily whole-wheat pizza but also offers vegetable and BBQ burgers, an organic salad bar, and an a la carte menu of rice, beans, and tofu meatballs. For vegans, Jimbo's prepares its own totally dairy-free (no casein!) tofu cheese. **Open daily. Full service, vegan options, fresh juice, organic coffee, non-alc. beer, beer/organic wine, take-out, $**

Jyoti Bihanga
3351 Adams Ave., San Diego, CA 92116   **(619) 282-4116**

Natural foods. Jyoti Bihanga offers excellent vegetarian and macrobiotic foods in a peaceful, serene atmosphere with a fountain, high arched ceiling, and fifteen-foot windows. Sample daily specials, homemade soups and desserts, and an all-you-can-eat Saturday breakfast buffet. **Closed Sunday. Full service, vegan/macrobiotic options, fresh juices, take-out, no credit cards, $–$$**

• Kung Food
2949 Fifth Ave., San Diego, CA 92103   **(619) 298-7302**

Vegetarian. Kung Food has been serving gourmet international vegetarian cuisine since 1975. The varied and extensive menu includes "Enchanting Desserts" with vegan options. Entrees include Layered Tofu Supreme, Greek Spinach Pie, and Spaghetti with Mock Italian Sausage. Dishes are prepared from scratch without the use of refined white or brown sugar. Most of the cheese is raw, vegetarian (rennetless), and undyed. The restaurant is located near Balboa Park and features an intimate dining room and garden patio. **Open daily. Full service, vegan options, wine/beer, take-out, VISA/MC/DISC, $**

La Fresqueria
1125 Suite B 6th Ave., San Diego, CA 92116   **(619) 235-0655**

Health-food-store deli. Healthy fresh foods with a Latin influence are offered on a limited menu featuring sandwiches and salads. Seasonal fruit salads and smoothies are also available. **Open Monday through Friday. Limited service, fresh juices, espresso/cappuccino, take-out, no credit cards, $**

Lotsa Pasta
1726 Garnet Ave., #7, San Diego, CA 92109   **(619) 581-6777**

Italian. Many different pastas are cut to order and served with different sauces for a total of more than 500 combinations. **Open daily. Full service, take-out, VISA/MC/AMX/DISC, $$**

• Lux Kahv'e
728 Fifth St., San Diego, CA 92101   **(619) 232-7700**

Vegetarian/bistro. This urban-style coffeehouse and sidewalk cafe has music every night as well as sandwiches, salads, Falafel, pasta, Hummus, blended juices (e.g., honeydew strawberry), and desserts. **Call for current hours. Full service, vegan options, blended juices, espresso/cappuccino, non-alc. beer and wine, beer/ wine, take-out, VISA/MC/AMX/DISC/DC, $$**

Mandarin Plaza
3760 Sports Arena Blvd., San Diego, CA 92110   (619) 224-4222
Mandarin/Cantonese Chinese. Mandarin Plaza's menu has both vegetable and special diet sections that include some unique dishes such as Braised Squash and Mushrooms and Subgum Vegetables. No MSG is used. **Open daily. Full service, vegan options, wine/beer, take-out, VISA/MC /AMX/DISC, $–$$**

Maria Isabella
1830 Sunset Cliffs Blvd., San Diego, CA 92107   (619) 298-2860
Mexican. A vegetarian menu is available. **Open daily. Limited service, vegan options, fresh juices, beer, take-out, $**

• Monsoon
3975 5th Ave., San Diego, CA 92103   (619) 298-3155
Vegetarian. Monsoon offers a wide variety of international vegetarian dishes including curries, lasagna, Greek salad, hummus sandwiches, Mexican pizza, vegetable burritos, and samosas. Be sure to sample the fresh juices, too. Outside dining is available. **Open daily for three meals. Limited service, fresh juices, cappuccino, VISA/MC/AMX, $**

•• Ocean Beach People's Natural Foods Market & Deli
4765 Voltaire St., San Diego, CA 92107   (619) 224-1387
Vegan deli. This deli in a health food store features vegan and raw foods. A great selection of organic produce and green salads, cold salads, soups, entrees, sandwiches, baked goods, and desserts are limited to take-out. **Open daily. Vegan options, fresh juices, take-out only, $**

Pasta Time Cafe
1417 University Ave., San Diego, CA 92103   (619) 296-2425
Italian. Pasta Time takes pride in creating dishes that are healthful and delicious. The menu lists twelve entrees, five of which are vegetarian. All of the sauces, soups, salads, and desserts are made from scratch. Daily pasta specials are joined by a different soup each day. No smoking. **Limited service, vegan options, non-alc. beer, take-out, $**

• Second Nature Vegetarian Cafe
4652 Mission Blvd., San Diego, CA 92109   (619) 272-7399

Vegetarian. Enjoy Tofu Fajitas, Blueberry Cornmeal Pancakes, enchiladas, and more at Second Nature Vegetarian Cafe. In the same location, you will find a fashion boutique offering recycled clothing. Smoking is not allowed. **Open Tuesday through Sunday for three meals. Closed Monday. Full service, vegan/macrobiotic options, espresso/cappuccino, fresh juices, smoothies, catering, take-out, VISA/MC, $**

Skinny Haven
4344 Convoy St., San Diego, CA 92111   **(619) 560-8151**

American. Skinny Haven features a vegetable platter, Quesadilla, Lasagna, a salad bar, and sandwiches. **Closed Sunday. Full service, take-out, VISA/MC, $**

• Zen Bakery
4920 Voltaire St., San Diego, CA 92107   **(619) 221-1220**

Vegetarian bakery. The bakery prepares all baked goods from scratch and uses fruit juice as a sweetener. It also serves fresh juices, tea, coffee, and cappuccino. **Open daily. Limited service, vegan options, take-out, $**

SAN FRANCISCO

(For more restaurants in the surrounding areas, see Berkeley, Burlingame, Campbell, Corte Madera, Cupertino, Emeryville, Foster City, Fremont, Larkspur, Los Gatos, Menlo Park, Mountain View, Oakland, Palo Alto, Redwood City, San Bruno, San Jose, San Rafael, San Clara, Saratoga, and Sunnyvale.)

A.J.'s Falafel King
420 Geary St., San Francisco, CA 94102   **(415) 776-2683**

Middle Eastern/kosher. Enjoy Falafel, Hummus, soups, salads, etc. **Open Sunday through Thursday all day, Friday morning and early afternoon. Counter service, take-out, $**

All You Knead
1466 Haight St., San Francisco, CA 94117   **(415) 552-4550**

American. Pasta, pizza, and soup are available. **Open Sunday through Saturday. $$**

• Amazing Grace
216 Church St., San Francisco, CA 94114   **(415) 626-6411**

Vegetarian. Sundry and simple vegetarian dishes include soups, baked potatoes, sandwiches, and a salad bar. The menu changes each day. **Closed Sunday. Cafeteria style, vegan options, fresh juices, $**

• Ananda Fuara
3050 Taraval St., San Francisco, CA 94102   **(415) 621-1994**

Vegetarian. This Sri-Chimnoy restaurant offers sandwiches, BBQ tofu burger, pizza, a curry dish, salads, and smoothies, plus a breakfast menu. The food has received an excellent rating from one of our members. **Open Monday through Saturday 7 A.M. to 7 P.M, except Wednesday until mid-afternoon. Full service, vegan/macrobiotic options, fresh juices, take-out, $–$$**

•• Chun Kang
608 Geary St., San Francisco, CA 94102   **(415) 771-3866**
Vegan. This vegan Chinese restaurant offers delicious soups, appetizers, and vegetable entrees such as Bean Curd with Black Mushrooms, Vegetables with Sweet and Sour Sauce, and Broccoli with Gluten. **Open for lunch and dinner daily. Full service, vegan only, take-out, $**

Cornucopia
114 Columbus, San Francisco, CA 94133   **(415) 398-1511**
Deli. No meat stock is used in the soups. Rigatoni Salad, Buckwheat Noodles, and Pasta Salad are also offered. **Open weekdays only. Cafeteria style, wine/beer, take-out, no credit cards, $**

Diamond Street Restaurant
737 Diamond St., San Francisco, CA 94114   **(415) 285-6988**
American. Diamond Street has some vegetarian options. **Open daily. Reservations accepted. Full service, wine/beer, take-out, VISA/MC/AMX, $$–$$$**

• The Ganges Restaurant
775 Frederick St., San Francisco, CA 94117   **(415) 661-7290**
Vegetarian/Indian. The vegetarian offerings are light but exotic, with distinct flavors from Gujarat, India. You can go à la carte or choose a special combination plate from the Ganges menu, which features dahl, curries, Saffron Rice, and other classic Indian appetizers. Enjoy a vegan dessert and, Thursday through Saturday, live Indian music. **Open for dinner Tuesday through Saturday. Full service, vegan options, wine/beer, take-out, $$**

Gaylord's India Restaurant
1 Embarcadero, San Francisco, CA 94111   **(415) 397-7775**
Indian. Gaylord's offers world-renowned Indian cuisine with bread baked fresh in clay ovens. Vegetarian appetizers and meatless specialties are listed on the menu. **Open daily for lunch and dinner. Full service, vegan options, fresh juices, wine/beer, take-out, VISA/MC/AMX/DISC, $$**

• Greens Restaurant
Fort Mason Building A, San Francisco, CA 94123   **(415) 771-6222**
Vegetarian. Greens is located in an old army warehouse with beautiful views of the San Francisco Bay and the Coastal Mountain Range. **Reservations suggested. Full service, limited vegan options, fresh juice, wine/beer, take-out, VISA/MC/DISC, $$$**

Haven Restaurant
One Post St., San Francisco, CA 94104   **(415) 397-1299**
Health food store. **Open daily 7 A.M. to 3 P.M. Fresh juices, wine/beer, catering, take-out, $**

• Josie's Cafe and Juice Joint
3583 16th St., San Francisco, CA 94114   **(415) 861-7933**
Vegetarian. Salads, soups, quiche, veggie burger, tofu burgers, tempeh burgers,

and baked goods are offered. This is a vegetarian restaurant during the day and a cabaret after 8 P.M. **Open daily. Counter service, fresh juices, take-out, $**

Joy Chinese Restaurant
3258 Scott St., San Francisco, CA 94123   **(415) 922-0270**
Szechuan/Mandarin. See entry under Foster City, CA.

Just Like Home
1924 Irving St., San Franciso, CA 94122   **(415) 681-3337**
Mediterranean. Enjoy Baba Ghanouj, Hummus, Falafel, Dolma, and Tabouleh. **Open daily for lunch and dinner. Full service, beer, take-out, VISA/MC/AMX/ DISC, $**

• Lotus Garden 🐄
532 Grant Ave. (between California and Pine)
San Francisco, CA 94108   **(415) 397-0707**
Vegetarian/Chinese. It is worth visiting this restaurant with its wide selection of vegetarian items ranging from Asparagus with Stewed Bean Gluten Puff to Vegetarian Won Ton to Almond Vegetarian Chicken Dices. The management is very supportive of vegetarian organizations. **Closed Monday. Full service, vegan options, wine/beer, VISA/MC/AMX, $$**

• Lucky Creation Vegetarian Restaurant
854 Washington St., San Francisco, CA 94108   **(415) 989-0818**
Vegetarian/Chinese. The phrase "Health is Wealth" is featured on the menu to let customers know Lucky Creation serves only vegetarian food because it is concerned about customers' health. The take-out menu is divided into appetizers, soups, entrees, clay pot dishes, pan fried noodles, noodles in soup, and rice plates. Entrees include Sauteed Black Mushrooms with Chinese Greens and Meatless Diced Almond Chicken, plus twenty-three other items. **Closed Wednesday. Full service, vegan option, wine/beer, take-out, $**

Maharani
1122 Post St., San Francisco, CA 94109   **(415) 775-1988**
Indian. See listing under Berkeley, CA.

•• Now and Zen
1826 B Buchanan St., San Francisco, CA 94115   **(415) 922-9696**
Vegan. Located in Japantown, this vegan restaurant and bakery features multi-ethnic entrees like tofu Bourgignonne, the Now and Zen burger, and seitan fillets— teriyaki-style. These creations are also found in the owner's cookbook called *The Now and Zen Epicure.* **Open daily for lunch and dinner. Brunch on Sunday. Full service, fresh juices, take-out, VISA/MC/AMX/DISC/DC, $–$$**

Real Good Karma
501 Dolores St., San Francisco, CA 94110   **(415) 621-4112**
Natural foods. Partake of various stir-fry dishes, salads, batter-dipped entrees, and fresh pasta with an Asian influence. Dine in a simple, sunny room with a piano open to anyone who is inspired to play. **Open daily for lunch and dinner. Full service, vegan/macrobiotic options, fresh juices, beer, take-out, $–$$**

Red Crane
1115 Clement, San Francisco, CA 94118   **(415) 751-7226**
Chinese. Mock meat entrees are featured. **Open daily. Full service, wine/beer, take-out, VISA/MC, $**

• Shangri-La
2026 Irving St., San Francisco, CA 94122   **(415) 731-2548**
Vegetarian/Northern Chinese. Eggs are used in some dishes, but no dairy. **Open daily. Full service, wine/beer, take-out, VISA/MC, $**

Tai Chi
2031 Polk St., San Francisco, CA 94109   **(415) 441-6758**
Chinese. Tai Chi features Spring Rolls, Chinese Pancakes, Vegetable Stir-Fry, Hot and Sour Cabbage, and Dry Braised Green Beans. **Open daily. Full service, wine/beer, take-out, VISA/MC/ AMX, $**

Taiwan Restaurant
445 Clement St., San Francisco, CA 94118   **(415) 387-1789**
Chinese. Enjoy vegetarian dishes such as Steamed Dumplings, Hot and Sour Fried Rice, Sweet and Sour Mock Pork, and other mock meat dishes. **Open daily for lunch and dinner. Full service, wine/beer, take-out, VISA/MC/AMX, $$**

Tortola
3521 20th Ave., San Francisco, CA 94132   **(415) 566-4336**

3640 Sacramento St., San Francisco, CA 94118   **(415) 929-8181**
Mexican. Features vegetarian tacos, burritos, and tostadas. No lard is used in the beans. **Sacramento St. closed Monday; 20th Ave. open daily. Full service, wine/ beer, full bar at Sacramento St., take-out, $$**

• Vegi Food
1820 Clement St., San Francisco, CA 94121   **(415) 387-8111**
Vegetarian/Chinese. No eggs, garlic, onions, or MSG is used in the varieties of mock meats. **Open Tuesday through Sunday for lunch and dinner. Full service, take-out, $–$$**

Vicolo Pizzeria
201 Ivy St., San Francisco, CA 94102   **(415) 863-2382**
Pizza. This pizzeria features corn-meal-crust pizza, wonderful salads, and vegetarian soups. **Open daily for lunch and dinner. Limited service, non-alc. beer, wine/beer, take-out, $–$$**

🍴 Reviewers' choice   • Vegetarian restaurant   •• Vegan restaurant
$ less than $6 $$ $6–$12 $$$ more than $12
VISA/AMX/MC/DISC/DC—credit cards accepted
Non-alc.—Non-alcoholic   Fresh juices—freshly squeezed

Wu Kong Restaurant
101 Spear St., San Francisco, CA 94105   **(415) 957-9300**
Chinese. "Vegetable Goose" (tofu stuffed with mushrooms) and various other bean curd and vegetable dishes are among the vegetarian options offered. **Full service, take-out, VISA/MC/AMX, $$**

SAN GABRIEL

• Diwana Restaurant
1381 E. Las Tunas Dr., San Gabriel, CA 91775   **(818) 287-8743**
Vegetarian/Indian. Diwana offers a unique dining experience—authentic Indian vegetarian dishes from all parts of India. Only the finest ingredients are used. Dishes are adapted from recipes handed down through generations. **Closed Tuesday. Full service, fresh juice, wine/beer, take-out, VISA/MC, $$**

•• Vegetarian Delight Restaurant
140 W. Valley #203, San Gabriel, CA 91776   **(818) 288-2698**
Vegan/Chinese. This restaurant is located on the second floor of the San Gabriel Mall, which is a Chinese shopping center. It offers a wide variety of vegan Chinese dishes. **Open daily for lunch and dinner. Full service, vegan options, take-out, $$**

SAN JOSE

Fresh Choice
1600 Saratoga Ave., San Jose, CA 95125   **(408) 866-1491**
American. The salad selection is extensive, and there is always one vegetarian soup and usually at least one vegetarian pasta. A fixed price includes everything from bread to dessert. **Open daily. Cafeteria style, wine/beer, VISA/MC, $$**

Hobee's Restaurant
920 Town & Country Village
Stevens Creek Blvd., San Jose, CA 95128   **(408) 244-5212**
Restaurant chain. See entry under Cupertino, CA.

• The Supreme Master Ching Hai International Meditation Association Vegetarian House
520 E. Santa Clara St., San Jose, CA 95112   **(408) 292-3798**
Vegetarian. Don't be fooled by the name, this restaurant features vegetarian fare of several ethnic flavors! Try one of the many Chinese, Thai, and Vietnamese dishes. If you're not in the mood for Asian food, have pizza, vegetarian lasagna, or French vegetable quiche. **Open daily for lunch and dinner. Full service, nonsmoking, VISA/MC/AMX/DISC, $–$$**

• White Lotus ❧
80 N. Market St., San Jose, CA 95113   **(408) 977-0540**
Vegetarian/ethnic. Mock meats make up a lot of the menu at this restaurant, so don't be surprised when you see beef, chicken, duck, pork, and fish dishes listed. Extremely flavorful fare, the foods are drawn from several cultures, especially

Vietnamese, and White Lotus utilizes many Eastern herbs and spices. The menu is mostly vegan. Absolutely no smoking. **Closed Monday. Full service, vegan options, take-out, VISA/MC/AMX, $$**

SAN JUAN CAPISTRANO

Natural Offering Cafe
San Juan Capistrano, CA   **(714) 472-1721**
This restaurant had yet to open at press time.

SAN LUIS OBISPO

Hobee's
1443 Calle Joaquin, San Luis Obispo, CA 93401   **(805) 549-9186**
Restaurant chain. One vegetarian and one vegan soup are offered daily. You can also partake of tofu burgers, Tofu Scramble, four vegetarian dinner specials daily, seven vegan veggie sautees with rice, Black Bean Chili, a salad bar, and baked goods. **Open daily. Full service, vegan options, fresh juice, wine/beer, take-out, VISA/MC/AMX, $$**

• Juice Club
17 Charro St., Suite C, San Luis Obispo, CA 93405   **(805) 549-8028**
Vegetarian juice bar. See description under Irvine.

• Santa Veggie
685 Higuera St., San Luis Obispo, CA 93401   **(805) 546-9700**
Vegetarian. Enjoy vegetarian Chinese dishes including Mushroom and Corn Soup, Stewed Bean Curd with Brown Sauce, Sautéed Wheat Gluten and Snow Peas, Curry Mushrooms, Chinese Cabbage with Black Mushrooms, and more. **Open daily for lunch and dinner. Full service, vegan options, take-out, $$**

SAN MATEO

The Good Earth
3190 Campus Dr., San Mateo, CA 94403   **(415) 349-0165**
Natural foods. See description under Palo Alto. This location is near the San Francisco Airport.

SAN RAFAEL

Bongkot Thai Express
857 Fourth St., San Rafael, CA 94901   **(415) 453-3350**
Thai. Bongkot Thai calls its vegetarian menu section "Vegie Deluxe" and offers seventeen vegetarian options including curries, noodle dishes, and veggies with various Thai seasonings. Prices are low. **Closed Sunday. Full service, vegan options, take-out, VISA/MC, $**

Healthy Gourmet Cafe
1132 4th St., San Rafael, CA 94901   **(415) 457-0132**
Natural foods. Enjoy freshly made soups, salads, sandwiches, muffins, daily specials,

and a juice bar. **Open Monday through Saturday. Cafeteria style, fresh juices, take-out, VISA/MC/DISC, $**

•• Milly's
1613 Fourth St., San Rafael, CA 94901   **(415) 459-1601**
Vegan. I haven't yet had the pleasure of sampling the gourmet vegan cuisine at Milly's, but it's definitely on my list of places to feast due to the rave reviews from various readers of *Vegetarian Journal.* One local patron of Milly's writes, "This is the finest, healthful, gourmet, low-fat, delicious food restaurant I have experienced in twenty years of vegetarian restaurant hunting around the world!" **Open for dinner daily except Monday. Full service, casual to formal, completely vegan, catering, wine/beer, take-out, MC, $$–$$$**

Szechuan Village Restaurant
720 "B" St., San Rafael, CA 94901   **(415) 454-2828**
Szechuan Chinese. Szechuan Village serves fresh vegetable pot stickers, spring rolls, assorted vegetarian soups, tofu salad, garlic and sweet and sour dishes. **Open daily. Full service, vegan options, wine/beer, take-out, VISA/MC/AMX, $**

SANTA ANA

Niki's Tandoori Express
3705 S. Bristol St., Santa Ana, CA 92704   **(714) 838-7615**

2031 E. 1st St., Santa Ana, CA 92705   **(714) 542-2969**
Indian. Niki's is a new concept in Indian fast food. Some vegetarian options are available. **Open daily. Cafeteria style, wine/beer, take-out, $–$$**

The Village Farmer
South Coast Plaza Village
3810 S. Plaza Dr., Santa Ana, CA 92704   **(714) 557-8433**
American. Vegetarian options are offered. **Open daily. Wine/beer, take-out, VISA/MC/AMX, $$**

SANTA BARBARA

• Follow Your Heart Natural Foods and Cafe 🦋
19 S. Milpas, Santa Barbara, CA 93103   **(805) 966-3694**
Vegetarian. See entry under Canoga Park, CA.

Galanga Thai Restaurant
507 State St., Santa Barbara, CA 93101   **(805) 899-3199**

🦋 Reviewers' choice   • Vegetarian restaurant   •• Vegan restaurant
$ less than $6 $$ $6–$12 $$$ more than $12
VISA/AMX/MC/DISC/DC—credit cards accepted
Non-alc.—Non-alcoholic   Fresh juices—freshly squeezed

Thai. Dine on more than twenty different vegetarian Thai dishes at this restaurant. Be sure to choose dishes that do not contain oyster sauce. **Open for lunch and dinner Thursday through Tuesday. Closed Wednesday. Full service, non-alc. beer, wine/beer, vegan options, take-out, $–$$**

Main Squeeze Cafe & Juice Bar
138 E. Canon Perdido, Santa Barbara, CA 93101   (805) 966-5365
Natural foods/macrobiotic. Homemade soups, salads, sandwiches, Mexican special-ties, and daily pasta specials are offered in addition to a vegetarian menu. Fresh squeezed juices, smoothies, shakes, and an espresso bar with fresh, homebaked desserts are also available. **Open daily. Limited service, vegan options, fresh juices, wine/beer, take-out, $**

The Natural Cafe and Juice Bar
508 State St., Santa Barbara, CA 93101   (805) 962-9494
Natural foods. The Natural Cafe is located in downtown Santa Barbara, five blocks away from the Pacific Ocean. Dine on items such as Vegetarian Chili, Guacamole with Chips, Spinach Salad, Falafel Pita, Veggie Stir-Fry, Tempeh Tacos, and more. **Open daily for lunch and dinner. Full service, fresh juices, vegan options, take-out, $–$$**

Sojourner Restaurant & Coffeehouse
134 E. Canon Perdido St., Santa Barbara, CA 93101   (805) 965-7922
Natural foods. Vegetarian options are scattered throughout the menu, which also includes non-vegetarian dishes. Some international themes are favored such as the Mediterranean Plate, curries, and Mexican fare. The Sojourner is now using vegetar-ian (rennetless) jack and cheddar cheese. Non-alcoholic specialty drinks such as Mocha Frosted and Carob Supreme are offered. Entirely non-smoking. **Open daily. Full service, vegan options, espresso/cappuccino, wine/beer, take-out, $$**

SANTA CLARA

Fresh Choice Restaurants
Corporate Offices
2901 Tasman Dr., Suite 109, Santa Clara, CA 95054   (408) 986-8661
American. There are over twenty-four Fresh Choice Restaurants in California, Washington, and Texas. Call for locations. An extensive salad selection is comple-mented by one vegetarian soup and usually at least one vegetarian pasta. A fixed price includes everything—even bread and dessert. **Open daily. Cafeteria style, wine/beer, VISA/MC, $$**

The Good Earth
2705 The Alameda, Santa Clara, CA 95050   (408) 984-0960
Natural foods. Enjoy wok dishes, Vegetarian Scramble, Tofu Scramble, Vegetarian Burger, burritos, tostadas, Eggplant Sandwich, salads, Pasta Primavera, Walnut Mushroom Au Gratin, Guatamalan Rice and Tofu. **Open daily. Full service, wine/beer, VISA/MC/AMX, $$**

Pasand India Cuisine
3701 El Camino Real, Santa Clara, CA 95051   (408) 241-5150

Indian. Authentic South Indian food is prepared with spices and herbs imported from India. Almost half of the menu lists various kinds of vegetarian dishes. Live classical Indian music is featured on Friday and Saturday evenings. **Open daily. Full service, vegan options, wine/beer, catering, take-out, VISA/MC/AMX/DISC/DC, $$**

Rooh's Cafe Salsa
2777 El Camino Real, Santa Clara, CA 95051   (408) 985-ROOH

University Plaza,
110 Homestead, Santa Clara, CA 95050   (408) 246-2455
Mexican/restaurant chain. See entry under Los Gatos, CA.

SANTA CLARITA

India's Tandoori
23360 Valencia Blvd., Unit I, Santa Clarita, CA 91355   (805) 288-1200
Indian. See entry under Los Angeles, CA.

SANTA CRUZ

• Asian Rose Cafe
1547 Pacific Ave., Santa Cruz, CA 95060   (408) 458-3023
Vegetarian. Customers can select one, two, or three items from about ten choices. All items are served with rice. The cafe also has a salad bar. **Open Monday through Saturday. Closed Sunday. Limited service, vegan options, take-out, $$**

The Bagelry
320 A Cedar St., Santa Cruz, CA 95060   (408) 429-8049

1636 Seabright Ave., Santa Cruz, CA 95060   (408) 425-8550
Bagel shop. Twenty kinds of bagels are baked daily. Dairy and non-dairy sandwiches are made with bagels and there are soups, salads, cookies, and a full selection of hot and cold beverages. Outdoor dining. **Open for three meals daily. Counter service, vegan options, fresh juices, take-out, $**

•• The Big Squeeze
605 Front St., Santa Cruz, CA 95060   (408) 459-0620
Vegan. Feast on Whole-Wheat Pancakes, Granola and Soymilk, Tofu Rancheros, and more for brunch. For lunch and dinner, try one of the many vegetarian burgers and sandwiches, as well as oil-free stir-frys, soups, salads, etc. **Open daily for three meals. Counter service, vegan/macrobiotic options, smoothies, fresh juices, take-out, $**

Guaranga's
503 Water St., Santa Cruz, CA 95060   (408) 427-0294
Vegetarian. This vegetarian self-service restaurant features an all-you-can-eat salad bar and entrees. An entree (choice of four), soup (choice of two), vegetables, bread, and dessert can be had for one low price. Some entrees are vegan, and there is a vegan night three times a week. **Open Monday through Saturday for lunch and dinner. Cafeteria style, vegan options, catering, take-out, $**

Hobee's Restaurant
The Galleria de Santa Cruz
740 Front St., Santa Cruz, CA 95060   **(408) 458-1212**
Restaurant chain. See entry under San Luis Obispo, CA.

India Joze Restaurant
1001 Center St., Santa Cruz, CA 95060   **(408) 427-3554**
Natural foods. On the menu, vegetarian selections are scattered amidst non-vegetarian dishes. The completely vegetarian category includes seven options such as
Tempeh Goreng and Coptic Chickpeas. India Joze hosts special food events
including "Fungi Festival" in January, "International Chickpea Festival" in Febru-
ary, and "Buddha's Birthday Celebration" in April. Patio seating. **Open for lunch
and dinner. Brunch on weekends. Full service, vegan options, fresh juices,
wine/beer, take-out, VISA/MC, $$–$$$**

Linda's Seabreeze Cafe
542 Seabright Ave., Santa Cruz, CA 95062   **(408) 427-9713**
American. Called a great restaurant by one of our reviewers, Linda's is a charming
place for breakfast or lunch on the way to the Santa Cruz beach. Breakfast features
pancakes, Tofu Scramble, and home fries. **Open daily for breakfast and lunch
only. Full service, vegan options, take-out, $**

• Malabar Cafe
1116 Soquel Ave., Santa Cruz, CA 95060   **(408) 423-1717**
Vegetarian. Malabar Cafe offers both Indian and Sri Lankan vegetarian dishes.
Open Monday through Saturday. Closed Sunday. Full service, $$

New Leaf Deli
2351 Mission St., Santa Cruz, CA 95060   **(408) 425-1306**
Health-food-store deli. While dining outdoors, you can enjoy approximately twenty
sandwiches plus hot foods, cold deli salads, soups, and green salads. **Open daily.
Cafeteria style, vegan options, fresh juices, wine/beer, take-out, VISA/MC, $**

•• Restaurant Keffi 🐾
2-1245-B East Cliff Dr., Santa Cruz, CA 95062   **(408) 476-5571**
Vegan. "Keffio" is a Greek word that shows you are enjoying the spirit of living;
the restaurant aims to help you do that by offering healthy, gourmet vegetarian
fare. The menu features appetizers, soups, salads, entrees, desserts, special drinks,
plus more. Dishes are artfully prepared. There's live music Wednesday through
Sunday. **Brunch on Sunday. Closed Monday. Full service, vegan options, fresh
juices, catering, take-out, $–$$**

🐾 Reviewers' choice   • Vegetarian restaurant   •• Vegan restaurant
$ less than $6 $$ $6–$12 $$$ more than $12
VISA/AMX/MC/DISC/DC—credit cards accepted
Non-alc.—Non-alcoholic   Fresh juices—freshly squeezed

Royal Taj India Cuisine
270 Soquel Ave., Santa Cruz, CA 95062   **(408) 427-2400**
Indian. See entry under Campbell, CA.

Saturn Cafe
1230 Mission St., Santa Cruz, CA 95060   **(408) 429-8505**
American. The cafe has its own bakery and serves soups, salads, burgers, sandwiches, chili, and ratatouille. **Open daily until midnight. Counter service, vegan options, espresso, wine/beer, take-out, $**

• Staff of Life Natural Foods Market
1305 Water St., Santa Cruz, CA 95062   **(408) 423-8041**
Vegetarian deli. This market includes a deli that offers burritos, falafels, sandwiches, and soups. The featured entree changes daily and is usually rice- or pasta-based. Some vegan options are available, and various salads and other items may be purchased separately. **Open daily. Cafeteria style, vegan options, fresh juices, take-out, $**

Whole Earth
University of California, Redwood Tower Bldg.
Santa Cruz, CA 95064   **(408) 426-8255**
Natural foods. Partake of muffins, scrambled tofu, soups, salads, and many vegan options. **Open daily. Cafeteria style, vegan options, take-out, $**

•• Zabib Deli
2340 Mission Ave., Santa Cruz, CA 95060   **(408) 429-8223**
Vegan. Enjoy a wide range of Ethiopian, East African, and Caribbean vegan dishes at this deli. **Open Monday through Saturday. Closed Sunday. Limited service, take-out, $$**

SANTA MONICA

Bistro of Santa Monica
2301 Santa Monica Blvd., Santa Monica, CA 90404   **(310) 453-5442**
Italian. The Bistro is a European-style restaurant featuring northern Italian cuisine. All items are prepared from scratch without salt, sugar, or preservatives. Vegetarian selections are offered in addition to items for guests with special dietary requirements. Fifteen types of pasta can be combined with numerous sauces listed under tomato, cream, olive oil, and specialty headings. **Open daily. Full service, vegan options, fresh juices, espresso/cappuccino, wine/beer/alcohol, take-out, VISA/MC/AMX/DISC, $$–$$$**

Get Juiced
1423 Fifth St., Santa Monica, CA 90401   **(310) 395-8177**
Juice bar. You can get fresh fruit and vegetable juices, wheatgrass, frozen fruit creams, and custom gift baskets. **Closed Sunday. Deli, fresh juices, VISA/MC/AMX**

• Mani's Bakery
2507 Main St., Santa Monica, CA 90405   **(310) 396-7700**
Vegetarian bakery/coffeehouse. See entry under Los Angeles, CA.

News Room Es-press-o Cafe
530 Wilshire Blvd., Santa Monica, CA 90401   **(310) 319-9100**
Natural foods. This cafe always has vegetarian specials including burritos, soups, sandwiches, and salads. There is also a vegan frozen dessert. **Open daily for three meals. Limited service, fresh juices, non-alc. beer, espresso, take-out, $**

•• Real Food Daily
514 Santa Monica Blvd., Santa Monica, CA 90401   **(310) 451-7544**
Vegan. Real Food Daily's philosophy is that healthy food prepared with gourmet style and hands-on care improves not only the health of the individual, but also that of the planet. You can dine on items such as Lentil-Walnut Pâté, Millet Croquettes, Seitan Fajitas, breads, and salads. **Open daily for lunch and dinner. Full service, vegan only, take-out, VISA/MC/AMX, $–$$**

Shambala Cafe
607 Colorado Ave., Santa Monica, CA 90401   **(310) 395-2160**
Ethnic. Sandwiches, pita, and pizza offerings are augmented by an international selection of Japanese, Mexican, Chinese, and Indian dishes. **Open daily. Cafeteria style, take-out, $$**

Tampico Restaurant
1025 Wilshire Blvd., Santa Monica, CA 90401   **(310) 451-1769**
Mexican. Tampico Restaurant added a special vegetarian menu to its offerings in 1993. Dishes include Tex-Mex Tempeh Tacos, Tofu Burritos, Tofu Fajitas, Veggie Mexican Burger, plus many other items. **Open daily for lunch and dinner. Full service, vegan options, wine/beer/alcohol, take-out, $$–$$$**

Zabie's
3003 Ocean Park Blvd., Santa Monica, CA 90405   **(310) 399-1150**
Natural foods. The menu is Provencal French and Italian with a Mediterranean influence. Zabie's daily fare is chosen from a list of seasonal dishes for breakfast, lunch, and dinner. The restaurant has its own bakery and uses organic produce and flours when available. **Open Monday through Saturday. Limited service, vegan options, fresh juices, espresso/cappuccino, wine/beer, catering, take-out, $$**

SANTA ROSA

East West Restaurant
2323 Sonoma Ave., Santa Rosa, CA 95405   **(707) 546-6142**

🍴 Reviewers' choice   • Vegetarian restaurant   •• Vegan restaurant
$ less than $6 $$ $6–$12 $$$ more than $12
VISA/AMX/MC/DISC/DC—credit cards accepted
Non-alc.—Non-alcoholic   Fresh juices—freshly squeezed

Natural foods. East West Restaurant serves international cuisine with a Middle Eastern flavor. It also offers non-dairy shakes and desserts. **Open daily for three meals. Full service, vegan/macrobiotic options, fresh juices, smoothies, take-out, VISA/MC/DISC, $$**

Fresh Choice
277 Santa Rosa Plaza, Santa Rosa, CA 95401   **(707) 525-0912**
American. See entry under Menlo Park, CA.

• Jump Start
1195 W. College Ave., Santa Rosa, CA 95401   **(707) 578-6151**
Vegetarian/deli. The food—soups, salads, breads, hot entrees, Vegetable Pot Pie, Lasagna, African Squash Stew, and Barley Loaf—meets McDougall guidelines. Jump Start also conducts cooking classes. **Open Monday through Saturday afternoon and evening. Deli/bakery, vegan options, fresh juices, catering, take-out, VISA/MC, $$**

• Revelation Original Sandwiches
645 Fourth St., Santa Rosa, CA 95404   **(707) 526-2225**
Vegetarian. Sandwiches, soups, and salads are available. **Open Monday through Saturday for breakfast and lunch. Counter service, take-out, $**

Ristorante Siena
1229 N. Dutton Ave., Santa Rosa, CA 95401   **(707) 578-4511**
Italian/natural foods. The menu for Ristorante Siena includes Antipasti, Insalata, Pasta/Polenta/Pizza, and specials. Lunch selections also include salads and sandwiches. Patio seating. **Open weekdays for lunch and dinner, weekends for brunch and dinner. Full service, wine, VISA/MC/DISC, $$**

Rooh's Cafe Salsa
3082 Marlow Rd., Santa Rosa, CA 95403   **(707) 544-ROOH**
Mexican/restaurant chain. See entry under Los Gatos, CA.

SARATOGA

Hobee's
14550 Big Basin Way, Saratoga Village, CA 95071   **(408) 741-1989**
Restaurant chain. See entry under Cupertino, CA.

SEBASTOPOL

• Nancy's Vegetarian
6970 McKinley St., Sebastopol, CA 95472   **(707) 829-6627**
Vegetarian. Vegetarian food is prepared without the use of eggs, white sugar, or preservatives; organic produce is used when available. Nancy's also features low-fat entrees. Soups and desserts are always dairy-free, and desserts are sweetened with barley malt, honey, date sugar, or Sucanat. Selections include grilled tofu, tempeh, or seitan; a nice variety of Mexican options; a veggie roll wrapped in whole-wheat tortilla; and steamed veggies over rice. **Open daily**

except Wednesday afternoon and evening. Vegan/macrobiotic options, organic coffees, fresh juices, $–$$

SHERMAN OAKS

Foods for Health
14543 Ventura Blvd., Sherman Oaks, CA 91403   **(818) 784-4033**
Natural foods. Enjoy healthy foods at low prices. Zesty salads, sandwiches, melts, and soups are made fresh every day. Fruit and vegetable juices, and protein drinks are available. **Closed Sunday. Full service, vegan options, fresh juices, take-out, VISA/MC, $**

SOLANA BEACH

Chung King Loh
552 Stevens Ave., Solana Beach, CA 92075   **(619) 481-0184**
Mandarin/Szechuan Chinese. An extensive vegetarian menu is offered at Chung King Loh with more than twenty veggie entrees plus appetizers and soups. Entrees include Broccoli and Carrots in Hot Peanut Sauce, Bean Curd with Ginger and Green Onions, and Mung Bean Noodle with Black Mushrooms. No MSG is used. Dishes made without oil, sugar, and salt are available upon request. **Open daily. Full service, vegan options, wine/beer/alcohol, take-out, VISA/MC/AMX/ DISC/DC/Carte Blanche, $$**

SOQUEL

The Bagelry
4763 Soquel Dr., Soquel, CA 95073   **(408) 462-9888**
Bagel shop. See entry under Santa Cruz, CA.

Tortilla Flats
4616 Soquel Dr., Soquel, CA 95073   **(408) 476-1754**
Mexican. Rice, beans, or the "Flatland Mix" (made from a nut mixture) can be substituted for meat in the burritos and tostadas. **Open daily. Full service, wine/beer, take-out, VISA/MC, $–$$**

SOUTH LAKE TAHOE

Sprouts
Hwy. 50 & Alameda Ave., South Lake Tahoe, CA 96153   **(916) 541-6969**
Natural foods. This small cafe offers a wide variety of vegetarian dishes including sandwiches, bagels, rice and beans, burritos, quesadillas, tempeh burgers, tostados, soups, and salads. **Open for three meals daily. Limited service, fresh juices, espresso/cappuccino, $**

SOUTH PASADENA

Grassroots Natural Food Market and Kitchen
1119 Fair Oaks Ave., South Pasadena, CA 91030   **(818) 799-0156**
Natural foods. Fast and fresh healthy food is made daily—from scratch. There's an unusual variety of salads, dairy-free soups, tasty hot entrees, sandwiches, and a

tempting selection of homemade muffins. **Closed Sunday. Cafeteria style, vegan options, fresh juices, take-out, VISA/MC/AMX, $**

STUDIO CITY

• Leonor's
12445 Moorpark St., Studio City, CA 91604   **(818) 762-0660**
Vegetarian. See entry under North Hollywood, CA. **Open for lunch and dinner Monday through Saturday. Closed Sundays.**

SUNNYVALE

The Country Gourmet & Co.
1314 S. Mary Ave., Sunnyvale, CA 94087   **(408) 733-9446**
Natural foods. The Country Gourmet features fresh baked goods, an extensive salad collection, and entrees that change daily. Everything is prepared from fresh ingredients with no preservatives or MSG. A couple of vegetarian entrees are featured nightly in addition to the regular menu selection, and there is a children's menu. No smoking. **Limited service, vegan options, fresh juices, wine/beer, take-out, VISA/MC, $$**

Dahlak Restaurant
1009 Duane Ave., Sunnyvale, CA 94086   **(408) 732-8444**
Eritrean. Low-fat dishes are a specialty of foods from Eritrea (formerly a region of Ethiopia). All dishes—including homemade breads and strict vegetarian offerings— are preservative- and additive-free. A special flax dressing is used on salads. **Closed Sunday. Full service, buffet lunches, vegan options, wine/beer/alcohol, VISA/ MC/AMX**

Royal Taj Indian Cuisine
889 E. El Camino Real, Sunnyvale, CA 94087   **(408) 720-8396**
Indian. See entry under Campbell, CA.

TARZANA

Armen & Salpy's
19014 Ventura Blvd., Tarzana, CA 91356   **(818) 343-1301**
Ethnic/natural foods. Falafel and salads are among the foods prepared daily for this smoke-free restaurant. **Closed Sunday. Full service, wine/beer, take-out, $$**

India's Cuisine
19006 Ventura Blvd., Tarzana, CA 91356   **(818) 342-9100**
Indian. See entry under Los Angeles, CA.

🍴 Reviewers' choice   • Vegetarian restaurant   •• Vegan restaurant
$ less than $6 $$ $6–$12 $$$ more than $12
VISA/AMX/MC/DISC/DC—credit cards accepted
Non-alc.—Non-alcoholic   Fresh juices—freshly squeezed

TOPANGA CANYON

Inn of The Seventh Ray
128 Old Topanga Rd., Topanga, CA 90290   **(310) 455-1311**
Gourmet Californian. This up-scale natural foods restaurant is willing to accommodate special requests. No smoking. **Open daily for dinner, Monday through Friday
for lunch, Saturday and Sunday for brunch. Full service, wine/beer, non-alc.
wine/beer, take-out, VISA/MC, $$$**

TUSTIN

Rutabegorz
158 W. Main St., Tustin, CA 92680   **(714) 871-1632**
International. See listing under Fullerton, CA.

UKIAH

Earthly Delight
415 Talmage Rd. #A, Ukiah, CA 95482   **(707) 462-4970**
Health-food-store deli. Located in the Pear Tree Shopping Center, Earthly Delight
offers homemade bread and soups, and sugar-free frozen yogurt. **Fresh juice,
take-out, $**

VENICE

A Votre Santé
1025 Abbott Kinney Blvd., Venice, CA 90291   **(310) 314-1187**
Natural foods. See entry under Brentwood, CA.

The Dandelion Cafe
636 Venice Blvd., Venice, CA 90291   **(310) 821-4890**
American/Californian. Vegetarians can dine on Vegetarian Chili Tostada, quiche,
Vegetable Garden Melt (with cheese), fresh fruit, and Avocado Melt at this patio
restaurant with a nice ocean breeze. **Open daily for breakfast and lunch. Full service,
vegan options, wine/beer/alcohol, VISA/MC/AMX/DISC, $$**

Fig Tree Cafe
429 Ocean Front Walk, Venice, CA 90291   **(310) 392-4937**
Natural foods. Any dish can be made vegetarian, or choose from Spinach Nutburger, Roasted Eggplant and Peppers, Santa Fe Tostada, and Stir Fry Pizzete (chapati
pizza). **Open daily. Full service, wine/beer, VISA/MC/AMX/DISC, $$**

VENTURA

Classic Carrot
1847 E. Main St., Ventura, CA 93001   **(805) 643-0406**
Natural foods. Enjoy international ethnic daily specials, homemade soups, vegetar-
ian chili, and sandwiches in a casual, friendly atmosphere. Garden, brick patio,
and indoor dining areas feature the work of local artists. All-weather patio dining.
**Open for three meals daily. Limited service, vegan options, fresh juices, es-
presso/cappuccino, wine/beer, take-out, VISA/MC/AMX, $**

• Garden Fresh
2833 A East Main St., Ventura, CA 93003 (805) 643-5627
Vegetarian. Homemade soups, salads, and desserts as well as an organic salad bar and non-dairy vegetarian burrito are available. Organic produce and purified water are used. **Open Monday through Saturday for lunch and dinner. Full service, fresh juices, take-out, VISA/MC, $**

Tipps Thai Cuisine
512 East Main St., Ventura, CA 93001 (805) 643-3040
Thai. Tipps has a full vegetarian menu featuring more than twenty entrees plus appetizers, soups, and salads. Entrees include standard vegetable dishes, mock meats, curries, and noodle and rice dishes. No MSG is used. **Open Monday through Saturday for lunch and dinner. Full service, vegan options, wine/beer, take-out, VISA/MC/AMX, $$**

WALNUT CREEK

Pita King
1607 Palo Verdes Mall, Walnut Creek, CA 94596 (510) 945-0386
Middle Eastern/pita bread bakery. Pita King serves falafel and other vegetarian sandwiches. **Open Monday through Saturday for breakfast and lunch. Counter service, take-out, $**

WESTLAKE VILLAGE

India House Restaurant
860 Hampshire Rd., Ste. Z, Westlake Village, CA 91361 (805) 373-6266
Indian. India House grinds its own spices, in addition to making its own cheese, yogurt, and breads. Only vegetable oil is used for cooking and no preservatives. The menu includes appetizers, clay oven entrees, curries, eight vegetarian items, breads, rice dishes, desserts, and beverages. **Closed Monday. Full service, vegan options, wine/beer, take-out, VISA/MC, $–$$**

WILLITS

• Harvest Bounty
39 S. Main, Willits, CA 95490 (707) 459-9647
Vegetarian. Fresh baked cornbread complements homestyle meals, and organic produce is used in salads. **Open for lunch. Full service, fresh juices, $**

Tsunami Restaurant
50 S. Main St., Willits, CA 95490 (707) 459-4750
Japanese/international. Dinner and lunch menu headings include Sushi, Salads, Side Orders, Grilled, Cajun, Colache, and Tempura. All categories list vegetable, tofu, fish, and chicken selections, and vegetarian specials are also offered. Dishes are all carefully prepared from scratch with natural ingredients, and most vegetables are locally and organically grown. Some dessert selections are prepared without dairy, sugar, or eggs. Beverages include local micro-brewery beers, coffee, and wine. Dine on the patio amidst Japanese maple trees, plum trees, and flowers. **Open daily. Reservations recommended. Full service, wine/beer, take-out, $$**

YREKA

Yreka Cafe
322 W. Miner, Yreka, CA 96097   **(916) 842-6010**
Natural foods. Fettucine, salads, and omelettes are featured. **Closed Sunday. Full
service, take-out, $**

COLORADO

ASPEN

• Explore Coffeehouse
221 E. Main St., Aspen, CO 81611   **(303) 925-5336**
Vegetarian. This sophisticated gourmet vegetarian restaurant and European-style
coffeehouse is located under the same roof as a contemporary bookstore. Each
week, a different ethnic specialty is featured in addition to the standard offerings
of soups, salad bar, tofu burger, and steamed veggies. **Open daily for lunch and
dinner. Full service, children's menu, vegan options, take-out, VISA/MC, $$**

AURORA

Denver Salad Co.
14201 E. Public Market, Aurora, CO 80012   **(303) 750-1339**
American. Features seventy-item salad bar, fresh soups, potato bar, and sandwiches.
Open daily. Cafeteria service, wine/beer, take-out, VISA/MC, $$

Fong Lynn
1780 S. Buckley Rd., Aurora, CO 80017   **(303) 745-9111**
Chinese. Fong Lynn features tofu dishes. **Open daily for lunch. Full service, wine/
beer/alcohol, take-out, VISA/MC/AMX, $**

Wild Oats Market
12131 East Iliff Ave., Aurora, CO 80014   **(303) 695-8801**
Health-food-store deli. Wholesome vegetarian dishes feature ethnic foods that are
prepared locally, salads, and baked goods. Wild Oats has recently added an
espresso/juice bar. **Open daily. Deli service, fresh juices, espresso, take-out,
VISA/MC/DISC, $**

ᕈ❧ Reviewers' choice   • Vegetarian restaurant   •• Vegan restaurant
$ less than $6 $$ $6–$12 $$$ more than $12
VISA/AMX/MC/DISC/DC—credit cards accepted
Non-alc.—Non-alcoholic   Fresh juices—freshly squeezed

BOULDER

Alfalfa's Market

1651 Broadway, Boulder, CO 80302   **(303) 442-0909**
Natural foods. Sandwiches, salads, and fresh baked goods are offered. **Open daily.**
Cafeteria style, catering, vegan options, take-out, VISA/MC, $

Attusso's Italian Cafe

1739 Pearl St., Boulder, CO 80302   **(303) 442-2262**
Italian. Imported pasta with fresh, organic veggies and everything else on the
menu is made to order. **Open daily for dinner. Full service, wine/beer/alcohol,
take-out, VISA/MC/AMX/DISC, $$$**

The Boulder Harvest Restaurant

1738 Pearl St., Boulder, CO 80302   **(303) 449-6223**
Natural foods. A natural foods restaurant for the 90s. The menu features healthy,
seasonal entrees, local produce, organic coffee, and environmentally friendly
products. Enjoy your meals inside or on the outdoor patio. **Open for three meals
daily. Full service, vegan options, fresh juice, wine/beer, take-out,
VISA/MC/AMX/DISC, $–$$**

Boulder Salad Co.

2595 Canyon Blvd., Boulder, CO 80302   **(303) 447-8272**
American. Features seventy-item salad bar, fresh soups, potato bar, and sand-
wiches. **Open daily. Cafeteria service, wine/beer, take-out, VISA/MC, $$**

Cafe Central

2100 Central Ave., Boulder, CO 80301   **(303) 443-8855**
Cafeteria. Cafe Central is an up-scale cafeteria serving pastries, salads, soups, specials,
and sandwiches prepared fresh daily. Vegetarian options. Carryout breakfast and box
lunches are available. **Open Monday through Friday for breakfast and lunch. Cafe-
teria style, fresh juice, wine/beer/alcohol, take-out, VISA/MC, $**

• Creative Vegetarian Cafe 🌿

1837 Pearl St., Boulder, CO 80302   **(303) 449-1952**
Vegetarian. Home-cooked foods are made with organic vegetables when in season.
The atmosphere is charming and the portions are good-sized. **Open daily. Sunday
brunch. Full service, take-out, VISA/MC, $$**

Dot's Diner

799 Pearl St., Boulder, CO 80302   **(303) 449-1323**
Natural foods. Dot's bases its reputation on its homestyle breakfasts, which are
served through lunchtime every day. The lunch menu includes daily specials,
Mexican dishes, grilled sandwiches, and a variety of vegetarian entrees. **Open
daily for breakfast and lunch. Full service, fresh juice, espresso/capuccino,
take-out, no credit cards, $**

Golden Buff

1725 28th St., Boulder, CO 80301   **(303) 442-2800**

Natural foods. **Open for three meals daily. Full service, fresh juice, wine/beer, take-out, VISA/MC, $–$$**

Healthy Habits
4760 Baseline, Boulder, CO 80303   **(303) 494-9177**
American. The restaurant features an extensive salad bar, with three vegetarian soups and three veggie pasta sauces that change daily, along with two veggie pizzas, bread, muffins, and desserts. **Open daily. Cafeteria service, wine/beer, VISA/ MC/AMX/DISC/DC, $$**

Himalaya's
2010 14th St., Boulder, CO 80302   **(303) 442-3230**
International. The cuisine here includes Indian, Nepali, and Tibetan food. Fresh breads are baked in the restaurant's Tandoor oven. Lunch is a buffet with four vegetarian dishes. **Open daily. Full service, wine/beer, take-out, VISA/MC, $$**

José Muldoon's
1600 38th St., Boulder, CO 80301   **(303) 449-4543**
Mexican. Blue corn, Santa Fe-style vegetarian and authentic Mexican fare includes appetizers, soups, salads, sandwiches, burgers, tostada bar, and vegetarian specials. Patio dining. **Open daily for lunch and dinner. Sunday brunch. Full service, vegan options, wine/beer/alcohol, take-out, VISA/MC/AMX, $–$$**

• Masala's International Creekside Cafe
2111-30th St., Boulder, CO 80301   **(303) 447-1776**
Vegetarian. Vegetarian Santa Fe sushi, artichoke enchiladas, and samosas as well as many other macrobiotic and international dishes are served at this restaurant featuring a different international cuisine nightly. **Open for lunch and dinner Monday-Saturday. Limited service, vegan options, espresso/cappuccino, take-out, VISA/MC, $–$$**

Nancy's
825 Walnut St., Boulder, CO 80302   **(303) 449-8402**
American/ethnic. Saturday and Sunday breakfast at Nancy's is a Boulder tradition. The restaurant also serves lunch and dinner, and in 1992 introduced four-course vegetarian specials nightly. **Open daily. Full service, vegan options, fresh juices, wine/beer/alcohol, take-out, VISA/MC/AMX, $–$$**

Narayan's Nepal Restaurant
921 Pearl St., Boulder, CO 80302   **(303) 447-2816**
Nepalese. A full menu of fine Nepali entrees is geared to the vegetarian diet. The menu includes vegetable curry, stuffed jumbo roti, pakodas, samosas, etc. **Full service, vegan options, wine/beer/alcohol, take-out, VISA/MC/AMX, $**

Pablo's New Mexican Cafe
2865 Baseline Rd., Boulder, CO 80303   **(303) 442-7512**
Mexican. Seven vegetarian options are on the menu at Pablo's. Tofu and tempeh are used in some of these dishes. **Open daily. Full service, vegan options, fresh juice, wine/beer/alcohol, take-out, VISA/MC/AMX/DISC/DC, $$**

Rocky Mountain Joe's Cafe & Espresso Bar
1410 Pearl St., Boulder, CO 80302 **(303) 442-3969**
Natural foods. Tempeh and garden burgers, vegetarian chili, salads, and some breakfast items make up the vegetarian offerings on Rocky Joe's menu. **Open daily for breakfast and lunch. Full service, fresh juice, espresso/cappuccino, take-out, VISA/MC, $**

Rudi's Restaurant
4720 Table Mesa Dr., Boulder, CO 80303 **(303) 494-5858**
Natural foods. Extended gourmet vegetarian menu along with ethnic specialties. All food is fresh and homemade. Bakery, cafe, espresso bar. **Open Tuesday through Sunday for lunch and dinner. Closed Mondays. Weekend brunch. Full service, wine/beer, catering, VISA/MC/DISC, $$**

Siamese Plate & Sumida's Sushi Bar
1575 Folsom, Boulder, CO 80302 **(303) 447-9718**
Thai. The vegetarian menu has a good selection of appetizers, soups, and entrees. Vegetarian versions of many of the regular menu items are available as well. **Open daily for lunch and dinner. Full service, wine/beer/alcohol, take-out, $$**

Walnut Cafe
3073 Walnut, Boulder, CO 80301 **(303) 447-2315**
Natural foods. Whether you're in the mood for a Boulder-sized muffin, Huevos Rancheros, or a veggie burger, the "Nut" has what you're looking for. The cafe cooks up a special soup, quiche, and omelette every day and has an espresso menu with sixteen drinks. No smoking. **Open daily for breakfast and lunch. Dinner served Tuesday through Saturday. Full service, fresh juices, take-out, VISA/MC/DISC, $**

Wild Oats Market
2584 Baseline, Boulder, CO 80303 **(303) 499-7636**
Health-food-store deli. Features Tabouleh, Hummus, Pasta Salad, and soup, with a full dinner menu. Some non-vegetarian items. **Open daily. Counter service, vegan options, take-out, VISA/MC/DISC, $**

• Wild Oats Vegetarian Market
1825 Pearl St., Boulder, CO 80302 **(303) 440-9599**
Vegetarian/health-food-store deli. Same as Wild Oats Market (above), except all vegetarian.

Young's Place Asian Cuisine
1083 14th St., Boulder, CO 80302 **(303) 447-9837**

ॐ Reviewers' choice   • Vegetarian restaurant   •• Vegan restaurant
$ less than $6 $$ $6–$12 $$$ more than $12
VISA/AMX/MC/DISC/DC—credit cards accepted
Non-alc.—Non-alcoholic   Fresh juices—freshly squeezed

Asian. Korean, Japanese, Chinese, and Mongolian cuisines are served at Young's Place. The Mongolian barbecue has tofu and vegetable options, and there are some other vegetarian selections. **Closed Sunday. Full service, take-out, $**

BRECKENRIDGE

Amazing Grace Natural Foods
213 Lincoln Ave., Breckenridge, CO 80424   **(303) 453-1445**
Health-food-store deli. Located in a historic building, Amazing Grace has a chalkboard menu that lists a soup du jour, veggie sandwiches, smoothies, garden salads, and fresh juice. **Open daily for lunch and dinner. Deli service, fresh juices, take-out, $**

The Red Orchid
206 N. Main St., Breckenridge, CO 80424   **(303) 453-1881**
Chinese. Szechuan, Hunan, and Mandarin cuisines are offered at the Red Orchid. Some vegetarian dishes include Braised Bean Curd, Moo Shu Vegetables, and Szechuan Eggplant. **Open daily for lunch and dinner. Full service, deck dining, vegan options, wine/beer/alcohol, take-out, VISA/MC, $$**

CHERRY CREEK

Alfalfa's
201 University, Cherry Creek, CO 80209   **(303) 442-0909**
Natural foods. See description under Boulder, CO.

COLORADO SPRINGS

Dale Street Cafe
115 E. Dale St., Colorado Springs, CO 80903   **(719) 578-9898**
Natural foods. All-natural freshly prepared foods include appetizers, salads, pasta, and some Mediterranean dishes. **Open daily for lunch and dinner. Full service, non-alc. beer, wine/beer/alcohol, take-out, VISA/MC, $$**

Golden Dragon Restaurant
903 S. 8th St., Colorado Springs, CO 80906   **(719) 632-3607**
Chinese/American. Vegetarian appetizers, soup, and entrees are available at the Golden Dragon. No MSG is used and the restaurant is willing to accommodate special diets (may require advance notice). **Open daily for lunch and dinner. Full service, vegan options, wine/beer/alcohol, take-out, VISA/MC/AMX/DISC, $$**

The Indian Palate
117 E. Bijou, Colorado Springs, CO 80903   **(719) 633-1080**
Indian. According to this restaurant's menu, "India is the cradle of vegetarianism," and this idea is supported with vegetarian Indian appetizers, lunch and dinner specials, and The Vegetarian Feast—a complete vegetarian meal. **Open Monday through Saturday for lunch and dinner. Full service, vegan options, wine/beer/alcohol, take-out, VISA/MC, $$**

José Muldoon's

222 N. Tejon St., Colorado Springs, CO 80903   **(719) 636-2311**

Mexican. See description under Boulder, CO.

The Olive Branch

333 N. Tejon St., Colorado Springs, CO 80903   **(719) 475-1199**

2140 Vickers Dr., Colorado Springs, CO 80918   **(719) 593-9522**

Natural foods. Vegetarian, "heart healthy," and other items are served. **Both locations open daily for three meals and Sunday brunch. Full service, fresh juices, take-out, VISA/MC/AMX/DISC, $**

DENVER

(For more restaurant listings in the surrounding areas, see Aurora, Englewood, Littleton, Westminster, and Wheatridge.)

Beau Jo's Pizza

2700 S. Colorado Blvd., Denver, CO 80222   **(303) 758-1519**

Pizza restaurant. Enjoy delicious pizza—sixteen vegetarian toppings and a vegan pizza topped with tofu and whatever else you'd like! A soup and salad bar is also available. **Open daily for lunch and dinner. Full service, vegan options, wine/beer/alcohol, take-out, VISA/MC/AMX/DISC, $**

City Spirit Cafe

1434 Blake St., Denver, CO 80202   **(303) 575-0022**

Natural foods. Everything served here is made from scratch. Organic items are available. The use of fats is minimal. Entrees include organic tamales, Cityburritas, and Urbanachos. Live music on weekends. **Open late daily. Full service, vegan options, wine/beer/alcohol, take-out, $**

Delhi Darbar

1514 Blake St., Denver, CO 80202   **(303) 595-0680**

Indian. Buffet lunch every day features primarily vegetarian foods, and the extensive vegetarian dinner menu includes fresh baked breads. **Open daily for lunch and dinner. Full service, wine/beer/alcohol, take-out, VISA/MC/AMX/DISC, $$**

Denver Salad Co.

2700 S. Colorado Blvd., Denver, CO 80207   **(303) 691-2050**

American. See description under Aurora, CO.

Golden Tempura Bowl

1448 Market St., Denver, CO 80202   **(303) 534-3370**

Japanese. Healthy Japanese food is served efficiently in a fast-food-restaurant atmosphere. **Closed Sunday. Counter service, BYOB, take-out, $**

Good Friends

3100 E. Colfax Ave., Denver, CO 80206   **(303) 399-1751**

Natural foods. "Fern bar" from the '70s offers a wide selection of moderately priced foods. Over half of the menu is vegetarian including dishes such as eggplant salad, stir-fry, Mexican food without lard, and salads. **Open daily for lunch and dinner. Full service, wine/beer/alcohol, take-out, VISA/MC/AMX/DISC, $–$$**

• Govinda's Vegetarian Buffet
1400 Cherry St., Denver, CO 80220   **(303) 333-5462**
Vegetarian buffet. Here's an all-you-can-eat vegetarian buffet in the Govinda's tradition. No eggs are used and only vegetarian (rennetless) cheese is served. Thursday is vegan day—all items are non-dairy. Salad bar, rice, breads, and steamed vegetables round out the international entrees. **Closed Sunday. Buffet, vegan options, take-out, VISA/ MC, $**

Harvest Restaurant & Bakery
430 S. Colorado Blvd., Denver, CO 80222   **(303) 399-6652**

7730 E. Belleview, Denver, CO 80111   **(303) 779-4111**
Mexican/healthy foods. See entry under Boulder, CO.

Healthy Habits
865 S. Colorado Blvd., Denver, CO 80206   **(303) 733-2105**
American. See description under Boulder, CO.

Jerusalem Restaurant
1890 E. Evans Ave., Denver, CO 80210   **(303) 777-8828**
Middle Eastern. The Middle Eastern food offered at this restaurant includes many vegetarian appetizers and a couple of $combo" dishes that make a satisfying meal. A special section of the menu lists the vegetable dishes. **Open daily, 24 hours on Friday and Saturday. Full service, vegan options, take-out, VISA/MC/AMX, $**

Josephina's
7777 E. Hampden Ave. #120, Denver, CO 80231   **(303) 750-4422**
Italian. Josephina's serves Northern and Southern Italian foods plus heart-healthy and vegetarian dishes. Heart-healthy items are indicated on the menu. **Open daily. Full service, vegan options, wine/beer/alcohol, take-out, VISA/MC/AMX/ DISC, $$**

Mediterranean Health Cafe
2817 E. 3rd Ave., Denver, CO 80206   **(303) 399-2940**
Kosher/Mediterranean. Various Middle Eastern vegetarian foods are available from the primarily vegetarian menu. Fish is the only non-vegetarian food served. On the menu are Falafel, Hummus, Veggie Burger, Vegetarian Chili, and sandwiches. The editors of the *Vegetarian Journal* give the food rave reviews. **Open daily. Full service, kosher, vegan options, take-out, VISA/MC/AMX, $**

Paul's Place
Cherry Creek Shopping Center
3000 E. 1st Ave., #115, Denver, CO 80206   **(303) 321-5801**
Gourmet fast food. This fast-food restaurant offers a wide selection of vegetarian and vegan dishes including veggie burgers and hot dogs, sandwiches, tamales, burritos, chili, baked potatoes, and tacos. **Open Monday through Saturday for three meals. Counter service, vegan options, catering, take-out, VISA/MC/DISC, $**

• Rosewood Cafe
Porter Hospital, 2525 S. Downing St., Denver, CO 80210   (303) 778-5881
Vegetarian. The Rosewood Cafe offers an exciting, varied menu that changes daily. Most food, including baked goods, is freshly prepared. The public is welcome! **Open every day. Cafeteria Style, kosher, some vegan options, fresh juice, take-out, no credit cards, $**

Seoul Food
701 E. 6th Ave., Denver, CO 80203   (303) 837-1460
Korean. Seoul Food serves authentic Korean cuisine with vegetarian and health-oriented selections. **Open daily for lunch and dinner. Full service, wine/beer, take-out, VISA/MC, $**

T-WA Inn Vietnamese Restaurant
555 S. Federal Blvd., Denver, CO 80219   (303) 922-4584
Vietnamese. Special vegetarian section on menu features fourteen entree options including Vegetables with Rice Noodles, Tofu with Lemongrass, curry, and eggplant dishes. **Open daily for lunch and dinner. Full service, vegan options, wine/beer/alcohol, VISA/MC/AMX, $$**

Walnut Cafe
338 E. Colfax Ave., Denver, CO 80203   (303) 832-5108
Natural foods. Open for breakfast and lunch. Tofu available as a meat, cheese, or egg substitute. **Open daily. Full service, take-out, $**

Wolfe's Barbecue
333 E. Colfax Ave., Denver, CO 80203   (303) 831-1500
Barbecue. Traditional hole-in-the-wall (their words, not ours!) barbecue offering vegan BBQ entrees and side dishes. Wolfe's even has coleslaw without mayonnaise! **Open Monday through Friday for lunch and dinner. Limited service, take-out, VISA/MC, $**

ENGLEWOOD

Paul's Place
Southgate Shopping Center
6818 S. Yosemite, Englewood, CO 80237   (303) 771-8855
Gourmet fast food. This fast-food restaurant offers a wide selection of vegetarian and vegan fast dishes including veggie burgers and hot dogs, sandwiches, tamales, burritos, chili, baked potatoes, and tacos. **Open daily for breakfast, lunch, and dinner. Counter service, vegan options, catering, take-out, VISA/MC/DISC, $**

Twin Dragon Restaurant
3021 S. Broadway, Englewood, CO 80110   (303) 781-8068

ϩ♥ Reviewers' choice   • Vegetarian restaurant   •• Vegan restaurant
$ less than $6 $$ $6–$12 $$$ more than $12
VISA/AMX/MC/DISC/DCcredit cards accepted
Non-alc.—Non-alcoholic   Fresh juices—freshly squeezed

Mandarin/Szechuan. Extensive menu offers approximately fifteen vegetable and tofu options. **Open daily for lunch and dinner. Full service, vegan options, wine/beer/alcohol, take-out, VISA/MC/AMX/DISC, $$**

ESTES PARK

Molly B's
200 Moraine Ave., P.O. Box 3280, Estes Park, CO 80517   (303) 586-2766
Natural foods. Vegetarian selections are available for both lunch and dinner. Examples include pasta, stir-fry, and lasagna. Various specials are offered daily. Baked goods are prepared on the premises. **Full service, vegan options, fresh juices, wine/beer, take-out, VISA/MC/AMX, $$**

EVERGREEN

Buckwheat's Natural Foods Store & Cafe
29011 Upper Bear Creek Rd., Evergreen, CO 80439   (303) 674-5843
Natural foods. Buckweat's Cafe offers daily specials, fresh soup, veggie burgers, and a spelt/whole-wheat soy pizza. Enjoy an incredible view of a lake and mountain as you dine. **Lunch served daily. Limited service, catering, vegan options, $**

River Sage Restaurant
4651 S. Hwy. 73, Evergreen, CO 80439   (303) 674-2914
Natural foods. The cuisine is described as "exuberant Rocky Mountain," and you can dine indoors surrounded by wonderful artwork, or on the streamside deck. Featured are homemade entrees such as Rainbow Garden Skillet for breakfast, Vegi Burritos and Southwestern Tempeh Sauté for lunch, and Oriental Nine Vegetable Wok or Indian Vegetable Curry for dinner. **Open daily. Full service, vegan options, wine/beer, take-out, VISA/MC, $$**

FORT COLLINS

Chow's Garden
23 Old Town Square #100, Fort Collins, CO 80524   (303) 484-6142
Chinese. There's a vegetarian section on the menu with nine selections including eggplant and tofu dishes. **Full service, wine/beer/alcohol, take-out, VISA/MC/AMX/ DISC, $–$$**

Cozzola's Pizza
241 Linden, Fort Collins, CO 80524   (303) 482-3557
Pizza restaurant. Cozzola's offers gourmet pizza with whole-wheat, herb, or white crusts plus a variety of sauces and toppings—even soy cheese! Some of the sauces do contain cheese, so vegans should inquire first. **Closed Monday. Full service, vegan options, take-out, no credit cards, $**

Cuisine! Cuisine!
130 S. Mason, Fort Collins, CO 80524   (303) 221-0399
International. Chalkboard menu changes daily, featuring regional and international theme weeks such as French, Caribbean, Southwestern, Pacific Northwest, Cajun, and Southeast Asian. There are vegetarian options. **Closed Mondays. Full service, formal, vegan options, take-out, VISA/MC/AMX, $$$**

Fort Collins Food Co-op
250 E. Mountain Ave., Fort Collins, CO 80524 **(303) 484-7448**
Natural foods deli. This small take-out deli is in a natural foods market. **Open Monday through Friday. Deli service, fresh juice, take-out, no credit cards, $**

• Govinda's Vegetarian Cafe and Juice Bar
105 E. Laurel Ave., Fort Collins, CO 80524 **(303) 484-4282**
Vegetarian. Govinda's offers an inexpensive all-you-can-eat vegetarian buffet as well as a juice bar. **Lunch served Tuesday through Saturday. Dinner served Thursday through Saturday. Closed Sunday. Limited service, fresh juices, vegan options, catering, take-out, $**

Rainbow Ltd.
212 W. Laurel, Fort Collins, CO 80521 **(303) 221-2664**
Natural foods. **Open daily. Full service, wine/beer, take-out, VISA/MC, $**

Rio Grande Mexican Restaurant
143 W. Mountain Ave., Ft. Collins, CO 80524 **(303) 224-5428**
Mexican. Rio Grande serves authentic Mexican foods with sauces made fresh daily. All bean dishes are made with black beans and without lard. **Open daily. Full service, vegan options, wine/beer/alcohol, take out, VISA/MC/DISC, $$**

GRAND JUNCTION

Good Pastures Restaurant & Lounge
733 Horizon Dr., Grand Junction, CO 81506 **(303) 243-3058**
International. Good Pastures takes pride in serving as natural a product as possible and therefore avoids using chemicals, dyes, and preservatives. The menu is varied and geared to please any appetite. **Open for three meals daily. Full service, vegan options, fresh juices, wine/beer/alcohol, take-out, VISA/MC/AMX/DISC, $$**

River City Cafe & Bar
748 North Ave., Grand Junction, CO 81501 **(303) 245-8040**
Natural foods. The menu features pasta, bean burgers, bean burritos, and enchiladas. **Open daily. Full service, vegan options, non-alc. beer, wine/beer/alcohol, take-out, VISA/MC/AMX/DISC, $$**

• Sundrop Grocery
321 Rood Ave., Grand Junction, CO 81501 **(303) 243-1175**
Vegetarian deli. The fare here is pre-made sandwiches including tofuna, guacamole, veggie pita, bagel sandwiches and more. **Closed Sunday. Take-out only, vegan options, $**

GREENWOOD VILLAGE

Harvest Restaurant & Bakery
7730 E. Belleview, Greenwood Village, CO 80111 **(303) 779-4111**
Mexican/healthy food. See Boulder, CO, listing for description.

IDAHO SPRINGS
Beau Jo's Pizza
1517 Miner St., Idaho Springs, CO 80452   **(303) 567-4376**
Pizza. A visit to Beau Jo's will undoubtedly be worth the trip, whether you eat or not. Seventeen years' worth of napkin art is displayed at the restaurant. But if you do want to eat, the pizza options are just as interesting. Sixteen vegetarian toppings are offered plus a tofu pizza, which is vegan. There is also a soup and salad bar. **Open daily for lunch and dinner. Full service, vegan options, wine/beer/alcohol, take-out, VISA/MC/AMX/DISC, $$**

LAFAYETTE
Efrain's Mexican Restaurante & Cantina
101 E. Cleveland, Lafayette, CO 80026   **(303) 666-7544**
Mexican. Mexican food is prepared fresh daily, and vegetarian items are indicated on the menu. **Open daily for lunch and dinner. Full service, vegan options, take-out, VISA/MC, $**

LITTLETON
Alfalfa's
5910 S. University, Littleton, CO 80121   **(303) 798-9699**
Natural foods/juice bar. A natural foods store with deli, bakery, pizza bar, and juice bar. **Open daily for three meals. Cafeteria style, fresh juices, cappuccino, take-out, catering, VISA/MC/DISC, $$**

Denver Salad Co.
2010 E. County Line Rd., Littleton, CO 80126   **(303) 798-3453**
American. See description under Aurora, CO.

Harvest Restaurant & Bakery
5056 S. Wadsworth Blvd., Littleton, CO 80123   **(303) 933-2011**
Natural foods. See description under Boulder, CO.

LONGMONT
Ichi Ban Japanese Restaurant
1834 N. Main St., Longmont, CO 80501   **(303) 772-6882**
Japanese. Ichi Ban features authentic Japanese foods with vegetarian options such as Egg Rolls, Vegetable Tempura, and noodle dishes. **Open Tuesday through Saturday. Full service, wine/beer, take-out, VISA/MC, $$**

🍴 Reviewers' choice   ● Vegetarian restaurant   ●● Vegan restaurant
$ less than $6 $$ $6–$12 $$$ more than $12
VISA/AMX/MC/DISC/DC—credit cards accepted
Non-alc.—Non-alcoholic   Fresh juices—freshly squeezed

LOUISVILLE

Karen's Kitchen
700 Main St., Louisville, CO 80027 **(303) 666-8020**
Natural foods. Features Eggplant Parmesan, burritos, Lasagna, and salads. **Open daily, only brunch served on Sunday. Full service, vegan options, wine/beer, take-out, $$**

MANITOU SPRINGS

Adam's Mountain Cafe
733 Manitou Ave., Manitou Springs, CO 80829 **(719) 685-1430**
Natural foods. This award-winning restaurant features Southwestern entrees including a breakfast burrito. Other dishes include the Small Planet Burger and Vegetarian Colorado. Scenic location. **Open daily. Full service, vegan options, wine/beer, take-out, $$**

TELLURIDE

Athenian Senate
123 S. Spruce, Telluride, CO 81435 **(303) 728-3018**
Greek/Italian. This is a friendly and comfortable family restaurant. Many Greek and pasta dishes are suitable for vegetarians. Children's menu. **Open daily. Full service, vegan options, wine/beer/alcohol, take-out, VISA/MC/AMX, $$$**

Gregor's Bakery & Cafe
217 E. Colorado Ave., Telluride, CO 81435 **(303) 728-3334**
Natural foods. This restaurant serves a variety of creative vegetarian foods and features a bakery. **Open daily. Limited service, beer, take-out, $$**

WESTMINSTER

La Casa Loma Cafe
710 W. 120th St., Westminster, CO 80234 **(303) 450-6906**
Mexican/American. La Casa Loma's menu features low-cholesterol foods that include many Mexican and American dishes. No lard is used in the beans or green chili. Vegetarian options are on the menu, and the restaurant is willing to accommodate special diets. **Closed Sunday. Full service, vegan options, wine/beer/alcohol, take-out, VISA/MC, $**

WHEATRIDGE

Gemini Restaurant
4300 Wadsworth Blvd., Loehmann's Plaza
Wheatridge, CO 80033 **(303) 421-4990**
Natural foods/ethnic. Extensive menu offers appetizers, salads, soups, sandwiches, quiche, pasta, and Mexican dishes—vegetarian and non-vegetarian foods. Children's menu. **Open for three meals daily, weekend brunch. Full service, vegan options, fresh juice, wine/beer/alcohol, take-out, VISA/MC, $$**

CONNECTICUT

BRIDGEPORT

• Bloodroot ✿

85 Ferris St., Bridgeport, CT 06605   **(203) 576-9168**

Vegetarian. Situated on an inlet in Long Island Sound, Bloodroot is "a feminist restaurant and bookstore with a seasonal vegetarian menu." This menu changes every three to four weeks to take advantage of foods in season. Outdoor dining on the herb terrace. **Open Tuesday and Thursday through Sunday. Limited service weekdays, full service on weekends, vegan options, wine/beer, no credit cards, $$**

CANTON

Tangiers Mediterranean Cafe

140 Albany Turnpike, Canton, CT 06019   **(203) 693-6668**

Middle Eastern. Savor vegetarian Middle Eastern specialties. **Closed Tuesday. Full service, vegan options, fresh juice, take-out, VISA/MC, $$**

DANBURY

Sesame Seed

68 W. Wooster St., Danbury, CT 06810   **(203) 743-9850**

Natural foods. Middle Eastern dishes, Broccoli Strudel, Spinach Dumplings, and Vegetable Pie are featured at Sesame Seed. **Closed Sunday. Full service, non-alc. beer, wine/beer, take-out, $–$$**

GLASTONBURY

Garden of Light Natural Foods Market

2858 Main St., Glastonbury, CT 06033   **(203) 657-9131**

Natural foods deli and juice bar. Award-winning vegan chef Ken Bergeron supervises this store's deli. Organic ingredients are used whenever possible. Enjoy a full salad bar, fresh baked goods, and hot dishes sold mostly by the pound. **Open daily. Counter service, vegan/macrobiotic options, fresh juices, catering, take-out, VISA/MC, $–$$**

HARTFORD

Cafe at Reader's Feast

529 Farmington Ave., Hartford, CT 06105   **(203) 232-3710**

Cafe and bookstore. Various international menu items and sandwiches are served. Breakfast includes granola, eggs, French toast, and omelettes. Reader's Feast has a monthly art exhibit by local artists, and readings on most Sundays. Menu changes seasonally. **Open for breakfast, lunch, and dinner Monday through Saturday; only for brunch on Sunday. Full service for dinner, cafeteria style for lunch, vegan options, wine/beer, take-out, VISA/MC, $–$$**

Congress Rotisserie
7 Maple Ave., Hartford, CT 06114 **(203) 560-1965**
Bistro. A stir-fry and a pasta dish make up the vegetarian selection on the menu at this bistro, but the restaurant notes that special diets can be accommodated. In general, the menu features eclectic fish and chicken dishes. **Open daily. Full service, wine/beer/alcohol, take-out, VISA/MC/AMX, $$**

Kashmir Restaurant
481 Wethersfield Ave., Hartford, CT 06114 **(203) 296-9685**
Indian. Sample classic Moghul cooking plus a wide variety of authentic dishes from various Indian traditions. The menu includes appetizers, soups, side dishes, entrees, breads, and desserts, all of which are prepared without artificial ingredients, additives, or saturated fats. **Full service, vegan options, take-out, $$**

MIDDLETOWN

•• It's Only Natural Restaurant
686 Main St., Middletown, CT 06457 **(203) 346-9210**
Vegan. This is a vegan restaurant serving international gourmet vegetarian and macrobiotic meals, and featuring fresh baked bread and desserts. **Open Tuesday through Saturday. Full service, completely vegan, fresh juices, catering, take-out, AMX, $$**

NEW HAVEN

Avanti's
45 Grove St., New Haven, CT 06511 **(203) 777-3234**
Italian. Avanti's is an Italian restaurant and pizzeria with several vegan options. **Closed Sunday. Full service, vegan options, espresso/cappuccino, wine/beer, take-out, VISA/MC, $$**

Claire's CornerCopia
1000 Chapel St., New Haven, CT 06510 **(203) 562-3888**
International. Claire's offers meatless Mexican, Italian, and Jewish fare. The wide variety of baked goods is made on the premises. **Open daily. Limited service, vegan options, fresh juices, take-out, no credit cards, $–$$**

Edge of the Woods
379 Whalley Ave., New Haven, CT 06511 **(203) 787-1055**
Health-food-store deli. Partake of vegetarian fare with some vegan choices and baked goods. **Open daily. Sunday brunch. Cafeteria style, fresh juices, take-out, $**

🏖 Reviewers' choice • Vegetarian restaurant •• Vegan restaurant
$ less than $6 $$ $6–$12 $$$ more than $12
VISA/AMX/MC/DISC/DC—credit cards accepted
Non-alc.—Non-alcoholic Fresh juices—freshly squeezed

House of Chao
898 Whalley Ave., New Haven, CT 06515   **(203) 389-6624**
Chinese. House of Chao offers many vegan options and is accustomed to adjusting the menu for vegetarians. **Open daily for lunch and dinner. Full service, vegan options, take-out, $$**

India Palace
65 Howe St., New Haven, CT 06511   **(203) 776-9010**
Indian. There's a vegetarian menu section plus vegetable pakora, samosas, soup, breads, and desserts. **Open daily for lunch and dinner. Full service, vegan options, wine/beer, take-out, VISA/MC, $$**

Mamoun's Falafel Restaurant
85 Howe St., New Haven, CT 06511   **(203) 562-8444**
Middle Eastern. Traditional Middle Eastern foods such as Hummus, Falafel, Baba Ghanouj, salads, and pastries are served. **Open daily. Limited service, vegan options, take-out, $**

Rainbow Garden
1022 Chapel St., New Haven, CT 06511   **(203) 777-2390**
Natural foods. Hot and cold vegetarian sandwiches along with ethnic entrees, daily specials, and soups are available at Rainbow Garden. Menu changes daily and has many vegan entrees. Smoke- and alcohol-free environment. **Open daily. Self-serve, vegan options, take-out, VISA/MC/AMX, $**

SOUTHBURY

Natural Merchant Cafe
142 Main St., Southbury, CT 06488   **(203) 264-9954**
Natural foods. Located in a historic building, this restaurant is accompanied by a natural foods store and offers soups, sandwiches, salads, quiche, and fresh baked desserts and muffins. Two entrees are offered daily. **Open daily for lunch. Fresh juices, BYOB, take-out, VISA/MC/AMX, $–$$**

Senior Pancho's Mexican Restaurants
Union Square Mall, Southbury, CT 06488   **(203) 262-6988**
Mexican. A separate vegetarian menu includes chimichangas, black bean soup, vegetable fajitas, as well as several other vegetarian items. **Open daily for lunch and dinner. Full service, espresso/cappuccino, smoothies, catering, take-out, VISA/MC/AMX/DC, $–$$**

WEST HARTFORD

Pacific Restaurant
206 Park Rd., West Hartford, CT 06119   **(203) 236-6639**
Vietnamese. Pacific Restaurant offers vegetarian fare and does not use MSG in the preparation of its meals. **Open daily for lunch and dinner. Full service, vegan options, take-out, VISA/MC/AMX, $**

Tapas
1150 New Britain Ave., West Hartford, CT 06040　　　**(203) 521-4609**
Mediterranean. Platters, eclectic pizzas, side orders, salads, and daily specials for lunch and dinner are offered at Tapas. Patio dining. **Open daily. Full service, vegan options, wine/beer, take-out, VISA/MC/AMX, $$**

DELAWARE

DOVER

El Sombrero
655 N. D Hwy., Dover, DE 19901　　　**(302) 678-9445**
International. Vegetarian menu includes vegetable fajita, lasagna, samosa, and other items. **Open daily for lunch and dinner. Vegan options, wine/beer/alcohol, take-out, VISA/MC/AMX/DISC, $$**

HOCKESSIN

Capriotti's
120 Lantana Square Shopping Center, Route 7 & Valley Rd.
Hockessin, DE 19707　　　**(302) 234-2322**
Deli. Capriotti's is more than just a regular deli as it features several options for vegetarians, including vegetarian turkey and ham hoagies, veggie burgers and hot dogs, and veggie tuna for subs and sandwiches. **Deli, vegan options, take-out, $**

NEW CASTLE

Capriotti's
708 W. Basin Rd., New Castle, DE 19720　　　**(302) 322-6797**
Deli. See description under Hockessin, DE.

Tribeni Indian Restaurant
216 N. Dupont Hwy., New Castle, DE 19720　　　**(302) 322-2260**
Indian. This friendly, family-owned restaurant takes special measures to offer fresh and healthful Indian food. All of the food is prepared with 100-percent vegetable oil and is free from preservatives. A large vegetarian selection is available, and on Sundays, a complete vegetarian dinner buffet is offered. Enjoy excellent food and friendly service. **Closed Monday. Full service, vegan options, take-out, VISA/MC/DISC, $$**

NEWARK

Capriotti's
614 Newark Shopping Ctr., Newark, DE 19711　　　**(302) 454-0200**
Deli. See description under Hockessin, DE.

King's Chinese Restaurant
2671 Kirkwood Hwy., Newark, DE 19711   **(302) 731-8022**
Chinese. Chef and owner Bob Chang invites you to explore his new menu of homemade soups, tasty appetizers, and vegetarian entrees. King's extensive vegetarian menu features many Chinese dishes including mock meat and exotic mushroom entrees. The restaurant is very flexible and willing to prepare whatever you request. King's is located in the Meadowood Shopping Center but is difficult to see from the highway as you must drive around to the side of the shopping center to find it. **Open daily for lunch and dinner. Full service, vegan options, wine/beer/alcohol, take-out, VISA/MC/AMX/DISC, $$**

Newark Co-op
280 East Main St., Newark, DE 19711   **(302) 368-5894**
Food co-op with deli. This successful food co-op offers a small deli where you can purchase pre-made cold salads and sandwiches. **Closed Sunday. Vegan options, take-out, $**

Satori Natural Food Restaurant
280 East Main St., Newark, DE 19711   **(302) 738-1975**
International. Satori Natural Food Restaurant offers a wide range of vegan food including a Bean Burger, a Hummus and Tabouli Pita Sandwich, Taco Salad, a Burrito Platter, Vegetable Stir-Fry, and a special macrobiotic platter each Wednesday. In addition to the regular menu, daily specials are offered. Entertainment is provided on Friday and Saturday evenings. **Open Monday through Saturday for lunch and dinner. Closed Sunday. Full service, fresh juices, catering, take-out, $–$$**

WILMINGTON

Capriotti's
510 N. Union St., Wilmington, DE 19805   **(302) 479-9818**

2124 Silverside Rd., Barba Plaza, Wilmington, DE 19810   **(302) 454-0200**
Deli. See description under Hockessin, DE.

DISTRICT OF COLUMBIA

(For more restaurant listings in the surrounding areas, see Arlington and Falls Church in Virginia; Bethesda, Capital Heights, College Park, Gaithersburg, Greenbelt, Olney, Riverdale, Rockville, Silver Spring, Spencerville, Tacoma Park, and Wheaton in Maryland.)

Aditi Indian Cuisine
3299 M St., NW, Washington, DC 20007   **(202) 625-6825**
Indian. Sample vegetarian appetizers, soup, entrees, breads, and dessert. **Open Tuesday through Sunday for lunch and dinner and on Monday for dinner only. Full service, vegan options, fresh juices, wine/beer/alcohol, take-out, VISA/MC/AMX/DISC, $$**

• Balajee

1379 K St., NW, Washington, DC 20005 **(202) 682-9090**

Vegetarian/Indian. Partake of a wide variety of vegetarian Indian dishes. **Open daily for lunch and dinner. Cafeteria style, vegan options, fresh juices, take-out, $–$$**

The Bombay Club

815 Connecticut Ave., NW, Washington, DC 20006 **(202) 659-3727**

Indian. Regional Indian cuisine is served in clublike ambiance. Varied vegetarian dishes from all of India. **Open daily for lunch and dinner. Full service, wine/ beer/alcohol, take-out, VISA/MC/AMX, $$**

City Cafe

2213 M St., NW, Washington, DC 20037 **(202) 797-4860**

Natural foods. The City Cafe serves multi-ethnic new American cuisine using all organic ingredients. Vegetarian appetizers, salads, and entrees are offered. Menu changes seasonally. **Closed Sunday. Open Monday through Friday for lunch and dinner and on Saturday for dinner only. Full service, vegan options, fresh juices, wine/beer/alcohol, take-out, VISA/MC, $$–$$$**

City Lights of China

1731 Connecticut Ave., NW, Washington, DC 20009 **(202) 265-6688**

Hunan/Szechuan. Request the special vegetarian menu at City Lights, and you'll be pleased to find a wide assortment of delicious vegetarian appetizers, entrees, and soups that include mock meat dishes as well as other vegetarian Chinese foods. **Open daily for lunch and dinner. Full service, vegan options, wine/beer/ alcohol, take-out, VISA/MC/AMX, $$**

•• Delights of the Garden

3285-1/2 M St., NW, Washington, DC 20007 **(202) 342-6407**

Vegan. Diners at this vegan, raw-food restaurant will enjoy a wide variety of dishes based on fruits, vegetables, grains, nuts, and seeds. We recommend that you try one of the sampler platters the first time you visit this establishment. Sunday brunch offered. **Open daily for lunch and dinner. Full and counter service, completely vegan, fresh juices, take-out, VISA/MC/AMX/DISC/DC, $$**

• Eat For Strength Vegetarian Cafe

1917 9th St., NW, Washington, DC 20001 **(202) 332-7604**

Vegetarian. Entrees, soups, side orders, "pitawiches" (pita bread sandwiches), eggless egg rolls, and salads priced per pound make up the offerings at the Eat For Strength Cafe. The food is mostly dairyless with a wide variety of tasty vegetarian dishes. Seven entrees and eight soups are listed on the menu. **Closed Saturday. Buffet, vegan options, fresh juices, take-out, $**

ᵏ🐾 Reviewers' choice • Vegetarian restaurant •• Vegan restaurant
$ less than $6 $$ $6–$12 $$$ more than $12
VISA/AMX/MC/DISC/DC—credit cards accepted
Non-alc.—Non-alcoholic   Fresh juices—freshly squeezed

Fasika's Ethiopian Restaurant
2447 18th St., NW, Washington, DC 20009   **(202) 797-7673**
Ethiopian. Fasika's has a vegetarian menu section featuring salads, vegetable, and
grain dishes. **Open daily for dinner. Full service, vegan options, wine/beer/alcohol, take-out, VISA/MC/AMX/DC, $$**

Food for Thought
1738 Connecticut Ave., NW, Washington, DC 20009   **(202) 797-1095**
Natural foods. The extensive menu features a wide assortment of creative sandwiches, salads, soups, light fare, and desserts. Several dinner entrees and daily
specials are also available. Live music nightly. **Open Monday through Saturday for
lunch and dinner; Sunday, dinner only. Full service, vegan options, fresh juices,
wine/ beer/alcohol, winter beverages, take-out, VISA/MC/AMX, $$**

Good Health Natural Foods
325 Pennsylvania Ave., SE, Washington, DC 20003   **(202) 543-2266**
Natural foods/macrobiotic. Macrobiotic and vegetarian sandwiches, soups, salads,
and snacks are available for take-out at Good Health Natural Foods. Menu items
include sushi, soba, hijiki, chiraci, various bean and grain soups, and veggie
burgers. **Closed Sunday. Vegan options, take-out only, VISA/MC, $**

• Govinda's
2471 18th St., NW, Washington, DC 20009   **(202) 332-5190**
Vegetarian. Govinda's is located in the Adam's Morgan area of Washington, D.C. It
features the "Endless Plate," which is an all-you-can-eat option. Dishes include
Kofta-Balls, Roasted Tofu, pakoras, Oriental Stir-Fry, Organic Brown Rice, Vegetable Soup, Dahl, Hummus Sandwiches, veggie burgers, salads, and more. **Open
Tuesday through Thursday for dinner. Open Saturday and Sunday for lunch and
dinner. Brunch served on Sunday. Full service, fresh juices, vegan options,
catering, take-out, $–$$**

Health Zone
1445 K St., NW, Washington, DC 20005   **(202) 371-2900**
Natural foods. This restaurant offers many vegetarian options including a multi-bean
burrito, veggie burger and dog, pizza, Vegetable Sushi, Middle Eastern Platter, and
black beans and rice. Low-fat cooking is emphasized. **Open Monday through Friday
for breakfast and lunch. Counter service, vegan options, take-out, $**

Ice In Paradise
615 Pennsylvania Ave., SE, Washington, DC 20003   **(202) 547-1554**
International deli. Various sandwiches, subs, entrees, and soups with an international flair are available at Ice In Paradise. **Open daily for lunch and dinner (call
on Sunday). Cafeteria style, vegan options, take-out, $**

India Gate Restaurant
2408 18th St., NW, Washington, DC 20009   **(202) 332-0141**
Indian. Enjoy various vegetarian appetizers, soups, entrees, homemade breads, and
salads. **Open daily for lunch and dinner. Full service, vegan options, wine/beer/alcohol, take-out, VISA/MC/AMX/DC, $$**

• Indian Delight

1100 Pennsylvania Ave., NW, Washington, DC 20004   **(202) 371-2295**

**Union Station Food Court, 50 Massachusetts Ave., NE,
Washington, DC 20002**   **(202) 842-1040**

2815 M St., NW, Washington, DC 20007   **(202) 338-6450**

Vegetarian/Indian. Eleven vegetarian entrees plus appetizers, soup, salad, and desserts are offered on the Indian Delight menu. Daily specials are also available. The Pennsylvannia Ave. restaurant is located inside an old post office, and the Georegetown restaurant (M St.) is next to Biograph Theater. **Open daily for lunch and dinner. Cafeteria style, vegan options, take-out, no credit cards, $**

Indian Kitchen

3506 Connecticut Ave., NW, Washington, DC 20008   **(202) 965-2541**

Indian. Indian cuisine with South Indian and exotic dishes of India is featured. Appetizers, vegetable entrees, special dishes, and breads are included on the menu. Indoor and outdoor seating. **Open daily for lunch and dinner. Limited service, vegan options, take-out, $**

Julia's Empanadas

2452 18th St., NW, Washington, DC 20011   **(202) 328-6232**

Latino. Try the spinach, broccoli, and cheese, or vegetarian-style empanadas. The ingredients in the vegetarian empanadas are changed weekly. **Open daily for lunch and dinner. Limited service, take-out, $**

Lebanese Taverna

2641 Connecticut Ave., NW, Washington, DC 20008   **(202) 265-8681**

Lebanese. Various Middle Eastern appetizers and salads plus approximately four vegetarian entrees are available. Outdoor cafe. **Full service, $$–$$$**

Madras Restaurant

3506 Connecticut Ave., NW, Washington, DC 20008   **(202) 966-2541**

Indian. This is a mostly vegetarian Indian restaurant. **Open daily for lunch and dinner. Cafeteria style, take-out, VISA/MC/AMX/DISC/DC, $**

• Madurai Vegetarian Room

3316 M St., NW, Washington, DC 20002   **(202) 333-0997**

Vegetarian/Indian. Madurai specializes in appetizers and soups. Eggs are not used. **Open daily, buffet on Sunday. Full service, VISA/MC/AMX, $$**

Paru's Indian Vegetarian Restaurant

2010 S St., SW, Washington, DC 20009   **(202) 483-5133**

⬥ Reviewers' choice   • Vegetarian restaurant   •• Vegan restaurant
$ less than $6 $$ $6–$12 $$$ more than $12
VISA/AMX/MC/DISC/DC—credit cards accepted
Non-alc.–Non-alcoholic   Fresh juices–freshly squeezed

Indian. Paru's is all vegetarian (except for one chicken dish) and features masala dosa in an inexpensive, informal atmosphere with a few tables. **Closed Sunday. Counter service, take-out, $$**

Red Sea Ethiopian Restaurant
2463 18th St., NW, Washington, DC 20009   **(202) 483-5000**
Ethiopian. Red Sea uses a rich variety of native herbs and spices to flavor the authentic Ethiopian cuisine. Diners eat in the traditional manner, using fingers and pieces of the Ethiopian bread, injera, in which to wrap and eat food. The menu clearly explains the various dishes. Several vegetarian appetizers and entrees are offered. **Open daily for lunch and dinner. Full service, vegan options, wine/beer/alcohol, take-out, VISA/MC/AMX, $$**

Restaurant Nora
2132 Florida Ave., NW, Washington, DC 20008   **(202) 462-5143**
Natural foods. Restaurant Nora is an organic and biodynamic restaurant serving multi-ethnic new American cuisine. The menu changes daily. Every evening, an organic, vegetarian plate is offered. There also is a selection of vegetarian appetizers and salads, and the restaurant is willing to accommodate special diets. **Open Monday through Saturday for dinner. Reservations recommended. Formal but no dress code, full service, fresh juices, wine/beer/alcohol, VISA/MC, $$$**

Sarinah Satay House
1338 Wisconsin Ave., NW, Washington, DC 20007   **(202) 337-2955**
Indonesian. Sarinah serves the internationally known Gado-Gado, a vegetarian dish with a special peanut butter sauce. Other vegetarian dishes include tofu and tempeh, noodles, and fried rice. **Closed Monday. Full service, vegan options, wine/beer/ alcohol, take-out, VISA/MC/AMX/DC/Carte Blanche, $$**

Skewers
1633 P St., NW, Washington, DC 20036   **(202) 387-4005**
Middle Eastern. Skewers features Vegetable Kabobs, Falafel, Hummus. **Open daily. Full service, vegan options, wine/beer/ alcohol, take-out, VISA/MC/AMX, $$**

•• Soul Vegetarian Cafe
2606 Georgia Ave., NW, Washington, DC 20010   **(202) 328-SOUL**
Vegan. The cover of the menu for Soul Vegetarian Cafe says it all, "All Vegan!!!, All the Time!!!" Try the Garvey Burger made from vegetable protein and spices, the Liberia Burger made from black eye peas and West African flavoring, a BBQ tofu sub, or one of the many other all-vegan choices, including desserts like tofu cheesecake. **Open Monday through Saturday for lunch and dinner, Sunday brunch. Limited service, smoothies, soy milk, VISA/MC, $–$$**

Stoup's of Athens
1825 Eye St., NW, Washington, DC 20006   **(202) 223-1169**
Greek. Authentic Greek cuisine is served along with vegetarian dishes such as Vegetable Platter, Spinach Pie, Stuffed Cabbage, and soups. **Closed Sunday. Vegan options, wine/beer, take-out, no credit cards, $**

Taj Mahal
1327 Connecticut Ave., NW, Washington, DC 20036   (202) 659-1544
Indian. Washington's oldest Indian restaurant has been serving the nation's capital since 1965. Vegetarian cuisine from North India is offered in a special section of the menu. Vegetarian appetizers, soup, and dessert are also on the menu. **Open daily for dinner, Monday through Friday for buffet lunch. Full service, vegan options, wine/beer/alcohol, take-out, VISA/MC/AMX/DISC, $$**

Yes! Natural Gourmet
1825 Columbia Rd., NW, Washington, DC 20009   (202) 462-5150

3425 Connecticut Ave., NW, Washington, DC 20008   (202) 363-1559
Natural foods. Soups, sandwiches, and fresh-squeezed juices are featured. **Open daily. Take-out service only, fresh juices, VISA/MC/AMX, $**

Zed's Ethiopian Cuisine
3318 M St., NW, Washington , DC 20007   (202) 333-4710
Ethiopian. As is customary with Ethiopian foods, no utensils are used at Zed's; the meal is eaten with the traditional bread, injera, which is used to pick up the food. Various vegetarian options are available. **Open daily. Full service, vegan options, wine/beer/alcohol, take-out, VISA/MC/AMX, $**

Zorba's Cafe
1612 20th St. NW, Washington, DC 20009   (202) 387-8555
Greek. Enjoy a variety of ethnic vegetarian dishes such as Fasolakia, Falafel, Spanakopita, and Fasolia. **Open daily for lunch and dinner. Deli style, vegan options, wine/beer, take-out, $**

FLORIDA

ALTAMONTE SPRINGS

Chamberlin's Natural Foods
Goodings Plaza, 1086 Montgomery Rd.
Altamonte Springs, FL 32714   (407) 774-8866
Natural foods. Salad bar, vegetarian deli, smoothies, homemade soup and veggie chili, frozen yogurt, hot and cold sandwiches, and hot vegetarian entrees are offered. **Open daily. Counter service, vegan options, fresh juices, take-out, no credit cards, $**

ATLANTIC BEACH

Heaven on Earth A Cafe
363-14 Atlantic Blvd., Atlantic Beach, FL 32233   (904) 249-6242
Natural foods. Enjoy dishes such as a Vegetarian Pâté Plate, chips and salsa or guacamole, beans and rice, or pasta of the day, and Carob Tofu Pie at this cafe featuring live folk music. **Open Tuesday through Sunday for dinner. Full service, fresh juices, beer/wine, VISA/MC, $$**

BOCA RATON
Wholly Harvest Market & Cafe
2200 W. Glades Rd., Boca Raton, FL 33461   **(407) 392-5100**
Natural foods. This natural foods cafe offers soups, pizza made with a whole-wheat crust, sandwiches, veggie burgers, steamed vegetables with rice, a macro platter, burritos, plus many other daily specials. **Open daily for three meals. Counter service, vegan/macrobiotic options, beer/wine/alcohol, catering, take-out, VISA/MC/DISC, $–$$**

CASSELBERRY
Chamberlin's Natural Foods
1271 Semoran Blvd., Ste. 105, Lake Howell Square
Casselberry, FL 32707   **(407) 774-8866**
Natural foods. See description under Altamonte Springs, FL.

CLEARWATER
Bunny Hop Cafe
1408 Cleveland St., Clearwater, FL 34615   **(813) 443-6703**
Natural foods. Located inside Nature's Food Patch, the Bunny Hop Cafe serves international vegetarian and macrobiotic foods in a casual atmosphere. High-fiber, low-fat cooking, fresh veggies and fruit, salad bar, veggie burgers, stir-fry, smoothies, desserts, and more are offered. Coffeehouse on Friday and Saturday nights. **Closed Sunday. Full service, vegan options, fresh juices, take-out, VISA/MC, $–$$**

Lonni's Sandwiches, Etc.
33 Garden Ave., Clearwater, FL 34616   **(813) 441-8044**
Natural foods. This restaurant offers several vegetarian options including sandwiches and salads, Wild Rice Soup, plus more. **Open Monday through Friday for lunch. Counter service, catering, take-out, cappuccino, beer/wine, $$**

COCONUT GROVE
The Last Carrot
3133 Grand Ave., Coconut Grove, FL 33133   **(305) 445-0805**
Natural foods/juice bar. Sandwiches, spinach pies, salads, and various fresh juices and smoothies are served. **Open daily for lunch and dinner. Deli style, vegan options, fresh juices, take-out, $**

Oak Feed Market & Restaurant
2911 Grand Ave., Coconut Grove, FL 33133   **(305) 448-7595**

🐾 Reviewers' choice   • Vegetarian restaurant   •• Vegan restaurant
$ less than $6 $$ $6–$12 $$$ more than $12
VISA/AMX/MC/DISC/DC—credit cards accepted
Non-alc.—Non-alcoholic   Fresh juices—freshly squeezed

Natural foods/macrobiotic. Oak Feed is a full-service restaurant featuring vegetarian and macrobiotic specialties plus a full range deli and bakery. **Open daily. Full service, vegan options, fresh juices, wine/beer/alcohol, take-out, VISA/MC/ AMX, $$**

DUNEDIN

Lonni's Sandwiches, Etc.
1153 Main St., Dunedin, FL 34698 **(813) 734-0121**
Natural foods. See description under Clearwater. **Take-out only.**

FORT LAUDERDALE

(For more restaurant listings in the surrounding areas, see Hollywood.)

Bread of Life Market and Restaurant
2388 N. Federal Hwy., Fort Lauderdale, FL 33305 **(305) 565-7423**
Natural foods. This gourmet natural foods restaurant and juice bar provides a beautiful art-deco, no-smoking environment. Bread of Life is willing to cater to special diets such as macrobiotic, fat-free, salt-free, etc. There's live jazz on Friday and Saturday nights. **Open daily for lunch and dinner. Full service, vegan options, fresh juices, wine/beer, VISA/MC/DISC/AMX, $$**

Nature Boy Health Foods
220 East Commercial Blvd., Fort Lauderdale, FL 33308 **(305) 776-4696**
Natural foods. Vegetable and fruit salads, sandwiches, soups, side orders, smoothies, and juices are served. **Open Monday through Saturday for lunch. Full service, limited vegan options, fresh juices, take-out, VISA/MC, $**

Nature's Delights
1544 E. Commercial Blvd., Fort Lauderdale, FL 33334 **(305) 776-7321**
Natural foods. The menu includes natural-style sandwiches, salads, soups, and dinner specials. **Closed Sunday. Full service, fresh juices, take-out, VISA/MC, $**

FORT MYERS

Great Harvest Bread Co.
7101-40 Cypress Lake Shopping Center
Fort Myers, FL 33907 **(813) 433-3363**
Natural foods bakery. Enjoy a wide variety of whole-wheat baked goods. **Open Monday through Saturday. Limited service, vegan options, $**

Thai Gardens
7091-15 College Pkwy., Fort Myers, FL 33907 **(813) 275-0999**
Thai. Enjoy several vegetarian entrees including Vegetable Curry, Sauteed Vegetables with Bean Curd, Veggie Fried Rice, and more. **Open daily for lunch and dinner. Full service, beer/wine, vegan options, VISA/MC/AMX/DISC, $$**

GAINESVILLE

(For more restaurant listings in the surrounding areas, see High Springs)

Falafel King Sandwiches
12 NW 13th St., Gainesville, FL 32601   **(904) 374-9830**

3252 SW 35th Blvd., Gainesville, FL 32608   **(904) 375-6342**
Middle Eastern. Middle Eastern specialties are provided in a deli-like atmosphere. Falafels, gyros, tabouleh, and other sandwiches are available for take-out. **Counter service, vegan options, take-out, $**

Ivey S. Grill
3303 W. University Ave., Gainesville, FL 32607   **(904) 371-4839**
Natural foods. Progressive menu with vegetarian entrees including tofu and pasta is featured. **Open for three meals Monday through Saturday, Sunday brunch. Full service, vegan options, fresh juices, wine/beer, VISA/MC/AMX, $$**

HIGH SPRINGS

The Great Outdoors Cafe
65 N. Main St., High Springs, FL 32643   **(904) 454-2900**
Natural foods. Located just off I-75 in north Florida, this cafe offers an eclectic array of foods: fresh salads, pastas, vegetarian entrees, and desserts. There is also a bed-and-breakfast inn serving vegetarian foods. Non-smoking. **Open daily. Full service, vegan options, wine/beer, take-out, VISA/MC/DISC/AMX, $$**

HOLLYWOOD

Harvest Village Natural Foods
1928 Harrison St., Hollywood, FL 33020   **(305) 921-5149**
Juice bar. Fruit and vegetable salads, sandwiches, and fresh fruit and vegetable juice are available. **Closed Sunday. Counter service, vegan options, take-out, VISA/MC, $**

JACKSONVILLE

Pattaya Thai Restaurant
10916 Atlantic Blvd., Jacksonville, FL 32225   **(904) 646-9506**
Thai. Choose from over twenty vegetarian Thai dishes including Spring Rolls, Vegetable Tofu Soup, Curry Fried Rice, Mixed Vegetables with Tofu, various curries, and Sweet and Sour Vegetables. **Open Thursday through Friday for lunch and dinner. Open Saturday and Sunday for dinner only. Closed Mondays. Full service, alc./beer/wine, VISA/MC/AMX/DISC/DC, $$**

MELBOURNE

Community Harvest Cafe
1405 Highland Ave., Melbourne, FL 32935   **(407) 242-2398**
Natural foods. Dine on multigrain pancakes, tempeh or tofu salad, hummus

sandwiches, veggie burgers, and more. **Open for three meals Monday through Friday. Open for breakfast and lunch Saturday. Closed Sunday. Full service, smoothies, fresh juices, vegan/macrobiotic options, VISA/MC, $**

Natureworks! Deli
461 N. Harbor City Blvd., Melbourne, FL 32935 (407) 242-0772
Natural foods. This is a mostly vegetarian deli. Natureworks! features a daily hot entree, soup, vegetarian chili, salad bar, and hot and cold sandwiches. The deli also offers vegetarian cooking classes and monthly vegan potluck dinner. **Closed Sunday. Limited service, vegan options, fresh juices, take-out, VISA/MC/AMX/DISC, $**

MIAMI

(For more restaurant listings in the surrounding areas, see Coconut Grove, Miami Beach, and Miami Springs.)

Granny Feelgood's
111 NW 1st. Street, Metro Dade Bldg., Miami, FL 33128 (305) 579-2104

190 SE 1st Avenue, Miami, FL 33131 (305) 358-6233
Natural foods. Granny Feelgood's makes a special effort to offer the freshest, healthiest foods available. Organic produce is offered and the menu selections (sandwiches, soups, salads, desserts, and international entrees) emphasize low-fat, low-cholesterol, and low-sodium foods. **Open Monday through Friday. Full service, vegan options, fresh juices, take-out, $**

Natural Eats
Dadeland Plaza, 9477 S. Dixie Hwy., Miami, FL 33156 (305) 665-7807
Natural foods. The Natural Eats menu is ahead of its time with a nutritional breakdown of the menu items. This rarely seen feature is quite handy and may be a more common addition to menus in the future. All foods are prepared with fresh ingredients and without refined sugar, saturated fats, preservatives, or chemicals. Salads, sandwiches, a veggie burger, and desserts are offered. Vegan muffins as well! **Open daily. Full service, fresh juice, take-out, $**

•• Natural Foods Express
Delivery Only (305) 672-FOOD
Vegan/delivery only. Although not a restaurant, this establishment delivers vegan meals in the Dade County area. Dishes include soups, whole-grain and bean dishes, seitan stew, stuffed butternut squash, salads, desserts, etc. **Delivery only; $37-minimum order**

☙ Reviewers' choice • Vegetarian restaurant •• Vegan restaurant
$ less than $6 $$ $6–$12 $$$ more than $12
VISA/AMX/MC/DISC/DC—credit cards accepted
Non-alc.—Non-alcoholic Fresh juices—freshly squeezed

Artichoke's Natural Cuisine
3055 NE 163rd St., N. Miami Beach, FL 33160   **(305) 945-7576**
International natural foods. Vegetarian, macrobiotic, and Pritikin dishes are served at this popular "neighborhood-type" restaurant. The menu includes appetizers, salads, entrees, and desserts. **Open for dinner nightly. Full service, vegan options, fresh juices, wine/beer, take-out, VISA/MC/AMX, $$**

Kebab Indian Restaurant
514 NE 167th St., N. Miami Beach, FL 33162   **(305) 940-6309**
North Indian. Kebab is recommended by the Vegetarian Gourmet Society in Florida as serving "the best Indian vegetarian foods that we have ever tasted." Dishes are made fresh and special diets are accommodated. **Open daily. Full service, vegan options, wine/beer, take-out, VISA/MC/AMX, $$**

•• Our Place
830 Washington Ave., Miami Beach, FL, 33139   **(305) 674-1322**
Vegan. Our Place features four or more daily specials, soups, and a wide variety of burgers and veggie sushi. **Open daily for lunch and dinner. Full service, vegan, wine/beer, take-out, VISA/MC, $–$$**

Pineapples
530 Arthur Godfrey Rd., Miami Beach, FL 33140   **(305) 532-9731**
Natural foods. This gourmet vegetarian and natural foods restaurant and market offers daily specials for lunch and dinner, weekend breakfast, and weekend brunch. **Open daily. Vegan options, take-out, $**

13th Street Cafe
227 13th St., Miami Beach, FL 33139   **(305) 532-8336**
Natural foods. Enjoy the "Carmen Miranda" motif at this cafe that serves fresh juices and smoothies, as well as vegetarian sandwiches and specialties. **Open daily for three meals. Full service, fresh juices, smoothies, take-out, $**

Unicorn Village
3565 NE 207th St., N. Miami Beach, FL 33180   **(305) 933-8829**
Natural foods. This three-story waterfront restaurant offers many vegetarian dishes including several creative salads, Spinach Lasagna, Roasted Eggplant, pasta, pizzas made with soy cheese, and a Veggie Burger. The chef tries to use as many organic ingredients as possible. **Open daily for lunch and dinner. Full service, fresh juices, organic wine/beer/alcohol, take-out, VISA/MC, $**

The Garden Restaurant
17 Westward Dr., Miami Springs, FL 33166   **(305) 887-9238**
Natural foods. A wide variety of appetizers, soups, salads, pastas, entrees, sandwiches, and burgers are listed on The Garden Restaurant menu. Many vegetarian

options are offered including a Veggie Burger, Vegetable Tempura, Zucchini Melt, and Tofu Marinara. **Open daily for lunch and dinner. Full service, vegan options, fresh juices, wine/beer, take-out, VISA/MC/AMX, $$**

NAPLES

Great Harvest Bread Co.
854 Neapolitan Way, Naples, FL 33940   **(813) 262-1887**
Natural foods bakery. See description under Fort Myers.

ORANGE PARK

Granary Deli
1738 Kingsley Ave., Orange Park, FL 32073   **(904) 269-7350**
Natural foods. The Granary Deli is located in the Granary Whole Foods store. This primarily vegetarian deli offers soups, sandwiches, salads, and much more. Organic ingredients are used when available. **Open for lunch and dinner Monday through Saturday. Closed Sunday. Limited service, fresh juices, vegan/macrobiotic options, take-out, $**

The Green Onion Cafe & Deli
459 Kingsley Ave., Orange Park, FL 32073   **(904) 264-4118**
Macrobiotic. This cafe offers a variety of macrobiotic/natural foods dishes including veggie burgers, Tabouli, Rice and Pasta Salad, vegetable platters, rice and beans, and soups. **Open Monday through Saturday for lunch. Closed Sunday. Full service, vegan/macrobiotic options, catering, take-out, $–$$**

ORLANDO

(For more restaurant listings in the surrounding areas, see Altamonte Springs, Casselberry, and Winter Park.)

Bee Line Diner
9801 International Dr., Peabody Hotel, Orlando, FL 32819   (407) 352-4000
International. This diner features a vegetarian section on the menu that includes Chili, Lasagna, Falafel, and veggie burgers. **Open 24 hours daily. Full service, non-alc. wine/beer, wine/beer/alcohol, take-out, VISA/MC/AMX/DISC/DC, $$**

Chamberlin's Natural Foods
Colonial Plaza Shopping Center
38 Colonial Plaza Mall, Orlando, FL 32803   **(407) 894-8452**

The Marketplace
7600 Dr. Phillips Blvd., Orlando, FL 32819   **(407) 352-2130**
Natural foods. See description under Altamonte Springs, FL.

• Florida Hospital Cafeteria
601 E. Rollins St., Orlando, FL 32803   **(407) 897-1793**
Vegetarian cafeteria. Deli and taco bar, soup and salad bar are featured; low-fat and low-salt entrees are available. **Open 24 hours every day. Cafeteria service, take-out, $**

4, 5, 6
657 N. Primrose Dr., Orlando, FL 32803   **(407) 898-1899**
Chinese. Vegetarian egg rolls, soups, and twenty non-dairy vegetarian dishes with brown rice are available. MSG is not used. **Open daily for lunch and dinner. Full service, vegan options, wine/alcohol, take-out, VISA/MC, $$**

Green Earth Health Foods
2336 W. Oakridge Rd., Orlando, FL 32809   **(407) 859-8045**
Natural foods. The cafe offers fresh soups, chili, sandwiches, salads, and smoothies. It is "dedicated to serving wholesome foods with no chemicals or preservatives" and uses organic products when possible. All food is prepared on the premises and is low-salt and low-fat. Green Earth is located in Oakridge Plaza. **Open Monday through Friday. Limited service, vegan options, fresh juice, VISA/MC, $**

Passage to India
5532 International Dr., Orlando, FL 32819   **(407) 351-3456**
Indian. The menu features vegetarian appetizers, soups, and twelve vegetarian entrees. **Open daily for lunch and dinner. Full service, non-alc. wine/beer, wine/beer, take-out, VISA/MC/AMX/DISC, $$**

PALM BEACH

• Sunrise Natural Foods
233 Royal Poinciana Way, Palm Beach, FL 33480   **(407) 655-3557**
Vegetarian/macrobiotic. Selections include soup, egg rolls, spinach pies, and artichoke pasta. **Open for lunch. Closed Sunday. Take-out only, non-alc. beer/wine, VISA/MC/AMX, $**

SARASOTA

• Froggy's
3025 North Tamiami Trail, Sarasota, FL 34234   **(813) 359-VEGE**
Vegetarian. This relatively new fast-food vegetarian restaurant is a must to visit if you find yourself along the Gulf Coast of Florida. The food is wonderful. The owners opened this restaurant due to their desire to help the environment and to promote low-fat eating. In fact, the local heart association recommends its patients dine at this establishment. Items featured on the menu include a wide variety of vegetarian burgers, sandwiches, delicious air-fried potatoes, burritos, and non-dairy banana smoothies. Saturday evenings there's a coffeehouse. **Open daily for lunch and dinner. Counter service, $**

Wildflower
5218 Ocean Blvd., Sarasota, FL 34242   **(813) 349-1758**
Macrobiotic. Diners enjoy a casual atmosphere near the beach. Daily specials include soups and creative vegetarian entrees. **Open daily for lunch and dinner. Full service, fresh juices, wine/beer, take-out, VISA/MC, $$**

ST. PETERSBURG

Lonni's Sandwiches, Etc.
133 1st St. N., St. Petersburg, FL 33701   **(813) 894-1944**
Natural foods. See description under Clearwater.

TALLAHASSEE

New Leaf Cafe
1146 E. Lafayette St., Tallahassee, FL 32301   **(904) 942-5643**
Natural foods. Enjoy several vegetarian selections at this cafe including pasta dishes, Ratatouille with Rice, Tofu-Barley "Meat Loaf," Seitan and Mushroom Sandwich, salads, soups, and much more. **Open for lunch Monday, lunch and dinner Tuesday through Friday, brunch and dinner Saturday, and brunch only on Sunday. Full service, take-out, VISA/MC, $$**

New Leaf Market
Parkway Shopping Center
1235 Apalachee Pkwy. Tallahassee, FL 32301   **(904) 942-2557**
Natural foods. The deli counter here offers a wide variety of salads and sandwiches including a rice salad, szechuan noodles, fruit salad, and hummus sandwiches. **Open Monday through Saturday. Fresh juices, smoothies, catering, take-out, $**

TAMPA

The Natural Kitchen, Inc. (The N.K. Cafe)
4100 W. Kennedy Blvd., Tampa, FL 33609   **(813) 287-1385**
Natural foods. Originally a vegetarian restaurant, the N.K. Cafe now offers meat and fish. There is still a decent selection of vegetarian fare, however, particularly for salads and sandwiches. There are three vegetarian entrees and many desserts. **Open Monday through Friday. Cafeteria style, limited vegan options, fresh juices, wine/beer, take-out, VISA/MC/AMX, $–$$**

WEST PALM BEACH

Wholly Harvest Market & Cafe
7735 S. Dixie Hwy., West Palm Beach, FL 33405   **(407) 585-8800**
Natural foods. See entry under Boca Raton. **Full service.**

WINTER PARK

Chamberlin's Natural Foods Restaurant
Winter Park Mall, 430 N. Orlando Ave.
Winter Park, FL 32789   **(407) 647-3330**
Natural foods. See description under Altamonte Springs, FL.

🐾 Reviewers' choice   ● Vegetarian restaurant   ●● Vegan restaurant
$ less than $6 $$ $6–$12 $$$ more than $12
VISA/AMX/MC/DISC/DC—credit cards accepted
Non-alc.—Non-alcoholic   Fresh juices—freshly squeezed

The Power House
111 E. Lyman Ave., Winter Park, FL 32789   **(407) 645-3616**
Natural foods. Enjoy sandwiches, salads, soup, vegetarian chili, and a wide variety
of shakes and smoothies. **Open daily. Limited service, vegan options, $**

GEORGIA

ATHENS

Bluebird Cafe
493 E. Clayton St., Athens, GA 30601   **(706) 549-3663**
Natural foods. Vegetarian dishes with a Mexican flair are included on the Bluebird
Cafe menu. Entrees such as burritos, quesadilla, enchiladas, plus salads, quiche,
sandwiches, and desserts are offered. **Open daily. Full service, vegan options,
take-out, no credit cards, $**

ATLANTA

(For more restaurant listings in the surrounding areas, see Decatur.)

•• Delights of the Garden
1081 Juniper NE, Atlanta, GA 30309   **(404) 876-4307**
Vegan. Diners at this vegan, raw-food restaurant will enjoy a wide variety of dishes
based on fruits, vegetables, grains, nuts, and seeds. We recommend that you try
one of the sampler platters the first time you visit this establishment. **Open daily.
Full and counter service, completely vegan, fresh juices, take-out, VISA/MC/
AMX/DISC/DC, $**

Eat Your Vegetables
438 Moreland Ave., NE, Atlanta, GA 30307   **(404) 523-2671**
Natural foods. Vegetarian and macrobiotic specials are available every day in
addition to the vegetarian entrees on the menu. **Full service, take-out, $$**

• Govinda's
1287 S. Ponce de Leon Ave., NE, Atlanta, GA 30306   **(404) 377-7205**
Vegetarian. Govinda's offers an all-you-can-eat vegetarian buffet. **Open Monday
through Saturday. Closed Sunday. Counter service, vegan options, take-out, $**

Lettuce Souprise You
Corporate offices in Atlanta, GA   **(404) 955-3999**

Loehmann's Plaza
2470-47 Briarcliff Rd., Atlanta, GA 30329   **(404) 636-8549**

Sandy Springs
5975 Roswell Rd., Atlanta, GA 30328   **(404) 874-4998**

Rio Mall
595 Piedmont Ave. #D200.1, Atlanta, GA 30308   **(404) 874-4998**

1109 Cumberland Mall, Atlanta, GA 30339   **(404) 438-2288**

245 Pharr Rd., Atlanta, GA 30305   **(404) 841-9583**
American/restaurant chain. All-you-can-eat salad-bar chain in the Atlanta area also
has muffins, soups, baked potatoes, and fresh fruit. Smoking is not allowed. **Open
daily. Buffet style, take-out, $–$$**

Nuts 'N Berries
4274 Peachtree St. NE, Atlanta, GA 30319   **(404) 237-6829**
Natural foods. This whole foods restaurant offers home-baked goods, sandwiches,
salads, and side dishes, chili, and soup. **Open daily. Limited service, vegan options,
fresh juices, take-out, VISA/MC, $**

Rio Bravo Cantina
3172 Roswell Rd., Atlanta, GA 30305   **(404) 262-7431**
Mexican. The cantina has an extensive Mexican menu offering appetizers, soups,
salads, sandwiches, specials, Mexican favorites, and vegetable entrees. Only pure
(100-percent) vegetable oil is used in cooking. **Open daily for lunch and dinner.
Full service, vegan options, fresh juices, wine/beer/alcohol, take-out, $$**

Shipfeifer on Peachtree
1814 Peachtree St., Atlanta, GA 30309   **(404) 875-1106**
Mediterranean. Wraps, salads, platters, side dishes, Mediterranean pizza, and
desserts are included on the Shipfeifer menu. All food is prepared fresh to order.
Outdoor patio dining. **Open daily for lunch and dinner. Full service, vegan
options, wine/beer, take-out, VISA/MC/AMX/DISC, $–$$**

•• Soul Vegetarian Restaurant
879 Abernathy Blvd., SW, Atlanta, GA 30310   **(404) 752-5194**

652 N. Highland Ave., Atlanta, GA 30306   **(404) 875-0145**
Vegan. Soul has its own unique gluten creation called "Kalebone" that is made into
burgers, "furters," steaks, and salads. Soul's many other original dishes—soups,
lentil burgers, veggie patties, tofu filet, veggie gyros, salads, and desserts—are sure
to keep your veggie taste buds happy. Children's dinner available. **Open daily for
lunch and dinner. Full service, totally vegan, fresh juice, catering, take-out,
VISA/MC/AMX, $**

• Veggie Delight
1051 Ponce de Leon Ave., Atlanta, GA 30306   **(404) 872-4539**
Vegetarian. Located in an area of Atlanta known as the Virginia Highlands, this
vegetarian restaurant offers excellent salads, sandwiches, burgers, stir-frys, pasta
dishes, plus much more. The food is primarily vegan, except for the soy cheese,
which contains caseine. **Open Monday through Saturday for lunch and dinner.
Closed Sunday. Full service, vegan options, take-out, $**

• Veggieland
211 Pharr Rd., NE, Atlanta, GA 30305   **(404) 231-3111**

220 Sandy Springs Cir., NW, Atlanta, GA 30328   **(404) 252-1165**

Vegetarian. This restaurant features delicious low-salt, low-calorie, sugar-free foods. Filtered water is used even for the ice cubes! Menu consists of starters, salads, veggie burgers and sandwiches, pasta, stir-fry, desserts, and specials. **Full service, vegan options, fresh juices, take-out, $$**

COLUMBUS

• Country Life Vegetarian Restaurant and Health Food Store
1217 Eberhart Ave., Columbus, GA 31906   **(706) 323-9194**
Vegetarian. A buffet lunch and a soup and salad bar are available Sunday through Thursday. The fare here is "Healthy foods that taste good" with a menu that changes daily. **Open for lunch Sunday through Thursday. Limited service, vegan options, take-out, VISA/MC, $**

DECATUR

• Indian Delights
1707 Church St., Decatur, GA 30030   **(404) 296-2965**
Vegetarian/Indian. Enjoy a wide variety of vegetarian Indian dishes including South Indian dishes. **Open Tuesday through Sunday for lunch and dinner. Closed Monday. Limited service, vegan options, catering, take-out, $**

Rainbow Natural Foods
2118 N. Decatur Rd., NE, Decatur, GA 30033   **(404) 636-5553**
Natural foods. Sandwiches and soups are featured along with daily special entrees. **Open daily for lunch and dinner. Sunday brunch. Full service, fresh juice, take-out, $**

DULUTH

Lettuce Souprise You
Gwinnett Esplanade
3525 Mall Blvd., Bldg. 6, Duluth, GA 30136   **(404) 418-9969**
American/restaurant chain. See entry under Atlanta.

ROSWELL

Lettuce Souprise You
Holcomb 400
1474 Holcomb Bridge Rd., #155, Roswell, GA 30076   **(404) 642-1601**
American/restaurant chain. See entry under Atlanta.

🐾 Reviewers' choice   • Vegetarian restaurant   •• Vegan restaurant
$ less than $6 $$ $6–$12 $$$ more than $12
VISA/AMX/MC/DISC/DC—credit cards accepted
Non-alc.—Non-alcoholic   Fresh juices—freshly squeezed

HAWAII

Chiang Mai Thai Restaurant
2239 S. King St., Honolulu, HI 96826 (808) 941-1151
Thai. Here you will find exotic northern Thai cuisine with a full vegetarian menu (and we mean full!). The front of the menu says, "Vegetarians Welcome," and what's offered on the inside reflects this. Appetizers, salads, soups, noodle and rice dishes, and other entrees of tofu and vegetables make up an excellent selection for vegetarians. **Open daily for lunch and dinner. Full service, vegan options, wine/beer, take-out, VISA/MC/AMX, $**

Crêpe Fever Restaurant
Ward Centre, 1200 Ala Moana Blvd.
Honolulu, HI 96822 (808) 521-9023
Natural foods. Crêpe Fever features an eclectic mixture of dishes for breakfast, lunch, and dinner. Salads, crêpe, sandwich, and croissant specialties are joined by soups, stir-fry, and side orders. **Open daily. Limited service, vegan options, fresh juices, espresso/cappuccino, wine/beer/alcohol, take-out, VISA/MC, $–$$**

• Down To Earth Deli
2525 S. King St., Honolulu, HI 96826 (808) 947-7678
Vegetarian. **Open daily. Cafeteria style, vegan options, fresh juices, take-out, VISA/MC, $**

• Guaranga's Vegetarian Dining Club
51 Coelho Way, Honolulu, HI 96817 (808) 595-3947
Vegetarian. Located on a lovely three-acre estate in the hills of Nuvano, Guaranga's is accompanied by the largest banyan tree on the island. The club features a full salad bar, homemade whole-grain bread, fresh baked cookies, mung dahl soup, brown and jasmine rice, and more. There are ethnic themes for each night. **Open for lunch and dinner Monday through Saturday. Buffet, vegan options, fresh juices, take-out, no credit cards, $$**

India Bazaar Madras
2320 S. King St., Honolulu, HI 96826 (808) 949-4840
Indian. India Bazaar features South Madras-style Indian cuisine. **Closed Sunday. Cafeteria style, BYOB, take-out, $**

Keo's Thai Cuisine
625 Kapahulu Ave., Honolulu, HI 96815 (808) 737-8240

1200 Ala Moana Blvd., Honolulu, HI 96814 (808) 533-0533

1486 S. King St., Honolulu, HI 96814 (808) 947-9988
Thai. Gourmet Thai cuisine is served in a casually elegant, tropical garden setting. Vegetarian appetizers, salads, entrees, and curry dishes are available on the menu. Any item can be made vegetarian because all food is cooked to order. **Dinner**

served nightly; also lunch, Monday through Saturday at the Moana Blvd. location. Full service, vegan options, wine/beer/alcohol, take-out, VISA/MC/AMX/ DISC/DC/Carte Blanche, $$

Mekong Restaurant
1295 S. Beretania St., Honolulu, HI 96814   **(808) 521-2025**
Thai. The oldest Thai restaurant in Hawaii, Mekong includes vegetarian dishes on the menu. No smoking. **Open daily for dinner; open Monday through Friday for lunch. Full service, BYOB, take-out, VISA/MC/AMX/DISC/DC, $–$$**

Pineland Chinese Restaurant
1236 Keeaumoku St., Honolulu, HI 96814   **(808) 955-2918**
Chinese. Pineland features a special vegetarian menu with dishes such as Hot and Sour Noodles in Soup, Fried Bean Curd with Szechuan Orange Flavor, and Eggplant with Spicy Hunan Garlic Sauce. **Open for dinner daily except Sunday. Full service, vegan options, BYOB, take-out, $**

Salsa Rita's
500 Ala Moana Blvd., Honolulu, HI 96813   **(808) 536-4828**
Mexican. Homemade tortillas, beans without lard, Mexican tofu, and meatless items make it easy for vegetarians to find a satisfying meal at Salsa Rita's. **Open daily for lunch and dinner. Full service, vegan options, wine/beer/alcohol, take-out, VISA/MC/AMX, $$**

Yen King Chinese Restaurant
4211 Waialae Ave., Kahala Mall, Honolulu, HI 96816   **(808) 732-5505**
Chinese. Szechuan, Mandarin, and Shanghai cuisines are featured. The back page of the Yen King menu lists thirty vegetarian dishes including soups, assorted vegetable and noodle entrees, mock meat, and gluten dishes. MSG is not used. **Open daily. Full service, vegan options, wine/beer/alcohol, take-out, VISA/MC/AMX, $$**

KAILUA

The Source Natural Foods & Juice Bar
32 Kainehe St., Kailua, HI 96734   **(808) 262-5604**
Natural foods. All salads, burgers, sandwiches, soups, and entrees are fresh and made to order. The Source serves a wide selection of vegetarian options, including chili, veggie burgers, sushi, and Mexican dishes. **Open daily. Limited service, vegan options, fresh juices, BYOB, take-out, no credit cards, $**

KAUAI

International Museum & Cafe
9875 Waimea Rd., Waimea, Kauai, HI 96796   **(808) 338-0403**
International. If you're looking for something unique, try this museum, where eating and drinking is not only allowed but encouraged. The menu is primarily vegetarian with appetizers, sandwiches, beverages, and desserts. You'll also enjoy the full Asian-Hawaiian museum, jewelry, clothing, and antiques for sale. No smoking. **Hours are seasonal. Full service, fresh juice, wine/beer/alcohol, take-out, AMX, $$**

Koloa Ice House & Deli
(Across from post office)
P.O. Box 1326, Koloa Town, Kauai 96756   **(808) 742-6063**
Natural foods. For fourteen years, Koloa Ice House has been working hard to spread aloha spirit with fresh sandwiches, salads, homemade soups, lasagna, quiche, and many other specialties. It also serves delicious smoothies and frozen desserts as well as homemade cookies. Outside dining. **Open daily. Counter service, fresh juices, take-out, AMX, $**

KEAAU TOWN

•• Tonya's Vegetarian Cafe
Across from Keaau Post Office, Keaau Town, HI 96749   **(808) 966-8091**
Vegetarian. An island-style vegetarian cafe with an international flair, this almost completely vegan cafe serves such items as tempeh burgers, varying international specials, and seasonal Hawaiian fruits and vegetables. **Closed Saturday and Sunday. Counter service, vegan options, BYOB, catering, $**

MAUI

Cheese Burger in Paradise
811 Front Street, Lahaina, Maui, HI 96761   **(808) 661-4855**
American. From the sound of its name, you would never expect Cheese Burger in Paradise to offer vegetarian food. But it does offer three vegetarian burgers—a Tofu Burger, Gardenburger, and a Spinach Nut Burger—as well as Lahaina Grilled Cheese. This restaurant is located on the beach and offers live music during the evening. **Open daily for lunch and dinner. Full service, fruit smoothies, wine/beer/alcohol, take-out, VISA/MC/AMX, $$**

Royal Thai Cuisine
Azeka Shopping Center, Kihei, Maui, HI 96753   **(808) 874-0813**
Thai. Although not a vegetarian restaurant, Royal Thai Cuisine offers more than twenty-five vegetarian entrees. **Open daily for dinner, Monday through Friday for lunch. Full service, take-out, VISA/MC/AMX, $-$$**

Saeng's Thai Cuisine
1312 Front Street, Lahaina, Maui, HI 96761   **(808) 244-1567**
Thai. Saeng's offers more than ten vegetarian entrees including several tofu dishes. **Open daily for lunch and dinner. Full service, take-out, $$**

Thai Chef Restaurant
Lahaina Shopping Center, Lahaina, Maui, HI 96761   **(808) 667-2814**
Thai. Authentic Thai cuisine is offered in a relaxed, cozy atmosphere. Thirteen vegetarian entrees including tofu, curry, and vegetable dishes are on the menu. The chef is willing to accommodate special diets and can prepare any of the regular dishes without meat. **Open seven days. Full service, vegan options, take-out, VISA/MC/DISC, $$**

PAIA

•• The Vegan Restaurant
115 Baldwin Ave., Paia, HI 96779   **(808) 579-9144**
Vegan. All of the vegan Thai food here is homemade. **Closed Monday. Limited service, completely vegan, fruit juices, non-alc. beer, take-out, VISA/MC, $$**

IDAHO

COEUR D'ALENE°

Coeur d'Alene Natural Foods Store and Cafe
301 Lakeside Ave., Coeur d'Alene, ID 83814   **(208) 664-3452**
Health-food-store cafe. **Open for lunch Monday through Saturday. Cafeteria style, fresh juices, take-out, VISA/MC, $**

ILLINOIS

ARLINGTON HEIGHTS

• Chowpatti Vegetarian Restaurant
1035 S. Arlington Heights Rd., Arlington Heights, IL 60005   **(708) 640-9554**
Vegetarian/ethnic. This family-owned vegetarian restaurant serves international fare—American, Italian, French, Mexican, and Middle Eastern dishes. Closed Monday. **Open for lunch and dinner. Full service, vegan options, fresh juices, non-alc. beer/wine, catering, take-out, VISA/MC/AMX/DISC/DC, $**

CHAMPAIGN

Fiesta Cafe
216 S. First St., Champaign, IL 61820   **(217) 352-5902**
Mexican. **Open daily for lunch and dinner. Full service, wine/beer/alcohol, take-out, VISA/MC/AMX/DISC, $**

CHICAGO

(For more restaurants in the surrounding suburbs, see Arlington Heights, Downers Grove, Evanston, Oak Park, Palatine, Rolling Meadows, St. Charles, Skokie, Villa Park, W. Dundee, and Westmont.)

The Bread Shop
3400 N. Halsted, Chicago, IL 60657   **(312) 528-8108**
Natural foods bakery and cafe. This full-line bakery, grocery, and cafe is famous for its whole-grain pizza and burritos. Menu changes. **Open daily for three meals. Full service, vegan options, fresh juices, take-out, VISA/MC, $**

Bukhara
2 E. Ontario St., Chicago, IL 60611 **(312) 943-0188**
Indian. Bukhara offers candlelight dinners and prepares its food in clay ovens. Vegetarian options include stuffed peppers with vegetables, nuts, and dried fruit; dal; potatoes with a rich stuffing of raisins, cashews, green chilies, and spices; and various Indian breads. **Open daily for lunch and dinner. Full service, vegan options, beer/wine/alcohol, catering, take-out, VISA/MC/AMX/DISC/DC, $$**

• Cafe Voltaire
3231 N. Clark St., Chicago, IL 60657 **(312) 528-3136**
Vegetarian. A cozy vegetarian restaurant that stays open late, the cafe occasionally features plays in a downstairs room. Organic produce is used in season. **Open daily for lunch and dinner. Full service, vegan options, fresh juices, espresso/cappuccino, non-alc. beer, wine/beer, VISA/MC, $$**

• The Chicago Diner
3411 N. Halsted, Chicago, IL 60657 **(312) 935-6696**
Vegetarian restaurant/juice bar. The Chicago Diner serves an eclectic assortment of international vegetarian fare without preservatives, processed, or artificial foods. Fresh organic produce is purchased whenever possible. The owners have traveled extensively and are dedicated to promoting healthy eating for the sake of humans, the planet, and animals. The diner serves delicious vegetarian fare and is the hub for the animal rights movement in the Midwest. Breakfast menu and kid's menu. Patio dining in summertime. **Open daily. Full service, vegan options, fresh juices, non-alc. beer, beer/organic wine, take-out, VISA/MC/AMX/ DISC, $$**

Gaylord India Restaurant
678 N. Clark St., Chicago, IL 60610 **(312) 664-1700**
Indian. Indian food is freshly prepared using no canned or processed ingredients. **Open daily for lunch and dinner. Full service, vegan options, wine/beer/alcohol, take-out, VISA/MC/AMX, $$**

• Govinda's Vegetarian Buffet & Salad Bar
1716 W. Lunt Ave., Chicago, IL 60626 **(312) 973-0900**
Vegetarian buffet. Consistent with Govinda's fashion, the buffet has a monthly menu with a different entree daily that is accompanied by bread, two types of rice, two vegetable dishes, a bean dish, large salad bar, ice cream, and sweets. All for one low price!! Vegan entrees are indicated on monthly menu. **Open Wednesday through Saturday for dinner. Buffet, vegan options, take-out, $**

Heartland Cafe
7000 N. Glenwood, Chicago, IL 60626 **(312) 465-8005**

ᕙᐤ Reviewers' choice   • Vegetarian restaurant   •• Vegan restaurant
$ less than $6 $$ $6–$12 $$$ more than $12
VISA/AMX/MC/DISC/DC—credit cards accepted
Non-alc.—Non-alcoholic   Fresh juices—freshly squeezed

Natural foods. "Good wholesome foods for the mind and body" are served in a comfortable environment. Starters, soups and salads, sandwiches, various entrees, and vegetarian specialties feature many Mexican and international dishes. There is late night music and dancing on winter weekends and outdoor dining during warm months. The cafe is accompanied by a general store that features wholistic and political magazines, and merchandise. **Open daily. Full service, vegan options, fresh juices, wine/beer/alcohol, take-out, VISA/MC/AMX, $$**

The Lo-Cal Zone
912 N. Rush St., Chicago, IL 60611   (312) 943-9060
Natural foods. The Lo-Cal Zone offers healthy fast food over half of which is vegetarian. This eatery does not serve red meat. Vegetarians can dine on veggie burgers, veggie chili burritos, pizza, various salads, plus much more. **Open daily for lunch and dinner. Counter service, espresso/cappuccino, smoothies, take-out, $**

Mama Desta's Red Sea
3216 N. Clark St., Chicago, IL 60657   (312) 935-7561
Ethiopian. The restaurant is decidedly decorated to create an African ambiance with crafts and paintings from Africa plus bamboo-and-reed-covered walls. **Open daily for lunch and dinner. Full service, wine/beer/alcohol, take-out, VISA/MC/AMX, $$**

• Natraj India Restaurant
2240 W. Devon Ave., Chicago, IL 60659   (312) 274-1300
Vegetarian/Indian. Natraj is a family restaurant with an emphasis on quality food. The menu includes a wide assortment of vegetarian appetizers, soups, salads, entrees, breads, rice, and desserts. **Open daily. Full service, vegan options, BYOB, catering, take-out, VISA, MC, $$**

A Natural Harvest
7122 S. Jeffery Blvd., Chicago, IL 60649   (312) 363-3939
Natural foods. Soups, salads, sandwiches, and other entrees are prepared on-site daily. The restaurant specializes in vegetable proteins; vegetarian burgers, steaklets, and hot dogs are sold by the pound. **Closed Sunday. Limited service, fresh juices, take-out, VISA/MC/AMX/DISC, $**

The Original Mitchell's Restaurants
101 W. North Ave., Chicago, IL 60610   (312) 642-5246

1953 N. Clybourn, Chicago, IL 60614   (312) 883-1157
Natural foods. Mitchell's prides itself on its delicious breakfasts known nationwide for such foods as vegetarian sausage, non-dairy whole-wheat pancakes, giant homemade muffins, and omelettes. Mitchell's has daily vegetarian lunch and dinner specials as well, including great chili and oatmeal walnut burgers. **Open daily. Full service, vegan options, fresh juices, wine/beer, take-out, VISA/MC, $**

Pattie's Heart-Healthy
520 N. Michigan, Chicago, IL 60614   (312) 645-1111

613 W. Diversey Pkwy., Chicago, IL 60657   (312) 248-1111

Heart-healthy fast food. Grams of fat and calories are listed for each menu item. Sandwiches, soups, pizza, calzones, vegetarian specials, and sweets are included on the menu. Breakfast menu, too. **Open daily. Counter service, vegan options, fresh juices, espresso/cappuccino, take-out, no credit cards, $**

Pegasus
130 S. Halsted, Chicago, IL 60606   **(312) 226-4666**
Greek. A local patron recommends Pegasus' excellent all-vegetable entrees and mentions that the restaurant has "more vegan selections than any other restaurant in Greek town." **Full service, $$**

•• Soul Vegetarian
205 E. 75th St., Chicago, IL 60619   **(312) 224-0164**
Vegan. Various ethnic dishes are featured at Soul Vegetarian, including African, Middle Eastern, and American fare. Examples include Vegetarian Ribs, Tofu Fish, Sunflower-Seed Burger, and Split Pea and Chickenless Noodle Soup. **Open daily. Reservations accepted. Full service, vegan options, fresh juices, take-out, VISA, $$**

Star of Siam
11 E. Illinois St., Chicago, IL 60611   **(312) 670-0100**
Thai. All dishes can be prepared without meat or with tofu or veggie substitutes. **Open daily for lunch and dinner. Full service, vegan options, wine/beer/alcohol, take-out, VISA/MC/AMX/DISC, $**

Sweet Pea Cafe
1367 W. Erie, Chicago, IL 60622   **(312) 829-4514**
Cafe. Vegetarian selections include corn fritters with tomato chutney, roasted red pepper and walnut dip with pita, marinated tofu with a cornmeal breading, and tagine—Moroccan stew. **Open daily for lunch and dinner, Saturday and Sunday brunch. Full service, fresh juices, espresso/cappuccino, VISA/MC/AMX/DC, $$**

• Udupi Palace
2543 W. Devon Ave., Chicago, IL 60659   **(312) 338-2152**
Vegetarian. This vegetarian restaurant features traditional southern Indian cuisine. They recommend the masala dosa as the "most popular item," but they also feature vegetarian appetizers, breads, soups, curries, rice specialties, and entrees. **Open daily for lunch and dinner. Full service, vegan options, fresh juices, catering, take-out, VISA/MC/AMX/DISC/DC, $$**

ELGIN

Al's Cafe & Creamery
43 Fountain Square, Elgin, IL 60120   **(708) 742-1180**
Cafe. Located in a historic building, Al's Cafe and Creamery provides a charming ambiance in which to sample many imaginative soups and sandwiches for vegetarians and non-vegetarians alike. The Creamery features special malts and shakes, and a fountain menu that lets you create your own sundaes. **Closed Sunday. Full service, wine/beer, take-out, VISA/MC/AMX, $$**

Jalapeños
7 Clock Tower Plaza, Elgin, IL 60120   **(708) 468-9445**
Mexican. The authentic, fresh-cooked Mexican cuisine is mostly vegeterian with a limited vegan selection. **Full service, vegan option, wine/beer/alcohol, takeout, $$**

EVANSTON

• Blind Faith Cafe ✿
525 Dempster St., Evanston, IL 60201   **(708) 328-6875**
Vegetarian. This cafe features a bakery, organic produce, and a filtered water system in an environmentally responsible, non-smoking environment. Savor the tempting flavors of pot stickers, seitan Francais, and corn and potato enchiladas verde. **Full service, vegan/macrobiotic options, fresh juices, wine/beer, catering, take-out, $$**

Dave's Italian Kitchen
906 Church St., Evanston, IL 60201   **(708) 864-6000**
Italian. Dave's serves homemade pasta and bread, salad, sandwiches, pizza, calzone, and Italian specialties. **Open daily. Full service, vegan options, wine/beer, take-out, no credit cards, $–$$**

MOLINE

Le Mekong Restaurant
1606 Fifth Ave., Moline, IL 61265   **(309) 797-3709**
Southeast Asian/French. Traditional curry dishes, tofu, and mock meats are featured in the vegetarian menu section. **Open daily. Full service, vegan options, wine/beer/alcohol, take-out, VISA/MC/AMX, $$**

NORMAL

• Coffee World Coffeehouse
114 E. Beaufort St., Normal, IL 61761   **(309) 452-6774**
Vegetarian. Everyone in the community enjoys this coffeehouse known as "a meeting place off the Illinois State University campus." Enjoy one of the many coffee blends and a creative, vegetarian meal of charbroiled tofu, falafel pita, or one of the many other vegetarian dishes on the menu. **Open daily for three meals. Limited service, vegan options, espresso/cappuccino, VISA/MC, $**

PEORIA

Main Street Nutrition and Cafe
537 Main St., Peoria, IL 61602   **(309) 676-1485**
Health-food-store deli. Several vegetarian sandwiches are on the menu of this deli located in a natural foods store. **Open Monday through Friday for lunch and dinner. Open Saturday for lunch only. Limited service, vegan options, fresh juices, VISA/MC/DISC, $**

One World Coffee and Cargo
1245 W. Main St., Peoria, IL 61606   **(309) 672-1522**

Coffeehouse. This restaurant's eclectic menu has vegetarian dishes marked with the symbol of one Earth and vegan dishes with two. Enjoy music from a live band, poetry, or theater—depending when you're there—and be sure to check out the international gift shop. **Open daily for three meals. Full service, vegan options, espresso/cappuccino, take-out, VISA/MC, $**

ROCKFORD

Dwaraka India Restaurant
6921 E. State St., Rockford, IL 61108   **(815) 397-2265**
Indian. Authentic Indian food from all parts of India. Boldly displayed on the menu are eleven vegetarian items including traditional curry and paneer (Indian cheese) dishes plus some more unique items such as Creamed Vegetable Balls and Spiced Eggplant Purée. **Open daily. Full service, vegan options, wine/beer/alcohol, take-out, VISA/MC/AMX, $$**

Keedi's
3231 N. Main St., Rockford, IL 61103   **(815) 877-5715**
American. A family restaurant and bakery, Keedi's offers a wide variety of vegetarian dishes including vegetable sandwiches on pita, Spinach Calzones, Falafel, vegetable burgers, vegetarian quiche, fresh breads, Cabbage Rolls, Tofu Stir-Fry, Vegetarian Chili, and Vegetable Lasagna. **Open daily for three meals. Full service, take-out, $**

SKOKIE

La Salad
3938 W. Dempster, Skokie, IL 60076   **(708) 679-6190**
American. This small restaurant features an all-you-can-eat self-serve buffet including a large variety of fruits, vegetables, and pasta salads. **Cafeteria style, take-out, $$**

Slice of Life
4120 W. Dempster, Skokie, IL 60076   **(708) 674-2021**
Kosher/natural foods. Slice of Life is an Italian/dairy kosher restaurant that serves fish and vegetarian foods. An eclectic menu lists a wide variety of appetizers, salads, soups, pasta, sandwiches, and vegetarian entrees. A children's section is on the menu. Monday is Mexican night. **Open daily. Full service, kosher, fresh juices, espresso/cappuccino, wine/beer/alcohol, take-out, $$**

ST. CHARLES

Al's Cafe & Creamery
105 N. 2nd Ave., St. Charles, IL 60174   **(708) 584-5120**
Cafe. See description under Elgin, IL. **St. Charles location open daily.**

ᘐ Reviewers' choice   • Vegetarian restaurant   •• Vegan restaurant
$ less than $6 $$ $6¥$12 $$$ more than $12
VISA/AMX/MC/DISC/DC—credit cards accepted
Non-alc.—Non-alcoholic   Fresh juices—freshly squeezed

URBANA

• Red Herring Vegetarian Restaurant
1209 W. Oregon, Urbana, IL 61801   **(217) 344-1176**
Vegetarian. The only vegetarian restaurant in Urbana is a nonprofit educational food service. All foods are made from scratch and organic ingredients are used when possible. A primarily vegan menu features international dishes and vegan baked goods. **Closed Sunday. Cafeteria style, vegan options, take-out, $**

VILLA PARK

•• Better Living
100-25 E. Roosevelt, Villa Park, IL 60181   **(708) 782-5433**
Vegan. Several entrees, a salad bar, and sandwiches are offered at this vegan establishment, which has introduced a Sunday brunch by reservation only. **Open Monday through Friday for lunch, Wednesday through Thursday for dinner, Sunday for brunch. Full service, completely vegan, fresh juices, non-alc. beer/wine, take-out, VISA/MC, $**

WEST DUNDEE

China Palace
840 W. Main St., W. Dundee, IL 60118   **(708) 428-8888**
Chinese. The management is willing to accommodate vegetarians and will substitute tofu for meat in any dish. **Open seven days. Full service, vegan options, wine/beer/alcohol, take-out, VISA/MC/AMX/DISC, $**

WESTMONT

• Shree Vegetarian Restaurant
655 N. Cass Ave., Westmont, IL 60559   **(708) 655-1021**
Vegetarian. A varied and extensive menu of well prepared Indian foods is served in a friendly, clean atmosphere. Incense and Indian music enhance the dining experience. **Open Thursday through Sunday. Reservations required Friday through Sunday. Full service, fresh juices, BYOB, take-out, AMX, $**

INDIANA

CROWN POINT

Twin Happiness Restaurant
1188 N. Main St., Crown Point, IN 46307   **(219) 663-4433**
Chinese. Twin Happiness offers a large variety of vegetable and tofu dishes. Corn oil is used for cooking, and the restaurant is very willing to accommodate requests for low-salt, low-fat foods, etc. **Open daily. Full service, wine/beer/alcohol, take-out, VISA/MC/AMX, $$**

Consulate House
245 S. Meriden St., Indianapolis, IN 46225   **(317) 637-1688**
Chinese. Features a vegetarian menu complete with appetizers, soups, and entrees.
**Open daily for lunch and dinner. Full service, non-alc. wine/beer, wine/beer/
alcohol, take-out, VISA/MC/AMX/DC, $$**

India Palace
4213 Lafayette Rd., Indianapolis, IN 46254   **(317) 298-0773**
Indian. Many vegetarian options including appetizers and side dishes are joined
by entrees such as paneer and brijani, and many breads. **Open daily for dinner,
and lunch on weekends. Full service, wine/beer, take-out, VISA/MC, $$**

Koerys Restaurant
1850 E. 62nd St., Indianapolis, IN 46220   **(317) 253-2252**
Greek. Koerys features Hummus, Baba Ghanouj, Falafel, and Spanakopita. **Open
daily for lunch and dinner. Full service, non-alc. beer/wine, wine/beer, take-out,
VISA/MC/AMX/DISC/DC, $$**

Mexicana Rose
1850 E. 62nd St., Indianapolis, IN 46220   **(317) 251-1355**
Mexican. At the same location as Koerys Restaurant (see above), this restaurant
features enchiladas and burritos, all with vegetarian beans. **Open daily for lunch
and dinner. Full service, non-alc. beer/wine, wine/beer, take-out, VISA/MC/
AMX/DISC/DC, $$**

Pesto
303 N. Alabama St., Indianapolis, IN 46204   **(317) 269-0715**
Italian. Pesto features Vegetable Casserole, Fettucine with Four Cheeses, Creamed
Spinach, pizza, and salads. **Closed Sunday. Full service, non-alc. beer, wine/beer/
alcohol, VISA/MC/AMX/DC, $$–$$$**

Cornucopia Restaurant
303 S. Michigan St., South Bend, IN 46601   **(219) 288-1911**
Natural foods. Homemade soups and daily specials are served in addition to
appetizers, salads, sandwiches, entrees, omelettes, sautéed tofu, and à la carte
items. Vegetarian Chili, Spinach Lasagna, and Mexican dishes are included on the
menu. **Closed Sunday. Full service, vegan options, fresh juices, wine/beer/alco-
hol, take-out, VISA/MC, $$**

Iowa

The Grubstake
2512 Lincoln Way, Ames, IA 50010   **(515) 292-9852**
Natural foods. The Grubstake offers a wide selection of vegetarian dishes, many of which feature Mexican fare and some other ethnic foods. The restaurant is located near Iowa State University. **Full service, $$**

The Pizza Kitchens
120 Hayward Ave., Ames, IA 50010   **(515) 292-1710**
Pizza. Among the gourmet pizza and Italian pasta dishes served here are two vegetarian pizzas and two pastas. Pizza Kitchens is located near Iowa State University. **Full service, espresso/cappuccino, take-out, $$**

The Greatest Grains On Earth
1600 Harrison St., Davenport, IA 52803   **(319) 323-7521**
Natural foods. Food, which can be ordered by the piece or by the pound, includes items such as pizza, enchiladas, burritos, Spinach Potato Pie, sandwiches, soups, side dishes, and desserts. **Open daily. Deli style, vegan options, fresh juice, take-out, $**

Campbell's Nutrition Center
4040 University Ave., Des Moines, IA 50311   **(515) 277-6351**
Health-food-store deli. Vegetarian pita sandwiches are featured here. **Closed Sunday. Deli, take-out, $**

El Patio
611 37th, Des Moines, IA 50312   **(515) 274-2303**
Mexican. **Closed Monday. Full service, wine/beer, VISA/MC, $$**

Sheffield's Restaurant
319 Court Ave., Des Moines, IA 50309   **(515) 246-8496**

2724 Ingersoll, Des Moines, IA 50312   **(515) 244-7733**

216 6th Ave., Des Moines, IA 50309   **(515) 288-7687**

10201 University, Des Moines, IA 50325   **(515) 224-6774**
Natural foods. Dine on vegetarian soup, sandwich, quesadilla, pizza, and salad. **Open daily. Full service, fresh juice, wine/beer, take-out, $**

Reviewers' choice   ● Vegetarian restaurant   ●● Vegan restaurant
$ less than $6 $$ $6–$12 $$$ more than $12
VISA/AMX/MC/DISC/DC—credit cards accepted
Non-alc.—Non-alcoholic   Fresh juices—freshly squeezed

A Taste of Thailand
215 E. Walnut St., Des Moines, IA 50309 **(515) 282-0044**
Thai. The authentic Thai cuisine includes an extensive vegetarian menu section. Vegetable soups, spring rolls, Thai salad, and various vegetarian entrees make up the selection at this restaurant. **Closed Sunday. Full service, vegan options, fresh juice, wine/beer, take-out, VISA/MC/AMX, $$**

FAIRFIELD

Bonnie's China Deli
51 N. Second St., Fairfield, IA 52556 **(515) 472-7587**
Natural foods. Traditional Chinese food includes a good vegetarian selection featuring dishes using tofu, wheat gluten, and veggie tempura. No MSG is used, and special diets can be accommodated (no oil, no salt, extra spicy, etc.). There is a wide range of international desserts and beverages. **Open Monday through Saturday for lunch and dinner. Limited service, vegan options, take-out, VISA/ MC, $**

IOWA CITY

Great Midwestern Ice Cream Co.
126 E. Washington St., Iowa City, IA 52240 **(319) 337-7243**
Ice cream/sandwich shop. Some vegetarian soups, sandwiches, and pastries are offered at this ice cream shop. No smoking. **Open daily. Cafeteria style, take-out, $**

URBANDALE

New Delhi Palace
3225 NW 86th St., Urbandale, IA 50322 **(515) 278-2929**
Indian. The palace features a special vegetarian menu section with eight entrees plus appetizers and soup. Fresh Indian breads are baked in clay ovens. **Open daily for lunch and dinner. Full service, vegan options, fresh juice, wine/beer, take-out, VISA/MC/AMX, $$**

KANSAS

LAWRENCE

Cornucopia Restaurant & Bar
1801 Massachusetts St., Lawrence, KS 66044 **(913) 842-9637**
Natural foods. Here you'll find a huge salad bar with homemade soups and breads. Some vegetarian appetizers, salads, stir-fry, pasta dishes, Avocado Sandwich, and Falafel make up the veggie selection. Children's menu has salad bar and veggie lasagna. **Full service, limited vegan options, wine/beer/alcohol, take-out, VISA/MC, $$**

Full Moon Cafe
803 Massachusetts St., Lawrence, KS 66044 **(913) 832-0444**

International. Full Moon Cafe uses a separate grill and utensils to prepare its vegetarian food. It features several vegetarian sandwiches and tofu and tempeh dishes. **Open daily for lunch and dinner. Limited service, vegan options, espresso/cappuccino, non-alc. beer, beer/wine/alcohol, $**

• Herbivores
9 E. 8th St., Lawrence, KS 66044   **(913) 749-2477**
Vegetarian. Herbivores offers an incredible vegetarian menu including Tempeh Reuben Sandwiches, Lentil Burgers, Tofu Salad, Hummus Pita Pocket Sandwiches, Veggie Burritos, salads, fresh juices, and smoothies. **Open for three meals daily. Limited service, fresh juices, smoothies, vegan options, catering, take-out, $**

Paradise Cafe
728 Massachusetts St., Lawrence, KS 66044   **(913) 842-5199**
Natural foods. "Good real food" is made from scratch and includes homemade breads and desserts, and entrees based on various ethnic dishes from Italy, India, and Mexico. Breakfast menu includes vegan options. **Open daily for three meals. Full service, vegan options, wine/beer/alcohol, take-out, VISA/MC/DISC, $$**

OVERLAND PARK

Mother India Restaurant Inc.
9036 Metcalf, Overland Park, KS 66212   **(913) 341-0415**
Indian. Family-style Indian dining includes many vegetarian specials. Spicewise, dishes are available mild, medium, hot, superhot, and flaming hot!! **Open daily for lunch and dinner. Full service, vegan options, wine/beer/alcohol, take-out, VISA/MC/AMX/DISC, $$**

PRAIRIE VILLAGE

Manna House Restaurant
5313 W. 94th Terrace, Prairie Village, KS 66207   **(913) 381-9615**
Natural foods. This homey cafe features heart-healthy foods and daily specials. It is located next to a health food store. **Closed Sunday. Limited service, fresh juices, take-out, VISA/MC/AMX, $**

SHAWNEE MISSION

Shawnee Mission Medical Center
9100 W. 74th St., Box 2923, Shawnee Mission, KS 66201   **(913) 676-2496**
Hospital cafeteria. Many vegetarian entrees and side dishes are available every day at this cafeteria. **Open daily. Cafeteria style, take-out, $**

KENTUCKY

LEXINGTON

Alfalfa
557 S. Limestone, Lexington, KY 40508   **(606) 253-0014**
International. A casual atmosphere surrounds a menu that varies daily, stressing international and regional fare. Vegetarian entrees, salads, home-baked bread and desserts are always offered. **Open daily. Full service, vegan options, wine/beer, take-out, $–$$**

Everybody's Natural Foods & Deli
503 Euclid Ave., Lexington, KY 40502   **(606) 255-4162**
Natural foods. Vegetarian sandwiches, Not Dogs, salads, and daily specials are featured and breakfast is served. Courtyard seating. **Open daily. Limited service, vegan options, fresh juices, take-out, VISA/MC/DISC, $**

LOUISVILLE

• Rainbow Blossom Natural Foods & Deli
106 Fairfax Ave., Louisville, KY 40207   **(502) 893-3626**
Vegetarian deli. Offering many vegan items, this vegetarian deli is take-out only. The foods are made with high-quality products using organic ingredients when possible. Rainblow Blossom is dedicated to providing an alternative to those people who seek healthy and convenient gourmet foods to go. **Open daily. Self-service, vegan options, fresh juices, take-out, VISA/MC, $**

LOUISIANA

METAIRIE

Nature Lovers
3014 Cleary Ave., Metairie, LA 70002   **(504) 887-4929**
Natural foods. Nature Lovers provides a deli and salad bar. **Full service, fresh juices, take-out, VISA/MC/AMX/DISC, $**

Smoothie King
2725 Mississippi Ave., Metairie, LA 70003   **(504) 885-1000**
Juice bar. Enjoy various smoothies at this juice bar. **Open daily. Counter service, take-out, VISA/MC/AMX, $**

?◆ Reviewers' choice   • Vegetarian restaurant   •• Vegan restaurant
$ less than $6 $$ $6–$12 $$$ more than $12
VISA/AMX/MC/DISC/DC–credit cards accepted
Non-alc.–Non-alcoholic   Fresh juices–freshly squeezed

Taj Mahal
923 C Metaire Rd., Metairie, LA 70005   **(504) 836-6859**
Indian. Taj Mahal offers several vegetarian dishes that are prepared in oil, not butter. Try curry, dal, fresh breads, and other items. The owner says that half the orders are vegetarian. **Open Tuesday through Sunday for lunch and dinner. Closed Monday. Full service, beer/wine/alcohol, take-out, VISA/MC/AMX/ DISC/DC, $$**

NEW ORLEANS

All Natural Foods & Deli
5517 Magazine St., New Orleans, LA 70115   **(504) 891-2651**
Natural foods deli. This deli is all vegetarian, except for tuna fish. It offers a wide variety of dishes including Hummus, Falafel, Tempeh Burgers, Tempeh Spread, Tofu Burgers, Vegetarian Sushi, smoothies, and daily special hot entrees. **Open daily. Counter service, fresh juices, smoothies, vegan/macrobiotic options, take-out, VISA/MC, $**

The Apple Seed Shoppe
346 Camp St., New Orleans, LA 70130   **(504) 529-3442**
Natural foods. Dig into salads, sandwiches, and specialties. **Open Monday through Friday. Limited service, fresh juices, BYOB, take-out, $**

Back to the Garden
920 St. Charles Ave., New Orleans, LA 70130   **(504) 522-8792**
Natural foods. Dine on a veggie stir-fry served over brown rice, bean chili, hearty salads, vegetarian tacos, and fruit smoothies at Back to the Garden, which is located in the YMCA Hotel. **Open Monday through Saturday for breakfast and lunch. Counter service, fresh juices, smoothies, vegan options, take-out, $**

•• Jack Sprat's Vegetarian Grill
3240 S. Carrollton Ave., New Orleans, LA 70118   **(504) 486-2200**
Vegan. The owners of this restaurant, which opened during the summer of 1994, are animal rights activists who want to promote veganism. Dine on creative salads, vegan burgers, sandwiches, and entrees such as Vegetable Stir-Fry, Red Beans and Rice, Middle Eastern Platter, and Mardi Gras Rice in a cozy, romantic old English decor. Enjoy candle-lit tables and Celtic music. **Open daily for lunch and dinner. Full service, vegan only, fresh juices, non-alc. beer/wine, beer/wine, catering, take-out, VISA/MC, $$**

Marty's Vegetarian Haven Cafe
207 Dauphine St., New Orleans, LA 70112   **(502) 522-5222**
Natural foods. Despite its name, Marty's is not a vegetarian cafe. Nevertheless, it does offer a number of interesting vegetarian dishes including red, lima, or black beans, or white beans with brown rice, and other items. Marty's is located in the French Quarter. **Open daily for lunch. Counter service, fresh juice, smoothies, vegan options, take-out, $**

Old Dog New Trick
307 Exchange Alley, New Orleans, LA 70130 **(504) 511-4569**
Natural foods. Vegetarian burgers, salads, tempeh sandwiches, veggie pizzas, and tofu entrees are offered at this New Orleans restaurant. It often has vegan desserts! **$**

Panda Riverview Chinese Restaurant
600 Decatur St., New Orleans, LA 70130 **(504) 523-6073**
Chinese. This Chinese restaurant offers a beautiful view of the Mississippi River. It is located in the French Quarter and is not too far from the convention center. It offers several vegetarian dishes and the management is quite accommodating. **Open daily for lunch and dinner. Full service, beer/wine/alcohol, VISA/MC/ AMX/DISC/DC, $$**

SHREVEPORT

Earthereal Restaurant & Bakery
3309 Line Ave., Shreveport, LA 71104 **(318) 865-8947**
Natural foods/macrobiotic. Salads, many unique sandwiches, and tacos with soymeat or avocado, plus daily specials are offered on the Earthereal menu. **Closed Sunday. Limited service, macrobiotic, fresh juices, take-out, VISA/MC, $**

MAINE

BAR HARBOR

Quiet Earth Restaurant
122 Cottage St., Bar Harbor, ME 04609 **(207) 288-3696**
International. Gourmet international cuisine is provided in a charming European-style atmosphere. Live music is featured regularly. Quiet Earth serves vegetarian, fish, and chicken dishes with non-dairy entrees available on request. **Open for dinner daily in summer, Thursday through Sunday in winter. Full service, wine/ beer, take-out, VISA/MC, $$**

BELFAST

Darby's
105 High St., Belfast, ME 04915 **(207) 338-2339**
Natural foods/macrobiotic. Darby's has operated continuously since 1845 with original walls, tin ceiling, and antique bar. Macrobiotic specials are offered daily. **Open daily. Full service, wine/beer/alcohol, take-out, VISA/MC, $$**

Kingsbury House Inn
35 Northport Ave., Belfast, ME 04915 **(207) 338-2419**
Macrobiotic bed-and-breakfast. This small New England bed-and-breakfast serves only macrobiotic fare. **Reservations required. Limited service, BYOB, take-out, $$**

90 Main Street
90 Main St., Belfast, ME 04915   **(207) 338-1106**
Natural foods/macrobiotic. Quality natural foods using organic produce are served when in season. Daily specials and desserts as well as black bean enchiladas, pasta dishes, salads, and vegetarian soups are featured. Outdoor dining in the summer. **Open daily for lunch and dinner. Full service, fresh juices, wine/beer/alcohol, take-out, VISA/MC, $$**

BIDDEFORD

New Morning Natural Food Market and Cafe
230 Main St., Biddeford, ME 04005   **(207) 282-1434**
Natural foods. The cafe offers an ever-changing selection of creative entrees. A wide variety of sandwiches is available on sourdough bread from a local bakery. There are also homemade soups and chili. **Open Monday through Friday. Full service, vegan options, fresh juices, take-out, $**

CAPE ELIZABETH

Basics Natural Foods Store
537 Shore Rd., Cape Elizabeth, ME 04107   **(207) 767-2803**
Natural foods deli. Basics has a deli with sesame noodles, soups, vegetable pot pies, veggie lasagna, sandwiches, and assorted desserts. Many dairy-free and wheat-free items are available. Most entrees are prepared for you to take home and heat. There are a few tables on the premises. **Open daily. Vegan options, wine/beer, mostly take-out, $**

FREEPORT

The Corsican Restaurant
9 Mechanic St., Freeport, ME 04032   **(207) 865-9421**
Natural foods. Homemade vegetarian soups, unique whole-wheat pizza, calzones, and fresh baked breads are offered daily. Delicious pies and cakes are also available. No smoking. **Open daily for lunch and dinner. Full service, wine/beer, take-out, $$**

PORTLAND

Bagel Works
15 Temple St., Portland, ME 04101   **(207) 879-2425**
Bagel deli. More than sixteen varieties of bagels are offered with various topping options including cream cheeses, tofutti spreads, salads, and vegetarian combinations. Only natural ingredients without preservatives are used. Bagel Works is environmentally conscious and socially active in its community. **Open daily. Counter service, vegan options, fresh juices, take-out, $**

Cafe No
20 Danforth St., Portland, ME 04101   **(207) 772-8114**
International. Cafe No's menu includes many salads, sandwiches, Middle Eastern specialties, fish dishes, and desserts with several vegetarian options. **Open Tuesday through Saturday. Full service, vegan options, wine/beer, take-out, no credit cards, $**

Good Day Market
155 Brackett St., Portland ME 04102   **(207) 772-4937**
Natural foods deli. Good Day Market is a food co-op that has take-out sandwiches, knishes, calzones, soup and chili, muffins, cakes, and tarts. **Deli open Monday through Friday. Take-out only, vegan options, wine/beer, no credit cards, $**

Pepperclub
78 Middle St., Portland, ME 04101   **(207) 772-0531**
Eclectic. The Pepperclub menu is about 50 percent vegetarian and 50 percent fish. There is always at least one vegan entree as well. **Open daily for dinner. Full service, wine/beer, take-out, VISA/MC, $$**

Raffles Cafe Bookstore
555 Congress St., Portland, ME 04101   **(207) 761-3930**
Natural foods. Raffles focuses on high quality, fresh, and nutritious food. The offering includes soup, salads, sandwiches, Middle Eastern foods, and daily vegetarian specials and homemade desserts. **Full service, fresh juices, espresso/cappuccino, take-out, VISA/MC, $**

Silly's
147 Cumberland Ave., Portland, ME 04102   **(207) 772-0360**
Natural foods. A small restaurant with a colorful and involving atmosphere, Silly's has delicious and surprising food, with a variety that includes Hummus, Falafel, Sesame Noodles, pizza, Jamaican Beans and Rice, and sandwiches. Patio for summer dining. **Open daily for lunch and dinner. Full service, vegan options, BYOB, take-out, $**

Victory Deli and Bake Shop
1 Monument Way, Portland, ME 04102   **(207) 772-7299**
Deli/cafe. This New York style deli, cafe, and bakery emphasizes preparation of food items from scratch. Veggie salads, sandwiches, Falafel, and veggie burgers are offered. There's a whole-grain bakery and organic vegetables in the summer. **Open for three meals Monday through Friday, for breakfast and lunch on weekends. Full service, fresh juices, wine/beer, take-out, $**

Walter's Cafe
15 Exchange St., Portland, ME 04101   **(207) 871-9258**
American. Walter's Cafe offers regional cuisine that is prepared fresh daily in the exhibition-style kitchen. Walter's offers friendly, courteous service in a casual but professional atmosphere. **Open for lunch and dinner daily. Full service, wine/beer, take-out, VISA/MC/AMX, $$**

🍴 Reviewers' choice   ● Vegetarian restaurant   ●● Vegan restaurant
$ less than $6 $$ $6–$12 $$$ more than $12
VISA/AMX/MC/DISC/DC—credit cards accepted
Non-alc.—Non-alcoholic   Fresh juices—freshly squeezed

West Side Restaurant
58 Pine St., Portland, ME 04102   **(207) 773-8223**
Gourmet/natural foods. Each entree is prepared to order at the West Side, a restaurant that prides itself on good quality, healthy food and is willing to accommodate special diets. Vegetarian dinner options include lasagna, a tofu dish, fettucine, stir-fry, a Mexican dish, and appetizers. **Open for three meals daily, Sunday for brunch only. Full service, vegan options, fresh juice, wine/beer, alcohol, limited take-out, $$–$$$**

The Whole Grocer
118 Congress St., Portland, ME 04101   **(207) 774-7711**
Natural foods deli. Two featured soups daily plus fresh baked muffins, sandwiches, salads, and sometimes desserts are offered here. **Open daily. Self-service, vegan options, wine/beer, take-out, $**

RAYMOND

• Northern Pines Health Resort
559 Route 85, Raymond, ME 04071   **(207) 655-7624**
Vegetarian/natural foods. The menu at Northen Pines is vegetarian but fish is occasionally served. Northern Pines offers a delicious variety of vegetarian dishes for breakfast, lunch, and dinner. Menu changes. **Open mid-June to Labor Day. Buffet, fresh juices, VISA/MC, $$**

SOUTH HARPSWELL

J. Hathaways
Rte. 123, S. Harpswell, ME 04079   **(207) 833-5305**
American. Recommended by a local patron, this restaurant has a terrific vegetarian lasagna and a meatless chili topped with cornbread. The bean soup is also delicious. **Full service, vegan option.**

MARYLAND

ANNAPOLIS

India Palace
186 Main St., Annapolis, MD 21401   **(410) 263-7900**
Indian. Enjoy several vegetarian dishes including Chickpeas, Onions and Tomatoes; Cauliflower and Potatoes; Mixed Vegetables; and more. **Open daily for lunch and dinner. Full service, vegan options, take-out, VISA/MC/AMX, $$**

Mexican Cafe
975 Bay Ridge Rd., Annapolis, MD 21403   **(410) 626-1520**
Mexican. This restaurant offers several vegetarian options. Beans do not contain lard. **Open daily for lunch and dinner. Full service, vegan options, beer/wine, take-out, VISA/MC, $–$$**

BALTIMORE

(For more restaurant listings in the surrounding suburbs, see Cockeysville, Columbia, Ellicott City, Owings Mills, Randallstown, and Towson.)

Adrian's Book Cafe
714 S. Broadway, Baltimore, MD 21231   **(410) 732-1048**

Natural foods. The menu at Adrian's Book Cafe changes daily; however, there are always several vegetarian dishes such as chili, quiche, spanikopita, calzones, salads, and soup. The cafe also offers a wide variety of coffee and desserts. Smoking is not allowed. **Open daily for three meals. Full service, espresso/cappuccino, take-out, VISA/MC/AMX, $**

Akbar
823 N. Charles St., Baltimore, MD 21201   **(410) 539-0944**

Indian. Akbar features authentic Indian cuisine with a wide variety of vegetarian dishes. The restaurant has consistently given great service. **Open daily. Full service, vegan options, wine/beer/alcohol, catering, take-out, VISA/MC/AMX/ DISC, $$**

Al Pacino Cafe
900 Cathedral St., Baltimore, MD 21201   **(410) 962-8859**

609 S. Broadway, Baltimore, MD 21231   **(410) 327-0005**

542 E. Belvedere Ave., (in the Belvedere Market)
Baltimore, MD 21212   **(410) 323-7060**

Middle Eastern/pizza. With a New-York-City-type atmosphere, this bustling cafe has great-tasting Middle Eastern food, steaming-hot pita bread, and unique pizza combinations such as the pizza served with curry. All pizza is available without cheese or with soy cheese. **Open daily. Full service, vegan options, take-out, VISA/MC, $$**

Bombay Grill
2 E. Madison St., Baltimore, MD 21202   **(410) 837-2973**

Indian. This cozy Indian restaurant offers Indian breads and many vegetarian entrees including Vegetable Kofta, potato dishes, Okra and Onions, Eggplant Stir-fry, and a grilled vegetable kabab. Dishes are prepared with vegetable or olive oil. Live music on weekends. **Open daily. Full service, vegan options, wine/ beer/alcohol, catering, take-out, VISA/MC/AMX/DISC/DC, $$**

Cafe Diana
3215 N. Charles St., Baltimore, MD 21218   **(410) 889-1319**

Natural foods. Cafe Diana is located near the Johns Hopkins University campus and is run and owned by a large group of women. The cafe does not serve red meat and offers many vegetarian dishes including Salsa and Chips, Pasta Salad, Veggie Sandwich, quiche, Lasagna, quesadillas, Noodle Pudding, soups, plus more. **Open daily for three meals. Counter service, espresso/cappuccino, vegan options, take-out, $**

Ding How
631-637 S. Broadway, Baltimore, MD 21231   **(410) 327-8888**
Chinese. This Fells Point Chinese restaurant offers many vegetarian items including appetizers, soups, tofu, and vegetable entrees. **Full service, vegan options, wine/beer/alcohol, take-out, VISA/MC/AMX/DISC/DC, $–$$**

Donna's Coffee Bar
2 W. Madison St., Baltimore, MD 21201   **(410) 385-0180**
Italian. Enjoy a wide variety of coffees along with delicious Italian cuisine and fresh breads at Donna's Coffee Bar. Half the food is vegetarian. **Open daily for three meals. Full service, espresso/cappuccino, catering, take-out, VISA/MC/AMX, $**

Funk's Democratic Coffee Spot
1818 Eastern Ave., Baltimore, MD 21231   **(410) 276-3865**
Coffeehouse. The bright colors, eclectic decor, occasional live music, and festive atmosphere make this casual cafe a great place to check out . . . besides that they have daily vegetarian and vegan meals. The menu differs daily and includes dishes like hummus sandwich, bulgur-lentil salad, ginger-carrot soup, falafel, and many other multi-ethnic creations. **Open daily for three meals. Counter service, vegan options, espresso/cappuccino, take-out, $**

• Golden Temple Cafe
2322 N. Charles St., Baltimore, MD 21218   **(410) 235-1014**
Vegetarian/natural foods. This natural foods store offers counter service and tables at which to sit, and a Mexican Fiesta salad bar. No meat, poultry, fish, or eggs are served. **Cafe open Monday through Saturday for lunch; salad bar available daily until dusk. Counter service, vegan options, fresh juices, catering, take-out, VISA/MC, $**

• Green Earth Natural Food Store & Deli
823 N. Charles St., Baltimore, MD 21201   **(410) 752-1422**
Natural foods/macrobiotic/health-food deli. This take-out-food store features gourmet homestyle cooking using mostly organic ingredients. **Open daily. Vegan/macro-biotic options, fresh juices, take-out only, VISA/MC, $**

Hacienda Mexican Restaurant
4840 Bel Air Rd., Baltimore, MD 21206   **(410) 488-9447**
Mexican. Enjoy vegetarian burritos, tacos, and quiche. **Open for dinner Tuesday through Sunday. Full service, wine/beer/alcohol, limited catering, take-out, VISA/MC/AMX, $$**

Henry & Jeff's
1220 N. Charles St., Baltimore, MD 21231   **(410) 727-3322**
American. Henry & Jeff's is located in midtown Baltimore and is close to several theaters. The eatery offers several vegetarian items including Hummus Sandwiches and Mexican dishes. **Open daily for three meals. Full service, espresso/cappuccino, beer/wine/alcohol, catering, take-out, VISA/MC/AMX/ DISC/DC, $–$$**

Jai Hind Indian Restaurant
5511 York Rd., Baltimore, MD 21212   **(410) 323-8440**

Indian. Jai Hind features formal dining with instrumental Indian music in the background. The restaurant is accommodating to vegetarians, with a nice vegetarian variety included on the menu. **Open Monday through Saturday for lunch, and Monday through Sunday for dinner. Full service, vegan options, wine/beer/alcohol, take-out, VISA/MC/AMX/DISC, $$**

Louie's Bookstore Cafe
518 N. Charles St., Baltimore, MD 21201 (410) 962-1224
Cafe/bookstore. Located downtown, Louie's is a fun, crowded, and popular combination of restaurant, bookstore, art gallery, and bakery. It features classical music performances every evening during dinner hours and at Sunday brunch. The menu is eclectic, with both local and international cuisine and a good number of options for vegetarians. **Open daily into night. Full service, vegan options, wine/beer/alcohol, take-out, VISA/MC, $$**

• Magic Lotus Catering
233 Blakeney Rd., Baltimore, MD 21228 (410) 455-6496
Vegetarian/caterer. Although not a restaurant, Magic Lotus caters vegetarian food only. Menu items include a choice of over twenty salads, ten appetizers, ten soups, chutneys and sauces, and entrees such as Spinach Lasagna, Eggplant Moussaka, Chili Con Tofu, Hungarian Potato Goulash, Philippine Vegetable Stew, Stuffed Peppers, Middle Eastern Potato and Chick Peas, plus more. You also can choose from a wide variety of rice dishes, breads, and desserts. **Catering. Full service or delivery only. Price varies according to number in party.**

Mencken's Cultured Pearl
1114-16 Hollins St., Baltimore, MD 21223 (410) 837-1947
Mexican. Located in a marginal neighborhood that is a hub of the local art scene, Mencken's features monthly art shows and kraft-paper table covers and crayons so you can draw. Fresh-squeezed limes are used in the margaritas, and animal fat is not used to fry the foods. There's a relaxed atmosphere and eclectic music. Weekend evenings, you often have a long wait to be seated. You can wait at the bar. **Open daily. Full service, wine/beer/alcohol, take-out, VISA/MC, $–$$**

Mike's
710 S. Broadway, Fells Point, MD 21231 (410) 342-6589
Mexican. Mike's is a small bar and tiny restaurant, but a fun place in the alternative-night-life section of Fells Point. Work by local artists is usually exhibited, and Mike's features Guacamole and Chips, Bean Tacos, and very large Bean Burritos made Mayan style. Refried beans are always made with peanut oil only. **Open daily. Full service, vegan options, wine/beer, take-out, $**

Mr. Chan Schechuan Restaurant ✿
1010 Reistertown Rd., Pikesville, MD 21208 (410) 484-1100

✿ Reviewers' choice • Vegetarian restaurant •• Vegan restaurant
$ less than $6 $$ $6–$12 $$$ more than $12
VISA/AMX/MC/DISC/DC—credit cards accepted
Non-alc.—Non-alcoholic Fresh juices—freshly squeezed

Chinese. Savor unique items for vegetarians. The chef is always experimenting to come up with new dishes and will cater to special needs, especially for vegans or macrobiotics. This top Baltimore choice offers great hot and sour soup, tempeh dishes, delicious orange spicy tofu, egg rolls or non-fried dumplings, mustard green treats, and more. **Open daily 10:30 A.M. to 10:30 P.M. Full service, vegan/ macrobiotic options, wine/beer/alcohol, catering, take-out, VISA/MC/AMX/ DISC, $$**

• One World Cafe
904 S. Charles St., Baltimore, MD 21230   **(410) 234-0235**
Vegetarian. Baltimore finally has a vegetarian cafe. One World Cafe, owned and run by three siblings, offers a wide variety of coffees, as well as vegetarian food including Chili, salads, soups, fresh breads and baked goods, Falafel, smoothies, plus more. The cafe is situated in a beautifully renovated town house in the Federal Hill area and is located a few blocks south of the Inner Harbor area and Baltimore Convention Center. **Open daily for three meals. Counter service, espresso/cappuccino, smoothies, vegan options, take-out, $**

Puffins Cafe
1000 Reistertown Rd., Pikesville, MD 21208   **(410) 486-8811**
Natural foods. Puffins bakes its own breads and desserts and features salads, pasta, and pizza. All soups and sauces are vegetarian. Vegetarian entrees are generally macrobiotic-style. Weekly specials are served in an art-filled atmosphere. No smoking. **Closed Sunday. Full service, non-alc. beer, wine/beer, catering, take-out, VISA/MC, $$$**

Sitar
Pace Plaza
1724 Woodlawn Dr., Baltimore, MD 21207   **(410) 265-5140**
Indian. Inexpensive Indian food is served in an informal atmosphere. **Open daily. Buffet/counter service, vegan options, take-out, $–$$**

Syrumie Cafe
3219 Eastern Ave., Baltimore, MD 21224   **(410) 563-2787**
Middle Eastern. Syrumie offers traditional Egyptian, Lebanese, and Syrian foods. Dinner and show (Egyptian dance) are featured once a month. **Open for dinner only Monday through Friday, lunch and dinner Saturday. Full service, vegan options, wine/beer, catering, take-out, $$–$$$**

The Tell Tale Hearth
1145 Hollins St., Baltimore, MD 21223   **(410) 234-0880**
American/ethnic. Enjoy hearth-baked pizza, Caribbean specialities, and pastas. **Open daily until 2:00 A.M. Full service, wine/beer/alcohol, catering, take-out, VISA/MC, $$**

Thai Restaurant
3316 Greenmount Ave., Baltimore, MD 21218   **(410) 889-7303**
Thai. Although the service and atmosphere are formal, dress is casual. There's a nice selection, and the restaurant will substitute tofu for meat in any of its dishes. The restaurant is located on a main street, but the neighborhood is

somewhat marginal. **Open daily. Full service, wine/beer/alcohol, catering, take-out, VISA/MC/AMX, $$**

Thairish Cafe
804 N. Charles St., Baltimore, MD 21201 (410) 752-5857
Thai. This family-run small operation offers delicious vegetarian curry dishes with or without tofu. The vegetables are steamed and crisp. The cafe also serves rice noodle dishes. Smoking is not permitted. **Open Tuesday through Sunday for lunch and dinner. Closed Monday. Counter service, vegan options, take-out, VISA/MC, $**

Tov Pizza
6313 Reisterstown Rd., Baltimore, MD 21215 (410) 358-5238
Kosher/dairy. This popular kosher dairy restaurant in Baltimore is primarily vegetarian with the exception of some fish dishes. Items available include pizzas and Falafel. **Counter service, vegan options, take-out, $**

Village Market Simply Delicious Deli
Colonial Village Shopping Center
7006 Reisterstown Rd., Pikesville, MD 21208 (410) 486-0979
Natural foods deli. Village Market Natural Grocer recently expanded and was able to add a deli section that offers a huge variety of salads and a salad bar, sandwiches, pizzas, burritos, and daily specials. **Open daily for three meals. Limited service, fresh juices, espresso/cappuccino, vegan options, VISA/MC, $**

BEL AIR

Hunan Chef
5 Bel Air South Parkway, Bel Air, MD 21014 (410) 838-2313
Chinese. **Monday through Saturday open late afternoon and evening, Sunday open from noon until 10:00 P.M. Full service, vegan options, take-out, VISA/MC/AMX, $$**

BETHESDA

(For more restaurant listings in the surrounding areas, see Washington, D.C.)

Bacchus
7945 Norfolk Ave., Bethesda, MD 20814 (301) 657-1722
Lebanese. This Lebanese restaurant offers several vegetarian items including Stuffed Grape Leaves, Hummus, Baba Ghanouj, Stuffed Eggplant, Eggplant Salad, Potato Salad, Cauliflower and Tahini Dip, and Falafel. **Open daily. Full service, vegan options, wine/beer/alcohol, catering, take-out, VISA/MC/AMX, $$–$$$**

• Green City Market and Cafe
4735 Bethesda Ave., Bethesda, MD 20814 (301) 652-0050
Vegetarian. This cafe offers a large number of raw, vegan dishes, as well as some cooked items. Options include a Quinoa Salad, Black Bean and Corn Salad, Walnut-Pate Sandwich, various soups, sweet and sour veggies with tempeh, etc.

The cafe offers a standard menu, as well as daily specials. Food is sold by the pound. **Open daily for three meals. Counter service, vegan options, take-out, VISA/MC, $$**

Tako Grill
7756 Wisconsin Ave., Bethesda, MD 20814   **(301) 652-7030**
Japanese. **Closed Sunday and for lunch on Saturday. Full service, wine/beer, take-out, VISA/MC/ AMX, $**

COCKEYSVILLE
The Natural Cafe
560 Cranbrook Rd., Cockeysville, MD 21030   **(410) 628-1262**
Health-food-store juice bar. This self-serve cafe has a chef on duty and offers home-made soup or chili daily. **Open for lunch Monday through Friday. Cafeteria style, vegan options, fresh juices, take-out, VISA/MC/AMX, $**

COLLEGE PARK

(For more restaurant listings in the surrounding areas, see Washington, D.C.)

• Berwyn Cafe
5010 Berwyn Rd., College Park, MD 20740   **(301) 345-6655**
Vegetarian. Berwyn Cafe is located in a natural foods store in a college town. It features two to three specials daily, one is usually vegan, and offers pita sand-wiches, veggie burgers, steamed vegetables, beans and rice, plus much more. **Open daily. Sunday brunch. Counter service, vegan/macrobiotic options, fresh juices, non-alc. beverages, take-out, VISA/MC/DISC, $**

COLUMBIA
Akbar
9400 Snowden River Pkwy., Columbia, MD 21045   **(410) 381-3600**
Indian. See description under Baltimore, Maryland.

Bombay Peacock Grill
10005 Old Columbia Rd., Columbia, MD 21046   **(410) 381-7111**
Indian. This cozy Indian restaurant offers Indian breads and many vegetarian entrees including Vegetable Kofta, potato dishes, Okra and Onions, Eggplant Stir-Fry, and a Grilled Vegetable Kabab. Dishes are prepared with vegetable or olive oil. **Open daily, with luncheon buffet. Full service, vegan options, wine/beer/alcohol, catering, take-out, VISA/MC/AMX/DIS/DC, $$**

꿍 Reviewers' choice   • Vegetarian restaurant   •• Vegan restaurant
$ less than $6 $$ $6–$12 $$$ more than $12
VISA/AMX/MC/DISC/DC—credit cards accepted
Non-alc.—Non-alcoholic   Fresh juices—freshly squeezed

• MELA
6476 Dobbin Center Way, Columbia, MD 21045   **(410) 997-2117**
Vegetarian/Indian. This new, small restaurant offers Indian vegetarian food made without eggs. Items may be prepared vegan upon request. Appetizers include samosas and Onion Pakoras. Various lentil soups are offered as well as a wide variety of entrees such as curries, rice-based dishes, and dals. **Open daily for lunch and dinner. Full service, vegan options, wine/beer, catering, take-out, VISA/MC, $–$$.**

CUMBERLAND

Gehauf's
1268 National Hwy., Cumberland, MD 21502   **(301) 729-3300**
American style. In a lovely airy setting, you'll find fresh-fruit plates in season, spinach salad, mixed salad with fresh vegetables, and a few vegetarian specials like vegetarian chili. **Open daily. Full service, wine/beer/alcohol, take-out, VISA/MC/AMX, $$**

L'Osteria
Rt 40, Cumberland, MD 21502   **(301) 777-3553**
Italian. The atmosphere is formal, and the food includes Eggplant Parmesan and Pasta Alfredo, imported pastas with vegetables, and a variety of salads and fruits. Some items can be made without cheese. **Open for dinner. Full service, reservations required, wine/beer/alcohol, catering, take-out, VISA/MC/AMX, $$**

The Melting Pot
Winchester Rd., Cumberland, MD 21502   **(301) 729-1960**
Ethnic foods. Various ethnic foods are featured, and the restaurant, which is very accommodating of special needs, will prepare low-fat entrees. There are many lacto-ovo choices. Lunch specials include vegetarian egg rolls. **Open daily. Full service, wine/beer/alcohol, take-out, $$**

ELLICOTT CITY

Han Sung Restaurant
3570 St. John Ln., Ellicott City, MD 21043   **410) 750-3836**
Korean/Japanese. Enjoy several vegetarian appetizers, steamed rice, and salads. **Wine/beer, $–$$**

FREDERICK

• Common Market (Frederick Co-op)
5813 Buckeystown Pk., Frederick, MD 21701   **(301) 663-3416**
Vegetarian/health-food-store deli. Enjoy sandwiches made with organically grown foods, and a juice bar. **Lunch hours. Limited service, fresh juices, take-out, $**

Health Express
1540 W. Patrick, Frederick, MD 21701   **(301) 662-2293**

Health-food-store deli. Sandwiches and homemade soups are the order of the day. **Lunch hours. Limited service, fresh juices, take-out, $**

Lotus Chinese Cuisine
107 Baughman's Ln., Frederick, MD 21702   **(301) 694-3388**
Chinese. Here's authentic Chinese cuisine in a relaxed atmosphere. There's a vegetarian section on the menu, and Lotus will gladly accommodate vegetarians/vegans. **Open daily. Full service, vegan options, wine/beer, take-out, VISA/MC/DISC, $$**

The Orchard
48 E. Patrick St., Frederick, MD 21701   **(301) 663-4912**
Natural foods. This natural foods restaurant serves chicken, seafood, and vegetarian items. It is completely non-smoking and has outdoor dining on the deck from April through October. **Closed Sunday and Monday. Open Tuesday through Saturday for lunch and dinner. Full service, vegan options, wine/beer, take-out, VISA/MC/AMX/DC, $$**

Taurasos
4 East St., Frederick, MD 21701   **(301) 663-6600**
American. This popular restaurant has an elegant formal dining room and a casual pub. A special vegetarian menu is available. **Open for lunch and dinner. $–$$$**

FROSTBURG

Giuseppe's
11 Bowery St., Frostburg, MD 21532   **(301) 689-2220**
Italian. This unique Italian restaurant in a small town near a ski area offers many lacto-ovo choices and a tasty plain sauce for vegans. Giuseppe's will accommodate special needs. **Open daily late afternoon and evening. Full service, wine/beer/alcohol, take-out, VISA/MC/AMX/DISC, $$**

GAITHERSBURG

Thai Sa-Mai Restaurant
8369 Snouffer School Rd., Gaithersburg, MD 20879   **(301) 963-1800**
Thai. On the menu are original spicy Thai foods and thirty vegetarian dishes made without MSG. *The Washingtonian* magazine named this restaurant's curry the best four-star. **Open Monday through Saturday. Full service, vegan options, wine/beer, take-out, VISA/MC, $$**

GREENBELT

China Pearl Restaurant
7701 Greenbelt Rd., Greenbelt, MD 20770   **(301) 441-8880**
Chinese. Enjoy Chinese dishes including vegetarian egg rolls. Tempeh is also available. **Open daily. Full service, alcohol, take-out, VISA/MC/AMX/DISC, $$**

Maharajah
8825 Greenbelt Rd., Greenbelt, MD 20770   **(301) 552-1600**

Indian. Here you'll find vegetarian appetizers, and main dishes that include eggplant, curries, and vegetable stir-fry. **Open daily for dinner, lunch served Tuesday through Friday. Full service, vegan options, wine/beer, take-out, VISA/ MC, $$**

• Udupi Palace
1329 University Blvd., Langley Park, MD 20873   (301) 434-1531
Vegetarian. This vegetarian restaurant opened in 1994 and serves Southern Indian food including dosai (crêpes filled with vegetables), uthappam (Indian-style pancakes), curries, and more. **Open for lunch and dinner daily. Full service, vegan options, take-out, VISA/MC/AMX, $$**

Mr. Wang Hunan
675 Main St., Laurel, MD 20707   (301) 317-8888
Chinese. A separate vegetarian menu offers a wide selection of mock meats including vegetarian egg rolls and crispy Sesame Chicken. **Open daily for lunch and dinner. Full service, vegan options, wine/beer, catering, take-out, $$**

Cafe Iguana
8201 Coastal Hwy., Ocean City, MD 21842   (410) 524-6300
Natural foods. The next time you visit Maryland's Ocean City beach resort area, check out Cafe Iguana. It offers several vegetarian items including a Veggie Pita Pocket Sandwich, several salads, Stuffed Grape Leaves, Hummus Platter, Mexican quesadillas, Vegetarian Chili, and Veggie Burger. **Open daily for three meals (hours change during winter months). Full service, vegan options, espresso/cappuccino, take-out, $**

Olney Ale House
2000 Olney Sandy Spring Rd., Olney, MD 20832   (301) 774-6708
Natural foods. This cozy restaurant with a fireplace during winter months offers several vegetarian dishes such as chili, tofu and sunburgers, salads, and homemade breads. It's very crowded on weekends, so expect a long wait. **Closed Monday. Full service, vegan options, wine/beer, take-out, VISA/MC/DISC, $$**

OWINGS MILLS

Sprouts
10027 Reisterstown Rd., Owings Mills, MD 21117   (410) 363-4222
Natural foods. This primarily vegetarian cafe is located in a natural foods market. Sprouts offers Vegetarian Chili, soups, salads, sandwiches, appetizers, and entrees including Stir-Fry Lo Mein, Pasta with Marinara Sauce, Steamed Vegetable Platter, Lasagna, and pita pizzas. Outdoor seating is available when weather permits. **Open for three meals daily. Full service, fresh juices, vegan options, catering, take-out, VISA/MC, $–$$**

RANDALLSTOWN

(For more restaurant listings in the surrounding areas, see Baltimore)

Akbar Restaurant 🐂
3541 Brenbrook Dr., Randallstown, MD 21133   (410) 655-1600
Indian. See description under Baltimore.

Szechuan Best
8625 Liberty Rd., Randallstown, MD 21133   (410) 521-0020
Chinese. This Chinese restaurant has an extensive vegetarian menu. **Full service, take-out, $$**

ROCKVILLE

Hard Times Cafe
1117 Nelson St., Rockville, MD 20850   (301) 294-9720
Ethnic. This old-fashioned Texas chili parlor cooks up vegetarian chili in a variety of ways. **Open daily. Full service, wine/beer, take-out, VISA/MC/AMX, $**

House of Chinese Gourmet
1485 Rockville Pk., Rockville, MD 20852   (301) 984-9440
Chinese. Savor the excellent and extensive vegetarian choices, such as Yellow Bird (made with bean curd skins), Crispy Eggplant, and Asparagus and Corn Soup. **Open daily for lunch and dinner. Full service, wine/beer/alcohol, take-out, VISA/MC/AMX, $$**

Natraj Restaurant
1327 F. Rockville Pk., Rockville, MD 20852   (301) 340-7373
Indian. No animal fat or MSG is used in cooking, and whole-wheat bread is always available. Natraj has Masala Dosas (large crêpe-like pancake with potato and onions) and a vegetarian all-you-can-eat-buffet. **Open daily. Full service, wine/beer, catering, take-out, VISA/MC/AMX/DISC, $**

•• The Vegetable Garden
11618 Rockville Pike, Rockville, MD 20852   (301) 468-9301
Vegan/Chinese. If you are in the D.C. area and you like Chinese food, this is a must-try restaurant. It has dozens of hard-to-find vegan and vegetarian dishes,

expecially seitan and wheat gluten items. It also offers such interesting soups as Sizzling Rice and Asparagus and Corn Soup, and a non-fat menu is available. **Open daily for lunch and dinner. Full service, vegan options, fresh juices, wine/beer/alcohol, take-out, VISA/MC/AMX, $$**

SILVER SPRING

• Siddhartha Vegetarian Restaurant
8241 Georgia Ave., Silver Spring, MD 20910   **(301) 585-0550**
Vegetarian/Indian. Savor a wide variety of Indian dishes. **Open daily for lunch and dinner. Cafeteria style, vegan options, fresh juices, take-out, $–$$**

Silver Palace Restaurant
11311 Lockwood Dr., Silver Spring, MD 20904   **(301) 681-9585**
Chinese. The Palace has a large banquet room. **Open daily. Full service, wine/beer/alcohol, VISA/MC/AMX, $$**

Thai Derm Restaurant
939 Bonifant St., Silver Spring, MD 20910   **(301) 589-5341**
Thai. The noodle specialities and all foods are made without MSG upon request. **Open Sunday. Full service, wine/beer, VISA/MC, $$**

Thai Orchid Restaurant
8519 Fenton St., Silver Spring, MD 20910   **(301) 587-2192**
Thai. MSG is left out upon request. **Open daily for lunch and dinner. Closed afternoons. Full service, wine/beer, take-out, VISA/MC, $$**

SPENCERVILLE

Edgewood Inn
16101 Oak Hill Rd., Spencerville, MD 20905   **(301) 421-9247**
American. Located in a historic house, Edgewood Inn offers a vegetarian buffet including soy products, Nut Loaf, Eggplant Parmesan, Lasagna, Rice Casserole, Potato Salad, homemade breads, Spinach Pie, Pineapple Cream Cake, and fruit. **Buffet, catering, $$$**

TAKOMA PARK

Royal Bengal
6846 New Hampshire, Takoma Park, MD 20912   **(301) 270-6054**
Indian/Pakistani/Bangladeshi. Diners have a choice of fourteen vegetarian dishes served with basmati rice. **Open daily for dinner, open for lunch Monday through Friday. Full service, vegan options, beer, $$**

TOWSON

Donna's Coffee Bar
22 W. Allegheny Ave., Towson, MD 21204   **(410) 828-6655**
Italian. See description under Baltimore.

China Chef Restaurant

11323 Georgia Ave., Wheaton, MD 20902   **(301) 949-8170**
Chinese. This Chinese restaurant offers several vegetarian entrees. **Open Daily. Full service, wine/beer/alcohol, catering, take-out, VISA/MC/AMX, $$**

Dusit Thai Cuisine

2404 University Blvd. West, Wheaton, MD 20902   **(301) 949-4140**
Thai. Dusit features vegetable and tofu dishes, noodle entrees, and vegetarian soup. **Open daily for lunch and dinner. Full service, wine/beer/alcohol, take-out, VISA/MC/AMX, $$**

• Nut House Pizza

11419 Georgia Ave., Wheaton, MD 20902   **(301) 942-5900**
Vegetarian (except tuna sometimes)/kosher/pizza. Experience pizza made with soy or kosher cheese, Falafel, vegetarian burgers, and Pita Chips. **Open Sunday through Thursday for lunch and dinner, open Friday until one hour before sundown, Saturday open one hour after sundown to 1:30 A.M. Limited service, catering, take-out, VISA/MC/AMX, $**

Sabang Indonesian Restaurant

2504 Ennali's Ave., Wheaton, MD 20902   **(301) 942-7859**
Indonesian. Sabang features vegetarian reistafel that includes soup, dessert, and about ten different vegetarian dishes. It's fun to go with a few friends. **Open daily for lunch and dinner. Full service, vegan options, wine/beer/alcohol, take-out, VISA/MC/AMX, $$-$$$**

MASSACHUSETTS

(For more restaurant listings in the surrounding areas, see Northampton)

The Raw Carrot

Carriage Shops, 9 E. Pleasant St., Amherst, MA 01002   (413) 549-4240
Juice bar. Vegan options are always available at this bright and cheery juice bar that offers a variety of lunch foods including soups, sandwiches, and salads. Organic produce is used when possible. **Limited service, fresh juices, take-out, $**

è Reviewers' choice   • Vegetarian restaurant   •• Vegan restaurant
$ less than $6 $$ $6–$12 $$$ more than $12
VISA/AMX/MC/DISC/DC—credit cards accepted
Non-alc.—Non-alcoholic   Fresh juices—freshly squeezed

ARLINGTON

Cafe Barada
161 Massachusetts Ave., Arlington, MA 02174   **(617) 646-9650**
Middle Eastern. Enjoy a wide variety of authentic Middle Eastern vegetarian and non-vegetarian dishes. **Closed Sunday. Full service, take-out, $–$$**

BOSTON

(For more restaurant listings in the Boston area, see Arlington, Braintree, Burlington, Cambridge, Concord [about 20 miles away], and Jamaica Plain.)

Acapulco Restaurant
266 Newbury St., Boston, MA 02116   **(617) 247-9126**
Mexican. Beans here are prepared without lard. **Open daily afternoon and evening. Full service, wine/beer/alcohol, take-out, VISA/MC/AMX/DC, $$**

Addis Red Sea Ethiopian Restaurant
544 Tremont St., Boston, MA 02118   **(617) 426-8727**
Ethiopian. Sample authentic Ethiopian cuisine with vegetarian appetizer and entree selections. **Open daily. Full service, vegan options, wine/beer, take-out, VISA/ MC/AMX, $**

•• Buddha's Delight ❧
5 Beach St., Boston, MA 02111   **(617) 451-2395**
Vegan/Chinese. The "delight" here is various tofu, vegetable, and mock meat dishes. **Full service, BYOB, take-out, $**

Buteco Restaurant
130 Jersey St., Boston, MA 02215   **(617) 247-9508**
Brazilian. The restaurant serves Brazilian cuisine with at least one vegetarian entree plus a few appetizers and soup. **Open daily. Full service, wine/beer, take-out, VISA/MC, $$**

•• Country Life Vegetarian Buffet
200 High St., Boston, MA 02110   **(617) 951-2462**
Vegan. An all-vegetarian buffet is offered by Seventh-day Adventists. **Open daily for lunch except Saturday. Call about dinner. Cafeteria style, vegan options, fresh juices, take-out, $**

India Quality
536 Commonwealth Ave., Boston, MA 02215   **(617) 267-4499**
Indian. Special breads baked freshly in clay ovens accompany an extensive vegetarian menu. **Open daily. Full service, vegan options, take-out, VISA/MC/ AMX/DISC, $$**

Kashmir
279 Newbury St., Boston, MA 02116 **(617) 536-1695**
Indian. Vegetable samosas, aloo palak, and several other vegetarian options available. **Open daily for lunch and dinner. Full service, vegan options, take-out, VISA/MC/AMX/DC, $$**

Kebab-N-Kurry
30 Massachusetts Ave., Boston, MA 02115 **(617) 536-9835**
Indian. Savor authentic Indian cuisine with vegetarian specials such as cauliflower curry, spinach with homemade Indian cheese, nine-vegetable curry, chickpea curry, and other veggie entrees. **Open daily. Full service, vegan options, wine/beer, take-out, VISA/MC/AMX, $$**

King & I
145 Charles St., Boston, MA 02114 **(617) 227-3320**
Thai. The vegetarian menu includes appetizers and chef's suggestions. Try the crispy fried tofu, tofu pad Thai, or Vegetable Vegetables. **Open daily for lunch and dinner. Full service, vegan options, take-out, VISA/MC/DISC, $-$$**

Milk Street Cafe
50 Milk St., Boston, MA 02109 **(617) 542-2433**

Post Office Square, Boston, MA 02109 **(617) 350-PARK**
Kosher. Features kosher dairy cuisine with daily specials including soups, quiche, and pizza. The Post Office Square cafe features both indoor and outdoor seating. **Closed weekends. Cafeteria service, take-out, $**

Souper Salad
103 State St., Boston, MA 02107 **(617) 227-9151**

102 Water St., Boston, MA 02109 **(617) 367-2582**

119 Newbury St., Boston, MA 02116 **(617) 247-4983**

82 Summer St., Boston, MA 02110 **(617) 426-6834**
Restaurant chain. Salad bar, soups, sandwiches, and entrees are all fresh and homemade with a decent selection of vegetarian options. Mexican dishes are featured. **Open daily. Full service, vegan options, fresh juices, wine/beer, take-out, VISA/MC/AMX, $**

Steve's Restaurants Inc.
316 Newbury St., Boston, MA 02115 **(617) 267-1817**
Greek. Steve's specializes in authentic Greek cuisine with a variety of vegetarian delights. Examples include Falafel, Grape Leaves, Spinach Pie, Hummus, Tabouleh, Eggplant Salad, Greek salads, etc. **Open daily. Full service, vegan options, take-out, no credit cards, $**

Taj Mahal at Kenmore
484 Commonwealth Ave., Boston, MA 02215 **(617) 247-7266**
Indian. Over a half-dozen vegetarian dishes are offered at this Indian restaurant.

Dine on curry, rice dishes, Indian breads, plus more. **Open daily for lunch and dinner. Full service, beer/wine, take-out, VISA/MC/AMX/DISC/DC, $$**

BRAINTREE

Souper Salad
South Shore Plaza, 250 Granite Ave., Braintree, MA 02184   (617) 843-4658
Restaurant chain. See entry under Boston for description.

BURLINGTON

Souper Salad
Burlington Mall, Burlington, MA 01803   (617) 229-2223
Restaurant chain. See entry under Boston for description.

CAMBRIDGE

Averof Restaurant
1924 Massachusetts Ave., Porter Square
Cambridge, MA 02140   (617) 354-4500
Mediterranean. A wide range of Mediterranean cuisine includes many traditional Middle Eastern dishes that are vegetarian. **Open daily. Full service, vegan options, wine/beer/alcohol, take-out, VISA/MC/AMX/DISC, $$**

Bombay Club
57 JFK St., Cambridge, MA 02138   (617) 661-8100
Indian. Authentic Indian cuisine with a vegetarian menu section features various curry dishes, dahl, and vegetable entrees. **Open daily. Full service, vegan options, wine/beer, take-out, VISA/MC/AMX, $$**

Bread & Circus Wholefood Supermarket
115 Prospect St. C, Cambridge, MA 02139   (617) 492-0070
Natural foods deli. Enjoy a wide variety of vegetarian and vegan options offered in Bread & Circus's deli and bakery. **Open daily for lunch and dinner. Counter service, macrobiotic/vegan options, non-alc. beer/wine, beer/wine, take-out, VISA/MC, $**

Christopher's Restaurant & Bar
1920 Massachusetts Ave., Cambridge, MA 02140   (617) 876-9180
Natural foods. Christopher's has combined mainstream American and Mexican fare with a variety of vegetarian dishes and a dedication to wholesome and healthful foods. (The owner is a long-time vegetarian!) The restaurant uses ingredients that are free of preservatives, artificial colors and flavors. All sauces, dressings, salsa, guacamole, etc., are homemade. Even the brewed decaf is prepared "Swiss water processed" and there are no dioxins in the coffee filters! In addition to quality food, Christopher's aims to be politically correct and supports 1% For Peace and other causes. **Open daily for lunch and dinner. Full service, vegan options, wine/beer/alcohol, take-out, VISA/MC/DISC, $-$$**

Gandhi Restaurant
704 Massachusetts Ave., Cambridge, MA 02139   (617) 491-1104
Indian. Traditional Indian cuisine includes eleven vegetarian entrees plus soups and appetizers. Also offers South Indian dishes. **Open daily. Full service, vegan options, wine/beer, take-out, VISA/MC, $$**

Joyce Chen Restaurant
390 Rindge Ave., Cambridge, MA 02140   (617) 492-7373
Chinese. See entry under Boston for description.

•• Masao's Kitchen
1815 Massachusetts Ave., Cambridge, MA 02140   (617) 497-7348
Vegan. Seitan, tofu, and tempeh dishes are served at this macrobiotic restaurant. Organic vegetables are used whenever possible. **Open Tuesday-Sunday for lunch and dinner. Full service, fresh juices, non-alc., take-out, VISA/MC/AMX, $$**

Passage to India
1900 Massachusetts Ave., Cambridge, MA 02140   (617) 497-6113
Indian. Authentic Indian cuisine includes a wide variety of vegetarian soups, appetizers, breads, entrees, and rice dishes. No eggs and only vegetable oil are used. **Open daily. Limited service, vegan options, wine/beer, take-out, VISA/ MC, $$**

Tandoor House
991 Massachusetts Ave., Cambridge, MA 02138   (617) 661-9001
Indian. Enjoy vegetarian authentic Indian cuisine. **Open daily for lunch and dinner. Full service, wine/beer/alcohol, take-out, VISA/MC/AMX, $$**

CAPE COD

(Restaurants in this area are those listed under Centerville, East Sandwich, Hyannis, Nantucket, Pocasset, Sandwich, and Woods Hole.)

CENTERVILLE

Sprouts Cafe at Cape Cod Natural Foods
Bell Tower Mall, 1600 Route 28, Centerville, MA 02632   (508) 771-8394
Natural foods cafe. Lunches feature many vegetarian sandwiches plus soups and salads. **Open daily for lunch. Limited service, vegan options, take-out, VISA/ MC, $**

CONCORD

The Natural Gourmet
98 Commonwealth Ave., Concord, MA 01742   (508) 371-7573

🍴 Reviewers' choice   • Vegetarian restaurant   •• Vegan restaurant
$ less than $6 $$ $6–$12 $$$ more than $12
VISA/AMX/MC/DISC/DC—credit cards accepted
Non-alc.—Non-alcoholic   Fresh juices—freshly squeezed

Natural foods deli. This deli serves everything, from exotic salads such as Quinoa with Pine Nuts and Apricots to soups and entrees such as Wild Rice & Sweet Potato Stew or Potatoes with Russian Walnut Sauce & Colored Peppers. **Open daily. Take-out, fresh juices, $**

EAST SANDWICH

The Beehive Tavern
406 Rte. 6A, E. Sandwich, MA 02537 **(508) 833-1184**
American. The Beehive features salads, sandwiches, dinner entrees, some Middle Eastern foods, and pasta. **Open daily, seasonal hours. Full service, non-alc. beer, wine/beer/alcohol, VISA/MC, $$**

GREAT BARRINGTON

Bronze Dog Cafe
Great Barrington Railroad Station
Great Barrington, MA 01230 **(413) 528-5678**
Natural foods. Bronze Dog Cafe offers several vegetarian dishes including Spicy Broiled Tofu; vegetarian curry with sweet potato, apple, red cabbage, couscous, and chutney; and Grilled Polenta with Wild Mushrooms. **Open Thursday and Friday for lunch and dinner, Saturday and Sunday for brunch and dinner. Full service, vegan options, take-out, VISA/MC/DISC, $$**

Dos Amigos Mexican Restaurant
250 Stockbridge Rd., Great Barrington, MA 01230 **(413) 528-0084**
Mexican. Vegetarian and vegan diets are easily accommodated at this restaurant serving excellent Mexican fare. Beans are vegetarian. The vegetarian sampler is delicious and can be made vegan. Dos Amigos is located in the Berkshires. **Open daily for lunch and dinner. Full service, vegan options, take-out, $$**

GREENFIELD

• Green River Cafe
24 Federal St., Greenfield, MA 01301 **(413) 773-3312**
Vegetarian. Enjoy a wide variety of vegetarian dishes at Green River Cafe, which features locally grown organic produce when in season and weekly musical performances. A community meal is offered each Sunday on a pay-what-you-can basis. No smoking. **Open Tuesday through Sunday for three meals. Closed for dinner on Mondays. Full service, vegan options, espresso/cappuccino, $–$$**

HADLEY

Bread & Circus Cafe
Rt. 9, Hadley, MA 01035 **(413) 586-9932**
Natural foods deli. See description under Cambridge.

HYANNIS

Pavilion Indian Cuisine
511 Main St., Hyannis, MA 02601 **(508) 790-0985**

Indian. This restaurant offers several vegetarian entrees including a mixed vegetable dish and a lentil dish. **Open for lunch and dinner. Full service, beer/wine, catering, take-out, VISA/MC/AMX, $$**

 JAMAICA PLAIN

Center Street Cafe
597 Center St., Jamaica Plain, MA 02130   (617) 524-9217
American/ethnic. This small, funky neighborhood restaurant serves no red meat but some chicken, fish, and vegetarian options. The eclectic collection of Mexican, Thai, Italian, and American cuisine is made fresh from scratch. **Brunch Wednesday through Sunday, dinner nightly. Full service, vegan options, fresh juices, BYOB, take-out, $$**

Five Seasons Restaurant
669A Centre St., Jamaica Plain, MA 02130   (617) 524-9016
Natural foods. This restaurant is often recommended by individuals living in the Boston area. Appetizers include Vegetable Tempura and Marinated Baked Tofu. Soups, salads, and sandwiches are offered, as well as a wide variety of entrees including pan-fried noodles with tofu, watercress, and scallions; a macrobiotic platter; a Mexican dish; and more. Reservations recommended. **Open for lunch and dinner Tuesday through Sunday. Open for dinner only on Monday. Full service, fresh juices, beer/wine, vegan/macrobiotic options, catering, VISA/MC, $$**

LEE

Cactus Cafe
54 Main St., Lee, MA 01238   (413) 243-4300
Mexican. Enjoy authentic Mexican dishes at Cactus Cafe including Guacamole and Chips, burritos, enchiladas, quesadillas, and salads. **Open for three meals Friday and Saturday. Open for lunch and dinner Sunday through Thursday. Full service, fresh juices, espresso/cappuccino, non-alc. beer/wine, beer/wine, catering, take-out, MC/AMX/DISC/DC, $$**

LENOX

The Garden Gourmet Deli & Bake Shop
8 Franklin St., Lenox, MA 01240   (413) 637-4156
Deli. This deli and bake shop offers a variety of vegetarian dishes with ethnic overtones. Examples include Stuffed Grape Leaves, pierogies, knishes, Falafel, and Chili. Many sandwiches, salads, and sweets are also offered. All soups are prepared with vegetable stock and organic ingredients are used when possible. **Open daily from May through October. Full service, vegan option, fresh juices, take-out, $$**

NANTUCKET

Something Natural
50 Cliff Rd., Nantucket, MA 02554   (508) 228-0504
Bakery and sandwich shop. Twenty varieties of breads are baked fresh daily. Large

sandwiches and salads are made to order. Garden seating. **Open daily in summer. Counter service, take-out, $**

Bela

68 Masonic St., Northampton, MA 01060 (413) 586-8011

Natural foods. Savor affordable eclectic vegetarian cuisine in a smoke-free environment. The chalkboard menu changes every one to two days and includes dishes from around the world. Many are dairy-free entrees. Desserts include honey- and sugar-sweetened, dairy and dairy-free. Local women's artwork is displayed in the restaurant. Outdoor cafe during nice weather. **Open Tuesday through Saturday. Full service, vegan options, take-out, $**

Fire & Water

5 Old South St., Northampton, MA 01060 (413) 586-8336

Natural foods. A majority of the food served at Fire & Water is vegetarian, including dishes like spicy peanut noodle, fantastic curried tofu, the sunshine burger, and falafels. This "community gathering point" also features nightly performances ranging from music to performance art to spoken word. **Open daily for lunch and dinner. Limited service, vegan options, fresh juices, espresso/cappuccino, smoothies, $**

Paul & Elizabeth's

150 Main St., Northampton, MA 01060 (413) 584-4832

Natural foods/macrobiotic. Vegetarian dishes are served at Paul & Elizabeth's, which is conveniently located downtown. Some entrees have dairy, but these are clearly labeled. The menu includes many vegan options. The food is excellent, generously portioned, and reasonably priced. The atmosphere is attractive but somewhat loud. **Full service, vegan/macrobiotic options, take-out, $$**

Stir Crazy

626 MacArthur Blvd., Pocasset, MA 02559 (508) 564-6464

Southeast Asian. The menu at Stir Crazy features Southeast Asian foods, specifically authentic Cambodian cuisine. It is clear that the restaurant caters to vegetarians and is willing to accommodate special diets. Foods are prepared with 100-percent pure olive oil using no artificial color or MSG. **Closed Mondays. Full service, vegan options, take-out, VISA/MC, $$**

ैं Reviewers' choice • Vegetarian restaurant •• Vegan restaurant
$ less than $6 $$ $6–$12 $$$ more than $12
VISA/AMX/MC/DISC/DC—credit cards accepted
Non-alc.—Non-alcoholic   Fresh juices—freshly squeezed

SANDWICH
Marshland Restaurant
Rte. 6A, Sandwich, MA 02563   **(508) 888-9824**
American. Marshland features salads, sandwiches, dinner entrees, some Middle Eastern foods, and pasta. **Open daily, seasonal hours. Full service, non-alc. beer, wine/beer/alcohol, VISA/MC, $$**

SHELBURNE FALLS
Copper Angel Cafe
2 State St., Shelburne Falls, MA 01370   **(413) 625-2727**
Natural foods. The atmosphere at Copper Angel Cafe is "heavenly," with over 100 angels in the dining room and a divine view of the famous Bridge of Flowers and Deerfield River. In addition to the atmosphere, enjoy vegetarian dishes like the Angel Burger made from a blend of grains, nuts, and seeds; grilled tofu sandwich; or lentil cutlets with vegetarian gravy. **Seasonal hours, call for information. Full service, vegan options, espresso/cappuccino, non-alc. wine/beer, take-out, VISA/MC, $-$$**

SOUTH ATTLEBORO
Fuller Memorial Hospital
231 Washington St., South Attleboro, MA 02703   **(508) 761-8500**
Cafeteria. This is a not-for-profit hospital owned and operated by the Seventh-day Adventist Church. **Open daily for lunch and dinner. Cafeteria style, vegan options, take-out, no credit cards, $**

WEST SPRINGFIELD
• Harvest Thyme
1312 Memorial Ave., West Springfield, MA 01089   **(413) 733-7375**
Vegetarian deli. Visit the juice bar or purchase vegetarian soups, stews, salads, sandwiches, and entrees sold by the pint. Low-cholesterol, yeast- and mold-free, and wheat- and dairy-free items are indicated on the menu. Daily selections rotate. **Open daily. Cafeteria style, vegan option, fresh juices, take-out, VISA/MC, $**

WEST STOCKBRIDGE
Truc Orient Express
2 Harris St., West Stockbridge, MA 01266   **(413) 232-4204**
Vietnamese. Truc Orient Express offers a separate vegetarian menu that includes dishes such as marinated tofu on fine rice noodles, Tofu with Lemon Grass, Sweet and Sour Mushrooms, Vegetarian Fried Rice, various soups and salads, plus more. **Open for lunch and dinner Monday through Friday; open only for dinner on weekends. Full service, beer/wine/alcohol, catering, take-out, VISA/MC/AMX/ DISC, $$-$$$**

WESTMINSTER
The 1761 Old Mill Restaurant
Rte. 2A East, Westminster, MA 01473   **(508) 874-5941**

Family dining. Salads and sandwiches are featured, and a children's menu is available. **Open daily. Full service, wine/beer/alcohol, VISA/MC/AMX/DISC, $$**

WOODS HOLE

Dome Restaurant
539 Woods Hole Road, Woods Hole, MA 02543　　　(508) 548-0800
New England fare. The restaurant is willing to accommodate vegetarians and offers dishes such as Pasta Primavera, Fusilli Pasta, and a steamed vegetable plate. **Open Tuesday through Sunday for dinner and Sunday for brunch as well. Full service, fresh juices, non-alc. beer/wine, wine/beer/alcohol, $$–$$$**

Fishmonger's Cafe
56 Water St., Woods Hole, MA 02543　　　(508) 540-5376
Natural foods. Along with a full range of vegetarian dishes, fish is served here and home-baked goods, too. **Open daily. Full service, wine/beer, VISA/MC, $$–$$$**

MICHIGAN

ANN ARBOR

The Blue Nile
317 Braun Ct., Ann Arbor, MI 48104　　　(313) 663-3116
Ethiopian. Authentic Ethiopian cuisine includes many vegetarian options. **Open daily. Full service, vegan options, wine/beer/alcohol, VISA/MC/AMX/DISC, $$–$$$**

Golden Chef
2016 Packard, Ann Arbor, MI 48104　　　(313)-741-0778
Chinese/vegetarian. Golden Chef serves delicious vegetarian pot stickers, spring rolls, and vegetarian entrees. Few dishes contain eggs. Only vegetarian food is served at dinner time. **Open daily for lunch and dinner. Full service, vegan options, take-out, VISA/MC/AMX, $$**

• Seva
314 E. Liberty, Ann Arbor, MI 48104　　　(313) 662-1111
Vegetarian/Mexican. We've been told Seva offers some of the best Mexican food in Michigan. The menu alone is certainly impressive. Vegan options are clearly indicated on the menu. Small Courses, Salads, Soups, Mexican Specialties, Oriental Specialties, Sandwiches, Omelettes, Beverages and Blended Drinks make up the menu headings. There's a blend of traditional and unique foods that sound delicious! **Open daily. Weekend brunch. Full service, vegan options, non-alc. beer, wine/ beer/alcohol, catering, take-out, VISA/MC/DISC, $$**

BERRIEN SPRINGS

• Andrews University
U.S. 31 North, Berrien Springs, MI 49104　　　(616) 471-3161

Vegetarian cafeteria. Cyclical menu changes feature soups, main dishes, hot food selections, plus extensive salad bar and desserts. Soy- and gluten-based meat analogs are utilized in many dishes. **Open daily during school year. Call for summer hours. Cafeteria style, $**

BIRMINGHAM

La Luna Grancafe
183 N. Woodward, Birmingham, MI 48009   **(313) 642-7070**
Italian. Delicious pizza selections include some without cheese. Pasta dishes are also available. **Full service, vegan options, fresh juices, non-alc. beer/wine, take-out, VISA/MC/AMX, $**

DEARBORN

La Shish
12918 Michigan Ave., Dearborn, MI 48126   **(313) 584-4477**
Lebanese. Several vegan dishes are available at La Shish. **Open daily for lunch and dinner. Full service, vegan options, take-out, VISA, $**

DETROIT

The Blue Nile
508 Monroe St., Detroit, MI 48322   **(313) 964-6699**
Ethiopian. See description under Ann Arbor, MI.

• Cosmic Cafe
87 West Palmer, Detroit, MI 48202   **(313) 832-0001**
Vegetarian. This smoke-free vegetarian cafe features fresh juices, salsa fries, vegetarian chili, several salads, pizza, Mexican dishes, veggie burgers, plus much more. **Open Monday through Friday for three meals and on Saturday for breakfast and lunch. Closed Sundays. Full service, vegan/macrobiotic options, fresh juices, take-out, $–$$**

Don Pedros
24366 Grand River, Detroit, MI 48219   **(313) 537-1450**
Mexican. Vegetarian dining is easy at Don Pedros as there is no lard in the beans and no chicken broth in the rice. There *is* a nice atmosphere. **Open daily for dinner. Lunch weekdays. Full service, vegan options, wine/beer/alcohol, take-out, VISA/MC/AMX/DC, $$**

• Govinda's at the Fisher Mansion
383 Lenox Ave., Detroit, MI 48215   **(313) 331-6740**

Vegetarian. Govinda's is located in the formal dining room of the Lawrence Fisher Mansion. The foods are prepared daily using only the freshest ingredients. **Open Friday through Sunday. Full service, vegan options, fresh juices, catering, take-out, VISA/MC/AMX, $$**

Traffic Jam and Snug
511 W. Canfield St., Detroit, MI 48201   **(313) 831-9470**

Natural foods. The menu changes weekly at this natural foods eatery, but there are always vegetarian entrees, usually vegan options as well. Seasonal and local foods are emphasized, and there are homemade breads, brews, and friendly service. **Closed Sunday. Full service, vegan options, fresh juices, wine/beer, take-out, VISA/MC/DISC, $$**

EAST LANSING

Hearthstone Bakery and Vegetarian Cafe
208 Mac, East Lansing, MI 48823   **(517) 333-EATS**

Vegetarian. Hearthstone is committed to providing the highest quality breads, baked goods, and ready-to-eat foods made from scratch with all natural ingredients. Organic ingredients are used whenever possible. Daily ethnic dinner and luncheon specials, full salad bar, pizza, egg rolls, deli sandwiches, and more are featured at Hearthstone. At least one of the daily specials is always vegan and there are several vegan options on the menu. **Open for three meals daily, Sunday for brunch and dinner only. Cafeteria style, vegan options, fresh juices, espresso/cappuccino, take-out, $**

Small Planet Food & Spirits
220 Mac Avenue, East Lansing, MI 48823   **(517) 351-6230**

Natural foods. Small Planet specializes in Jamaican, Mexican, vegetarian, and ethnic cuisines. You'll enjoy fine dining in a relaxed and unique atmosphere. **Open daily for lunch and dinner. Full service, fresh juices, non-alc. beer, wine/beer/alcohol, take-out, VISA/MC, $$**

FARMINGTON HILLS

Anita's Kitchen
31005 Orchard Lake, Farmington Hills, MI 48018   **(313) 855-4150**

Middle Eastern/Lebanese. The menu features Falafel and Hummus, as well as Black Bean Soup and Vegetarian Chili. **Open daily for breakfast, lunch, and dinner. Full service, vegan options, take-out, VISA/MC/AMX/DISC, $–$$$**

Shalimar
29200 Orchard Lake Rd., Farmington Hills, MI 48018   **(313) 626-2982**

Indian/Mexican. Vegetarian options are available at this restaurant offering Indian and Mexican foods. **Open for lunch and dinner. Full service, vegan options, non-alc. beer, wine/beer/alcohol, take-out, VISA/MC, $**

Om Cafe
23136 N. Woodward Ave., Ferndale, MI 48220   **(313) 548-1941**
Macrobiotic. Terrific macrobiotic food includes a good range of vegetarian and vegan dishes. **Open for lunch and dinner Monday through Saturday. No smoking. Full service, vegan options, $**

Apple Jade
505 Frandor, Lansing, MI 48912   **(517) 332-8010**
Chinese. This Chinese restaurant offers vegetarian pot stickers as well as many vegetarian entrees. **Open daily for lunch and dinner. Full service, take-out, VISA/ MC, $$**

Clara's
637 E. Michigan, Lansing MI 48912   **(517) 372-7120**
Italian/Mexican/American. Located in a refurbished train station with beautiful stained glass windows, Clara's offers excellent vegetarian sandwiches, calzones, and Mexican food. **Open daily for lunch and dinner; Sunday for brunch as well. Full service, take-out, VISA/MC/AMX/DISC/DC, $$**

• Hearthstone Bakery & Vegetarian Cafe
2003 E. Michigan, Lansing, MI 48912   **(517) 485-8600**
Vegetarian. See description under East Lansing, MI.

Dimitri's Rendezvous
36247 Gratiot, Mt. Clemens, MI 48043   **(313) 792-2200**
Greek. A local reader informed us about Dimitri's. It is difficult to find vegetarian food in this area, and Dimitri's has a vegetarian stir-fry and will meet special requests. **Open for lunch and dinner. Full service, vegan option, wine/beer/alcohol, take-out, $–$$**

Down To Earth Country Buffet
10025 Belding Rd., NE, Rockford, MI 49341   **(616) 691-7288**
Natural foods. Everything at this whole-foods restaurant is prepared on the premises. Fresh bread is baked daily. Organic fruits and vegetables are used in summer. **Closed Monday. Full service, BYOB, take-out, no credit cards, $$**

• Inn Season Cafe 🍃
500 E. Fourth St., Royal Oak, MI 48067   **(313) 547-7916**
Vegetarian. Inn Season has built its reputation on uncompromising, creative regional cuisine with old-world roots. Vegetarian or not, the clientele come for

the dining experience. There's a full menu with pizza, pasta, Mexican, Japanese, and Middle Eastern foods plus daily specials. Sugar-free desserts are also served. **Closed Sunday and Monday. No smoking. Full service, vegan options, fresh juices, non-alc. beer, organic coffee, take-out, VISA/MC/DISC, $$**

Les Auteurs
222 Sherman, Washington Square, Royal Oak, MI 48067   (313) 544-2887
American. Vegetarian entrees are served at lunch and dinner in this elegant but expensive establishment. **Full service, wine/beer/alcohol, $$–$$$**

UNION CITY

• Creative Health Institute
918 Union City Rd., Union City, MI 49094   (517) 278-6260
Living foods. Sample a living foods buffet that includes assorted sprouts, organic indoor greens, seed cheeses, and raw vegetable dishes, soups and salads. **Open Sunday only for open house and buffet. Reservations required for large groups only. Buffet, vegan options, $**

MINNESOTA

ANOKA

Anoka Co-op Grocery & Cafe
1917 2nd Ave. S., Anoka, MN 55303   (612) 427-3552
Natural foods cafe. Various international vegetarian foods include veggie burgers, Spanakopita, quiche, Wild Rice Stir-fry, soups, salads, sandwiches, pies, cookies, cakes, and more. **Open for lunch weekdays. Cafeteria style, vegan options, fresh juices, take-out, $**

BLOOMINGTON

Sawatdee Thai Restaurant
8501 Lyndale Ave., Bloomington, MN 55420   (612) 888-7177
Thai. Vegetarian spring rolls, a noodle dish, and a few vegetable entrees are offered. Tofu can be substituted in most meat dishes as well. **Open daily for lunch and dinner. Full service, vegan options, take-out, VISA/MC/AMX, $–$$**

DULUTH

Taste of Saigon
DeWitt-Seitz Marketplace, 94 Lake Ave. S.
Duluth, MN 55802   (218) 727-1598
Vietnamese. The Taste of Saigon offers a selection of vegetarian dishes including tofu and mock meat items. **Closed Sunday. Full service, vegan options, take-out, $–$$**

MINNEAPOLIS

Azur Restaurant
651 Nicollet Ave., S., Minneapolis, MN 55402   **(612) 342-2800**
Fine dining. The Azur Restaurant normally has vegetarian items but is also willing to take special requests. The menu changes frequently. **Reservations required for special meals. Formal, full service, wine/beer/alcohol, VISA/MC/AMX/DISC, $$$**

Cafe Brenda
300 1st Ave., N., Minneapolis, MN 55401   **(612) 342-9270**
Natural foods. Located in a restored warehouse in a historic district of downtown Minneapolis, Cafe Brenda prepares a good selection of vegetarian appetizers, sandwiches, and entrees. There are daily specials plus a full à la carte menu and a children's menu. **Closed Sunday. Full service, vegan options, fresh juice, organic coffee, espresso, non-alc. beer, wine/beer/alcohol, take-out, VISA/MC/AMX/ DC/Carte Blanche, $$**

• Delites of India ༈
1123 West Lake St., Minneapolis, MN 55408   **(612) 823-2866**
Vegetarian/Indian. Delites is the only vegetarian Indian restaurant in the Twin Cities. The menu consists of a wide selection of Indian foods plus some Middle Eastern and American dishes such as Hummus and Chili. No MSG or other chemicals are used in the food. Owners and service are "delites," too. Books on Indian philosophy, yoga, and vegetarian cooking line the walls and are for sale along with some Indian food products and tea. Even reading the menu is educational! **Closed Monday. Open daily for lunch and dinner. Full service, vegan options, wine/beer, take-out, VISA/MC/AMX/DC/Carte Blanche, $$**

The Good Earth Restaurant & Bakery
3001 Hennepin Ave. S., Calhoun Square
Minneapolis, MN 55408   **(612) 824-8533**
Natural foods. The Good Earth is a family-style natural foods chain with four restaurants in the Minneapolis/St. Paul area. The menu features many home-baked goods, soups, salads, sandwiches, and entrees. **Open daily. Full service, fresh juices, non-alc. beer/wine, beer/wine, take-out, MC/VISA/AMX, $–$$**

Loring Cafe
1624 Harmon Place, Minneapolis, MN 55403   **(612) 332-1617**
Cafe. Salads, appetizers, sandwiches, and vegetarian specials are available at the Loring Cafe. **Open daily. Full service, limited vegan options, wine/beer/alcohol, take-out, VISA/MC, $$–$$$**

༈ Reviewers' choice   • Vegetarian restaurant   •• Vegan restaurant
$ less than $6 $$ $6–$12 $$$ more than $12
VISA/AMX/MC/DISC/DC—credit cards accepted
Non-alc.—Non-alcoholic   Fresh juices—freshly squeezed

The Lotus of Campus
313 Oak St., SE, Minneapolis, MN 55414 **(612) 331-1781**
Vietnamese. The Lotus has a vegetarian section on its menu. **Full service, beer, take-out, no credit cards, $**

Lotus to Go Grant Mall
113 W. Grant St., Minnepolis, MN 55403 **(612) 870-1218**
Vietnamese. Vegetarian options include tofu, vegetable, and mock meat dishes. No eggs are used. **Take-out, vegan options, no credit cards, $**

Lotus Uptown
3037 Hennepin Ave. S., Minneapolis, MN 55408 **(612) 825-2263**
Vietnamese. The vegetarian menu section includes vegetable, tofu, and mock meat dishes. **Open daily. Full service, vegan options, wine/beer, take-out, no credit cards, $**

• Mudpie Vegetarian Restaurant �］
2549 Lyndale Ave. S., Minneapolis, MN 55405 **(612) 872-9435**
Vegetarian. No vegetarian should leave Minneapolis (or even Minnesota!) without visiting the Mudpie. It is certainly a heavenly experience and a trip worth making as often as possible. The menu consists of a variety of creative and traditional international dishes along with some standard vegetarian favorites served in ample portions. There's an extensive breakfast menu on weekends plus salads, soups, pizza, appetizers, sandwiches, entrees, and wonderful desserts for lunch and dinner. Items that cannot be prepared without dairy are clearly indicated on the menu. There's also an enclosed patio dining area. **Open daily for lunch and dinner, breakfast on weekends only. Full service, vegan options, fresh juices, wine/beer, take-out, VISA/MC/AMX, $–$$**

Nam Restaurant
1005 Nicollet Mall, Minneapolis, MN 55403 **(612) 332-3666**
Vietnamese. Located in the Nicollet Mall in downtown Minneapolis not too far from the Convention Center, Nam has a large vegetarian section on the menu. Various tofu, vegetable, and mock meat dishes are offered. **Open Monday through Saturday for lunch and dinner. Full service, vegan options, take-out, $**

New French Cafe
128 N. Fourth St., Minneapolis, MN 55401 **(612) 338-3790**
Ethnic/natural foods. The New French Cafe has a vegetarian lunch plate and is willing to tailor-make vegetarian meals. **Open daily. Full service, wine/beer/alcohol, take-out, VISA/MC/AMX/DC, $$–$$$**

• New Riverside Cafe
329 Cedar Ave., Minneapolis, MN 55454 **(612) 333-4814**
Vegetarian. This worker-owned-and-managed cafe with its funky, informal coffeehouse atmosphere has been a hub for alternative ideas and a center for community activism since 1970. The cafe is set up cafeteria style with a chalkboard menu that lists daily specials including Mexican dishes, stir-fry, and many vegan options. All of the dishes are made from quality whole foods using local organically grown ingredients and served very inexpensively. There is live music five nights a week.

Menu changes monthly. **Open daily (except Sunday) for three meals, Sunday for brunch only. Cafeteria style, vegan options, organic coffee, espresso/cappuccino, take-out, $**

Odaa Restaurant
408 Cedar Ave. S., Minneapolis, MN 55454   **(612) 338-4459**
Ethiopian. Authentic East African Oromo cuisine is prepared on-site from scratch. African decor and multi-ethnic music provide a soothing atmosphere for diners. Food is served in a traditional communal tray and eaten with bread and fingers. Several vegetarian options are available, and no preservatives are used. **Open daily for lunch and dinner, Sunday for dinner only. Full service, vegan options, beer, take-out, VISA/MC/AMX, $$**

Organica Cafeteria
Aveda Corporation
4000 Pheasant Ridge Dr., Minneapolis, MN 55434   **(612) 783-4000**
Natural foods. Located at Aveda Corporation headquarters, this employee cafeteria is open to the public and offers many vegetarian entrees, soups, salads, and sandwiches. **Open weekdays for lunch only. Cafeteria style, take-out, $**

Organica Deli
400 Central Ave., SE, Minneapolis, MN 55414   **(612) 378-7413**
Natural foods deli. Located in an educational center, this deli serves organic bean burritos, sandwiches, and special entrees each day. **Closed Sundays. Counter service, fresh juices, take-out, $**

Ping's Szechuan Bar & Grill
1401 Nicollet Ave., Minneapolis, MN 55403   **(612) 874-9404**
Chinese. Ping's serves Chinese food with a Szechuan emphasis in addition to Cantonese, Hunan, and Mandarin cuisines. Several vegetarian entrees appear on the menu and the restaurant is willing to make substitutions for any dish. Mock duck is available. Located near the Convention Center. **Open daily for lunch and dinner. Full service, vegan options, wine/beer/alcohol, take-out, VISA/MC/AMX/DISC/DC/CB, $$**

Seward Community Cafe
2129 E. Franklin Ave., Minneapolis, MN 55404   **(612) 332-1011**

1521 University Ave., SE, Minneapolis, MN 55414   **(612) 623-0388**
Natural foods cafe. The Seward Cafe is located on the corner across from the Seward Co-op and offers sandwiches, soups, salads, and desserts in a cafeteria/cafe atmosphere. Seward Co-op just recently celebrated its twentieth anniversary. Patio dining. **Franklin Ave. cafe open daily for three meals. University Ave. location open for lunch only Monday through Friday. Cafeteria style, vegan options, take-out, $**

St. Martin's Table
2001 Riverside Ave., Minneapolis, MN 55454   **(612) 339-3920**
Natural foods. St. Martin's Table is a nonprofit restaurant/bookstore with various political titles and resources on peace. The chalkboard menu has two soups daily,

three sandwiches, and special salads. Fresh baked goods made from scratch are also featured. Bring your own container for take-out. **Closed Sunday. Full service, take-out (you provide container), no credit cards, $**

Tao Natural Foods and Books
2200 Hennepin Ave., S., Minneapolis, MN 55405   (612) 377-4630
Juice bar/deli. The Tao has a small juice bar and deli in the front of its natural foods store. Daily sandwich and soup specials are offered along with a great selection of books. Tao is located next to an eco-store. **Closed Sunday. Limited service, fresh juices, take-out, $**

Wedge Community Co-op Deli
2105 Lyndale Ave. S., Minneapolis, MN 55405   (612) 871-3993
Natural foods deli. The Wedge Co-op has a deli counter in the back with a wide selection of salads, sandwiches, and some soups. **Counter service, take-out only, $**

MINNETONKA

The Marsh Restaurant
15000 Minnetonka Blvd., Minnetonka, MN 55345   (612) 935-2202
Health club restaurant. The Marsh Restaurant serves some vegetarian foods. All muffins and breads are baked on site from scratch using the freshest ingredients possible with a minimum of processed foods. **Open daily. Cafeteria style, fresh juice, wine/beer, take-out, VISA/MC, $$**

NEW BRIGHTON

Los Banditos
2321 Palmer Dr., New Brighton, MN 55112   (612) 636-5858
Mexican. Los Banditos offers authentic Mexican food with vegetable or guacamole as fillings. Beware—beans contain ham soup base. **Open daily for lunch and dinner, Sunday for dinner only. Full service, wine/beer/alcohol, take-out, VISA/MC/AMX, $**

ST. PAUL

Lotus Victoria Crossing
867 Grand Ave., St. Paul, MN 55105   (612) 228-9156
Chinese. See Lotus to Go entry under Minneapolis, MN, for description.

• The Old City Cafe
1571 Grand Ave., St. Paul, MN 55105   (612) 699-5347

🐾 Reviewers' choice   • Vegetarian restaurant   •• Vegan restaurant
$ less than $6 $$ $6–$12 $$$ more than $12
VISA/AMX/MC/DISC/DC—credit cards accepted
Non-alc.—Non-alcoholic   Fresh juices—freshly squeezed

Vegetarian. The only kosher restaurant in the Twin Cities, this cafe offers various Middle Eastern foods in addition to pizza, salads, veggie burgers, knishes, stuffed peppers, mock meats, and other items. **Closed Saturday. Limited service, vegan options, take-out, wine/beer, $**

ST. PETER

St. Peter Food Co-op Sandwich Shop
100 S. Front St., St. Peter, MN 56082   **(507) 931-4880**
Natural-food-store deli. The shop offers self-serve soups and entrees, plus a cooler stocked with pre-made sandwiches and salads. Fresh baked goods are also available. Here you will find low prices in a relaxed atmosphere. **Open daily. Cafeteria style, vegan options, take-out, $**

MISSISSIPPI

JACKSON

•• High Noon Cafe
4147 Northview Dr., Jackson, MS 39206   **(601) 366-1602**
Primarily vegan. The High Noon Cafe serves only vegan food every day except Saturday, which is a vegetarian day. The menu changes daily. **Open Monday through Saturday for lunch. Vegan, take-out, $–$$**

OXFORD

• Harvest Cafe & Bakery
1112 Van Buren Ave., Oxford, MS 38655   **(601) 236-3757**
Vegetarian. Harvest Cafe & Bakery supports sustainable agriculture, recycling, and local artists. The completely vegetarian menu offers whole-wheat pancakes and waffles for Sunday brunches; Black Bean Chili, soups, salads, hummus sandwiches, Tempeh Reubens, pasta dishes, and more for lunch and dinner. **Open for breakfast and lunch Sunday through Friday. Open for dinner Tuesday through Friday. Closed Saturdays. Full service, non-alc. beer/wine, beer/wine/alcohol, vegan options, take-out, $–$$**

MISSOURI

CHESTERFIELD

Lettuce Leaf Restaurants
444 Chesterfield Ctr., #130, Chesterfield, MO 63017   **(314) 537-1808**
Natural foods. Entrees, salads, gourmet sandwiches, pizza, homemade soups, and quiche. The menu is changed four times a year with the season in order to have the freshest ingredients available. **Open daily. Full service, wine/beer, take-out, VISA/MC/AMX/DISC, $$**

CLAYTON

Candicci's
7910 Bonhomme, Clayton, MO 63105   **(314) 725-3350**
Italian. Candicci's has a good selection of vegetarian pasta dishes and appetizers.
**Open daily. Full service, vegan option, fresh juice, wine/beer/alcohol, take-out,
VISA/MC/AMX, $$**

COLUMBIA

International Cafe
209 Hitt St., Columbia, MO 65201   **(314) 449-4560**
International, primarily Middle Eastern. One local patron recommends the appe-
tizer combo as the best-bet dish. Patio dining. **Limited service, $**

Mixed Company
1025 E. Walnut, Columbia, MO 65201   **(314) 449-1141**
Coffeehouse. This coffeehouse has a limited but expanding vegetarian menu. **Full
service, vegan options, $**

KANSAS CITY

Amber Waves
4305 Main St., Kansas City, MO 64111   **(816) 931-8191**
Macrobiotic. Amber Waves has a limited menu, but the Grainburger Platter is
excellent. Specials are offered. **Open Tuesday and Thursday for dinner, Saturday
for lunch. Full service, vegan options, take-out, $$**

Blvd. Cafe
703 SW Blvd., Kansas City, MO 64108   **(816) 842-6984**
Middle Eastern. Falafel, tabouleh, and matabel—an eggplant dip—are served at this
restaurant that features a variety of Mediterranean, Spanish, and Greek dishes.
**Open Monday-Friday for lunch and dinner. Open Saturday for dinner only.
Sunday Brunch. Full service, espresso/cappuccino, VISA/MC/DC, $$**

Daily Bread
4501 Genessee, Kansas City, MO 64111   **(816) 531-1452**
Natural foods. This restaurant's menu changes daily; however, it always offers some
vegetarian soups, salads, entrees, sandwiches, and desserts. Every meal includes a daily
special bread. No smoking is allowed. **Open for lunch Tuesday through Saturday,
also for dinner Thursday through Saturday. Closed Sunday and Monday. Take-out
dinners available Tuesday through Thursday. Limited service, vegan options, es-
presso/cappuccino, take-out, $–$$**

Food for Thought
1808-1/2 W. 39th, Kansas City, MO 54111   **(816) 756-5304**
International. At Food for Thought, you can dine on a wide variety of international
vegetarian dishes including Hummus with Pita Bread, Wheat Berry Tabouli,
crepes, Polenta with Tomato Sauce, Tofu with Black Beans, Stir-Fry Vegetables,
etc. Local art is displayed. **Lunch and dinner served Monday through Friday;**

open only for dinner on Saturday and only for brunch on Sunday. **Full service, vegan options, espresso/cappuccino, take-out, VISA/MC/AMX, $$**

ST. LOUIS

Al Baker's
10 Upper Barnes Rd., Saint Louis, MO 63124   **(314) 863-8878**
Italian. There is a "Heart-Smart" menu section at Al Baker's with a Vegetarian Plate, Linguini, and Pasta Primavera. Other vegetarian pasta dishes are also on the menu. Enjoy elegant dining with live entertainment and dancing. **Open Monday through Saturday for dinner. Formal, full service, vegan options, wine/beer/alcohol, VISA/MC/AMX/DISC, $$$**

California Pizza Kitchen
1493 St. Louis Galleria, St. Louis, MO 63117   **(314) 863-4500**
Pizza. In the Galleria, a large up-scale shopping center, you'll find good cheeseless pizzas, vegetarian pastas, and salads. **Full service, $$**

• The Golden Grocer Cafe
335 N. Euclid, St. Louis, MO 63108   **(314) 367-0405**
Vegetarian. The Golden Grocer features a fresh salad bar with mostly organic produce. There's also Hummus, Curried Tofu, Rice Salad, veggie pizza, and vegan burritos, and a deli case full of vegetarian items, and eggless baked goods, most of which are vegan. **Open Monday through Saturday. Limited service, vegan options, fresh juices, take-out, VISA/MC/DISC, $**

• Govinda's
3926 Lindell Blvd., St. Louis, MO 63108   **(314) 535-8085**
Vegetarian. Govinda's features a wide variety of vegetarian foods. **Closed Saturday. Buffet, vegan options, fresh juices, take-out, $**

Koh-i-noor
608 Eastgate Ave., St. Louis, MO 63130   **(314) 721-3796**
Pakistani. Vegetarian appetizers and main dishes are served here. **Full service, $–$$**

La Patisserie
6269 Delmar Blvd., St. Louis, MO 63130   **(314) 725-4902**
Ethnic. La Patisserie has a vegetarian sausage for breakfast plus soups, sandwiches, and barbecued tofu. **Full service, catering, $–$$**

---

*🍴 Reviewers' choice   • Vegetarian restaurant   •• Vegan restaurant
$ less than $6 $$ $6–$12 $$$ more than $12
VISA/AMX/MC/DISC/DC—credit cards accepted
Non-alc.—Non alcoholic   Fresh juices—freshly squeezed*

Lettuce Leaf Restaurants
107 N. 6th St., St. Louis, MO 63101 (314) 241-7773
Natural foods. See Chesterfield, MO, entry for description. **Open on weekends in spring and summer only.**

Red Sea
6511 Delmar Blvd., St. Loius, MO 63130 (314) 863-0099
Ethiopian. Many vegetarian dishes are served in the traditional style with injera bread. **Full service, vegan options, $–$$**

Saleem's Restaurant
6501 Delmar, St. Louis, MO 63130 (314) 721-7947
Lebanese. Vegetarian appetizers, platter, and eggplant dish are offered. **Closed Sunday. Full service, wine/beer/alcohol, take-out, VISA/MC/DISC, $$**

Star of India
4569 LaClede Ave., St. Louis, MO 63108 (314) 361-6911
Indian. Many vegetarian options are available. **Open daily. Full service, vegan options, beer, take-out, VISA/MC/AMX, $$**

Sunshine Inn ❧
8¹/₂ S. Euclid, St. Louis, MO 63108 (314) 367-1413
Natural foods. Vegetarian options include veggie burgers, soy foods, dairy-free dishes, and homemade soups. Sunday brunch offers an à la carte menu featuring omelettes, multi-grain pancakes, potato pancakes, fresh fruit and juices. **Closed Monday. Full service, vegan options, fresh juices, non-alc. wine/beer, take-out, VISA/MC/AMX/DISC, $$**

UNIVERSITY CITY

Brandt's Market & Cafe
6525 Delmar, University City, MO 63130 (314) 727-3663
Natural foods. Eggplant Parmagiana, Veggie Burger, Black Bean Chili, Spring Rolls, pizza, and other options are available. There is live music nightly. **Open daily. Full service, vegan options, fresh juice, wine/beer/alcohol, VISA/MC/AMX/DISC, $$**

Red Sea
6511 Delmar, University City, MO 63112 (314) 863-0099
Ethiopian. Red Sea offers several vegetarian Ethiopian dishes. **Open daily for dinner, Wednesday through Saturday for lunch. Full service, non-alc. wine/beer, wine/beer/alcohol, catering, take-out, VISA/MC/AMX/DISC, $$**

WEBSTER GROVES

The Webster Grill and Cafe
8127 Big Bend Blvd., Webster Groves, MO 63119 (314) 962-0564
New American. Vegetarian Stir-Fry, Falafel, salads, and sandwiches are offered here. **Open daily for lunch and dinner, breakfast on weekends. Full service, vegan**

options, non-alc. beer, wine/beer/alcohol, take-out, VISA/MC/AMX/DISC/ DC, $$

MONTANA

BOZEMAN

Community Food Co-op
908 W. Main St., Bozeman, MT 59715   **(406) 587-4039**
Natural foods. Indoor and outdoor seating is available at this deli, which offers an incredible view of the Bridger Mountains in a parklike setting. Vegetarian options are seasonally and locally based. Smoking is not allowed. **Open daily for lunch and dinner. Counter service, macrobiotic/vegan options, catering, fresh juices, organic coffee and tea, take-out, $**

The Hearthstone Cafe & Bakery
1211 E. Main St., Bozeman, MT 59715   **(406) 586-4031**
Natural foods. This smoke-free cafe is located just off Interstate 90 and has a great view of the Bridger Mountains. Whole-grain baked goods and a wide variety of vegetarian dishes are offered. **Open daily for three meals. Full service, non-alc. beer/wine, fresh juices, espresso, smoothies, catering, vegan options, take-out, VISA/MC, $–$$**

CORWIN SPRINGS

The Ranch Kitchen
Hwy. 89, Corwin Springs, MT 59021   **(406) 848-7891**
Natural foods/American. Offers miso soups, seitan dishes, soy burgers, Mexican vegetarian dishes, and fruit-sweetened desserts. Features a weekend buffet and a dinner theater behind the restaurant. **Open May through mid-September for breakfast, lunch, and dinner. Full service, non-alc. wine/beer, take-out, VISA/MC/AMX, $$–$$$**

MISSOULA

• The Black Dog
138 W. Broadway St., Missoula, MT 59802   **(406) 542-1138**
Vegetarian. The Black Dog features a menu with daily specials, and includes organic ingredients whenever possible. Two or three soups, at least three entrees, sandwiches such as tempeh or lentil burgers, many vegan options, and desserts are offered. **Closed Sunday, open for lunch during the week, for dinner only on Saturday. Full service, vegan options, catering, no credit cards, $$**

China Garden
2100 Stephens Ave., Missoula, MT 59801   **(406) 721-1795**
Chinese. This restaurant uses no MSG. Vegetarian options include vegetable

sautées, soups, vegetable and noodle dishes, Vegetarian Foo Young, and Vegetable Fried Rice. **Open for lunch and dinner, closed Monday. Full service, take-out, VISA/MC/AMX, $$**

Mammyth
131 W. Main St., Missoula, MT 59802 (406) 549-5542
Natural foods cafe. This comfortable cafe features a great salad bar *and* the work of local artists and live music during lunches. The menu has many options in sandwiches, soups, and entree specials that change daily. **Closed Sunday. Cafeteria style, fresh juices, take-out, VISA/MC/AMX, $**

The Mustard Seed
419 W. Front St., Missoula, MT 59802 (406) 728-7825
Contemporary Oriental. The Mustard Seed offers a separate vegetarian menu that includes sushi, spring rolls, wok dishes, and tofu and vegetable dishes with various sauces. Smoking is not allowed. **Open daily for lunch and dinner. Full service, non-alc. wine/beer, wine/beer/alcohol, take-out, VISA/MC/AMX/DISC, $**

NEBRASKA

LINCOLN

Asian Palace
3031 "O" St., Lincoln, NE 68510 (402) 435-8884
Chinese. Partake of a good selection of Chinese vegetarian fast food. **Open daily. Limited service, take-out, $**

Open Harvest Natural Foods Grocery
1618 South St., Lincoln, NE 68502 (402) 475-9069
Natural-foods-store deli. This natural foods deli has a good selection of vegetarian items and a whole-grain bakery. **Open daily. Deli, take-out, $**

The Oven
201 N. 8th, Ste. 117, Lincoln, NE 68508 (402) 475-6118
Indian. Enjoy fine dining and Indian food with a very good selection for vegetarians. **Open daily. Full service, vegan options, wine/beer/alcohol, VISA/MC/ AMX, $$**

Taste of India
1320 "O" St., Lincoln, NE 68508 (402) 475-1642

🐾 Reviewers' choice   • Vegetarian restaurant   •• Vegan restaurant
$ less than $6 $$ $6–$12 $$$ more than $12
VISA/AMX/MC/DISC/DC—credit cards accepted
Non-alc.—Non-alcoholic   Fresh juices—freshly squeezed

Indian. Enjoy authentic Northern Indian cuisine from family recipes handed down for generations. Taste of India offers a wide variety of vegetarian entrees, fresh baked breads, desserts, and beverages. **Open daily. Full service, vegan options, wine/beer/alcohol, take-out, VISA/MC/AMX/DISC, $$**

OMAHA

The Food Gallery
312 S. 72nd St., Omaha, NE 68114   (402) 393-4168
Middle Eastern. This is a deli featuring Middle Eastern/Lebanese foods with several vegetarian selections. **Closed Sunday. Cafeteria style, vegan options, take-out, $–$$**

Indian Oven
1010 Howard St., Omaha, NE 68102   (402) 342-4856
Indian. The hallmark of Indian Oven's cuisine is its "Tandoori Cuisine," cooking in its clay oven. Included on the menu are stuffed and plain tandoor breads, pakoras, papadums, and samosas as well as various other vegetarian options. **Open daily. Full service, fresh juices, wine/beer/alcohol, take-out, VISA/MC/AMX, $$**

McFoster's Natural Kind Cafe
302 South 38th St., Omaha, NE 68131   (402) 345-7477
Natural foods. Enjoy Falafel, almond-milk-based soups, a juice bar, and more. Acoustic music and patio service are provided. **Open for lunch and dinner Monday through Saturday. Closed Sunday. Full service, vegan options, take-out, VISA/MC, $–$$**

NEVADA

LAS VEGAS

Beijing Restaurant
3900 Paradise Rd., Las Vegas, NV 89109   (702) 737-9618
Chinese. Be sure to request the vegetarian menu, which is quite large. **Open daily for lunch and dinner. Full service, vegan options, take-out, $$**

The Health Connection
4750 S. Eastern Ave., Las Vegas, NV 89121   (702) 458-8058
Natural foods. This natural foods restaurant is located in a World Gym fitness center. It offers a wide variety of veggie burgers, Mexican dishes, sandwiches, salads, pizza, and more. **Open for three meals daily. Counter service, vegan options, fresh juices, take-out, $**

Kokmol Restaurant
953 E. Sahara Ave., Las Vegas, NV 89104   (702) 731-6542
Thai. This Thai restaurant offers an extensive vegetarian menu including seitan and tofu dishes. **Open for lunch and dinner daily. Full service, take-out, $**

Shalimar Fine Indian Cuisine
3900 Paradise Rd., Las Vegas, NV 89109 **(702) 796-0302**

2605 S. Decatur Blvd., Las Vegas, NV 89102 **(702) 252-8320**
Indian. Shalimar offers more than twenty vegetarian Indian dishes prepared in a Tandoor oven. **Open for dinner daily and for lunch weekdays. Full service, non-alc. beer, beer/wine/alcohol, VISA/MC/AMX/DISC/DC, $$**

RENO

• Blue Heron Natural Foods Restaurant & Bakery
1091 S. Virginia, Reno, NV 89502 **(702) 786-4110**
Vegetarian. Partake of sandwiches, salads, soup specials, side orders, and numerous vegetarian entrees; 75 percent of all soups and meals are vegan. There's a bookstore at the same location. **Open daily for lunch and dinner. Full service, vegan/macrobiotic options, fresh juices, wine/beer, take-out, no credit cards, $$**

Sapna Indian Restaurant
3374 Kietzke Center, Reno, NV 89502 **(702) 829-1537**
Indian. Sapna specializes in the cooking of North and South India. Various vegetable soups, appetizers, side orders, and curry entrees are offered. **Open Monday through Saturday for lunch and dinner. Full service, vegan options, wine/beer, take-out, VISA/MC/AMX, $$**

NEW HAMPSHIRE

DURHAM

The Bagelry
45 Mill Rd. Plaza, Durham, NH 03824 **(603) 868-1424**
American. In addition to bagels, The Bagelry offers several vegetarian dishes. **Open daily. Counter service, vegan options, take-out, $**

KEENE

Bagel Works Inc.
120 Main St., Keene, NH 03431 **(603) 357-7751**
Bagel deli. Sample more than sixteen varieties of bagels with various topping options, including cream cheeses, tofutti spreads, salads, and vegetarian combinations. Foods are prepared with all-natural ingredients without preservatives. Bagel Works is environmentally conscious and socially active in its community. **Open daily. Counter service, vegan options, fresh juices, take-out, $**

MEREDITH

For Every Season
67 Main St., Meredith, NH 03253 **(603) 279-8875**
Whole-foods deli. This restaurant located in the beautiful Lakes Region of New

Hampshire offers homemade soups and salads in a casual, kid-friendly environment. Breakfast is served all day. Garden deck. **Open daily for breakfast and lunch during summer. Open Tuesday through Saturday during winter. Limited service, vegan options, BYOB, take-out, $**

NORTH CONWAY
Cafe Chimes
Norcross Pl., Main St., North Conway, NH 03860   (603) 356-5500
Natural foods. "Homemade" and "natural" are the passwords at Cafe Chimes, which features soups, salads, quiche, pizza, grain dishes, and specials. The cafe's wheat mill grinds wheat berries daily to create unique whole-wheat bread.

PORTSMOUTH
The Bagelry
19 Market St., Portsmouth, NH 03801   (603) 431-5853

Woodbury Ave., Portsmouth, NH 03801   (603) 436-2244
American. See description under Durham.

NEW JERSEY

CLEMENTON
New Japan
Blackwood-Clementon Rd., Laurel Plaza
Clementon, NJ 08021   (609) 435-5630
Japanese. New Japan features Vegetable Sushi and Vegetable Tempura. **Open daily for lunch and dinner. Closed for dinner Monday. Full service, take-out, VISA/ MC/AMX/DISC/DC, $$**

Tandoor Palace Restaurant
Plaza 30
328 White Horse Pike, Clementon, NJ 08021   (609) 435-1234
Indian. Dine on vegetable samosas, freshly baked Indian breads, and a choice of more than ten vegetarian entrees. **Open daily for lunch and dinner. Full service, take-out, VISA/MC/AMX/$$**

COLONIA
• Siddhartha Authentic Indian Vegetarian Restaurant
1133 St. Georges Ave., Colonia, NJ 07067   (201) 750-0231
Vegetarian/Indian. **Closed Tuesday. Full service, vegan options, fresh juice, take-out, $**

EAST BRUNSWICK

Bombay Gardens
1020 Rt. 18, East Brunswick, NJ 08816 (908) 613-9500
Indian. Bombay Gardens offers a wide variety of vegetarian Indian dishes including many South Indian dishes. **Open daily for lunch and dinner. Full service, vegan options, take-out, $$**

EAST RUTHERFORD

Park and Orchard Restaurant 🍲
240 Hackensack St., East Rutherford, NJ 07073 (201) 939-9292
Extensively vegetarian. Park and Orchard was voted best restaurant in Northern New Jersey by readers of *New Jersey Magazine*. There's an award-winning wine list, and an excellent eclectic menu. **Full service, fresh juice, wine/beer/alcohol, take-out, VISA/MC/AMX/DISC, $$$**

EDISON

• Subras
1679 Oak Tree Rd., Edison, NJ 08820 (908) 549-9424
Vegetarian. Subras is a vegetarian Indian restaurant serving Gujarati and South Indian dishes. **Open daily for lunch and dinner. Full service, vegan options, take-out, $–$$**

ELIZABETH

Jerusalem Restaurant
150 Elmora Ave., Elizabeth, NJ 07202 (908) 289-0291
Natural foods/kosher. Enjoy kosher Middle Eastern vegetarian food, as well as pizza, salads, and more. **Open Sunday through Thursday for lunch and dinner. Open only for lunch Friday. Call for Saturday hours. Limited service, vegan options, catering, take-out, $**

FRANKLIN PARK

Aashiana Exotic Indian Cuisine
3191 Rt. 27, Franklin Park, NJ 08823 (908) 940-0662
Indian. Enjoy freshly baked Indian bread, as well as several different vegetarian entrees at this restaurant. **Open Tuesday through Sunday for lunch and dinner. Closed Monday. Full service, catering, vegan options, take-out, VISA/MC/AMX, $$**

🍲 Reviewers' choice   • Vegetarian restaurant   •• Vegan restaurant
$ less than $6 $$ $6–$12 $$$ more than $12
VISA/AMX/MC/DISC/DC—credit cards accepted
Non-alc.—Non-alcoholic   Fresh juices—freshly squeezed

HAINESPORT

Hainesport Health Haven
Rt. 38 and Lumberton Rd., Hainesport NJ 08036   (609) 267-7744
Lunch bar. Enjoy the pleasant atmosphere in this fully stocked natural foods store. The lunch bar is very willing to accommodate special diets, and there are many vegetarian options. **Lunch only. Limited service, take-out, VISA/MC, $**

HOBOKEN·

Hoboken Farm Boy
229 Washington St., Hoboken, NJ 07030   (201) 656-0581
Primarily vegetarian deli. Farm Boy offers deli-style service with an extensive vegetarian menu—sandwiches, burgers, Baked Tofu, soups, Black Bean Chili, plus more. Seating is very limited. **Open daily for lunch and dinner. Fresh juice, catering, take-out, VISA/MC/AMX, $**

ISELIN

• Udupi Authentic Indian Vegetarian Cuisine
1380 Oak Tree Rd., Iselin, NJ 08830   (908) 283-0343
Vegetarian/Indian. Udupi offers vegetarian Indian specialities. **Open daily for lunch and dinner. Full service, take-out, VISA/MC/DISC, $–$$**

LIVINGSTON

Jerusalem Restaurant
16 E. Mt. Pleasant Ave., Livingston, NJ 07016   (201) 533-1424
Natural foods/kosher. See description under Elizabeth.

MARLTON·

Mexican Food Factory
State Hwy. 70 and Cropwell Rd., Marlton, NJ 08053   (609) 983-9222
Mexican. The refried beans are made without lard or animal products. Patio for outdoor dining in season. **Full service, vegan options, take-out, beer/wine/alc., VISA/MC/AMX, $$**

TGI Friday's
970 Route 73 N., Marlton, NJ 08053   (609) 596-9117
Restaurant chain. A few vegetarian entrees are offered, and a no-smoking section is available. **Open daily for lunch and dinner. Full service, vegetarian options, beer/wine/alcohol, $$**

Zagara's
501 Route 73 S., Marlton, NJ 08053   (609) 983-5700
Natural foods. Hot bar selections differ daily, but have included mushroom barley soup with vegetable stock, vegetarian navy bean soup, rice tempeh with pineapple

salsa, and seitan and broccoli. **Open daily for three meals. Take-out, vegan options, fresh juices, smoothies, catering, VISA/MC/AMX, $$**

MONTCLAIR

Clairmont Health Food Centre

515 Bloomfield Ave., Montclair, NJ 07042 (201) 744-7122
Health-food-store deli. Clairmont offers Hummus, Brown Rice with Steamed Vegetables, veggie burgers, sandwiches to go, and daily specials. **Open daily for lunch. Counter service, vegan/macrobiotic options, fresh juices, take-out, VISA/MC, $**

MOORESTOWN

Homestyle Family Buffet

Moorestown Shopping Center
Route 38 and Lenola Road, Moorestown, NJ 08057 (609) 234-7542
American. Four or five vegetarian options are available at every meal, and there's a salad bar. **Cafeteria Style. Vegetarian options, $$$.**

MORRISTOWN

Chand Palace

79 Washington St. (Rt. 24W), Morristown, NJ 07960 (201) 539-7433
Indian. Chand Palace offers a wide variety of vegetarian Indian food including baked breads, vegetable curries, rice specialties, and more. The restaurant does not use eggs in its dishes. **Open Wednesday through Monday for lunch and dinner. Closed Tuesday. Full service, vegan options, take-out, $$**

Mayflower Restaurant

74 Morris St., Morristown, NJ 07960 (201) 267-3794
Chinese. This smoke-free Chinese restaurant offers a wide variety of vegetarian items including soups, rice and noodle entrees, tofu, gluten, and vegetable dishes, plus much more. **Open Tuesday through Sunday for lunch and dinner. Full service, fresh juices, vegan options, take-out, VISA/MC/AMX/DISC/DC, $–$$**

MOUNT LAUREL

Garden of Eden Natural Foods & Country Kitchen

1155 N. Route 73, Ramblewood Center
Mt. Laurel, NJ 08054 (609) 778-1971
Natural foods/deli. This deli-style restaurant has an extensive vegetarian menu, a daily vegetarian entree, and soup du jour. Organic foods are used as much as possible. Enjoy the friendly atmosphere, natural groceries, juice bar, and cooking classes in this recently expanded establishment. **Lunch and dinner Monday through Saturday, brunch on Sunday. Full service, fresh juices, catering, take-out, VISA/MC/DISC, $–$$**

NORTH ARLINGTON

• **The Lotus Light Cafe**
77 Ridge Rd., North Arlington, NJ 07031   **(201) 991-5858**
Vegetarian. Lotus Light Cafe offers international vegetarian dishes including
Mexican, Asian, Italian, Chinese, and Middle Eastern. Organic ingredients are
used when available. Local artists' work is exhibited. **Open Monday through
Saturday for lunch and dinner. Open Sunday for brunch. Limited service, vegan
options, catering, take-out, $$**

OCEAN CITY

Bashful Banana Cafe & Bakery
944 Ocean City Boardwalk—Colony Walk
Ocean City, NJ 08226   **(609) 398-9677**
Natural foods/extensively vegetarian. Offering a contemporary full-service menu
using only healthy, fresh ingredients, the cafe focuses on low-fat, sugar-free,
low-calorie, and some dairy-free items. Grams of fat, calories, and cholesterol are
listed on the menu for each item. This restaurant and bakery offers outdoor dining
with an ocean view. **Open daily Memorial day through Labor Day; open weekends
in April, May, September, and October. Full service restaurant and bakery,
vegan options, fresh juice, catering, VISA/MC, $**

OCEAN GROVE

The Raspberry Cafe
60 Main Ave., Ocean Grove, NJ 07756   **(908) 988-0833**
Natural foods. The Raspberry Cafe is located in Ocean Grove, a quaint seaside
Methodist town of beautifully painted Victorian houses. The cafe has both indoor
and outdoor seating and offers several vegetarian dishes including a veggie burger,
salads, Middle Eastern Platter, quiche, pita sandwiches, and daily specials. **Open
for breakfast and lunch weekdays, except Tuesday; open for dinner on Friday
and Saturday and for brunch on Sunday. Full service, espresso/cappuccino,
smoothies, fresh juices, vegan options, take-out, $–$$**

PARSIPPANY

Chand Palace
257 Littleton Rd., Parsippany, NJ 07054   **(201) 334-5444**
Indian. See description under Morristown.

PENNSAUKEN

New China Star
5201 Route 38, Pennsuaken, NJ 08109   **(609) 662-7711**

🍴 Reviewers' choice   • Vegetarian restaurant   •• Vegan restaurant
$ less than $6 $$ $6–$12 $$$ more than $12
VISA/AMX/MC/DISC/DC—credit cards accepted
Non-alc.—Non-alcoholic   Fresh juices—freshly squeezed

Chinese. Choose from a large vegetarian menu of appetizers, soups, and entrees. **Open daily for lunch and dinner. Full service, vegan options, VISA/MC/AMX/ DISC/DC, $$**

PLAINSBORO

Lee's Castle I

660 Plainsboro Rd., Plainsboro, NJ 08536   **(609) 799-1008**
Chinese. Choose from the "Happy Vegetarian Paradise" menu, which includes a large selection of vegetarian soups, appetizers, and entrees. **Open daily for lunch and dinner. Full service, vegan options, catering, take-out, VISA/MC/AMX, $$**

PRINCETON

Mykonos Greek Restaurant

22 Witherspoon St., Princeton NJ 08542   **(609) 921-2200**
Greek. Mykonos is a Greek restaurant with an extensive vegetarian menu. **Open for lunch and dinner daily except Sunday. Full service, vegan options, take-out, $–$$**

RED BANK

The Eurasian Eatery

110 Monmouth St., Red Bank, NJ 07701   **(908) 741-7071**
European/Asian. Along with eclectic European and Asian offerings, there's an extensive vegetarian menu. **Closed Monday, open Tuesday through Saturday for lunch and dinner, Sunday for dinner only. Full service, vegan options, BYOB, take-out, AMX, $$**

• Garden Vegetarian Restaurant

7 E. Front St., Red Bank, NJ 07701   **(908) 530-8681**
Vegetarian. Garden proudly serves vegetarian foods, including unique and original combinations of the finest fresh vegetables. All food on the extensive lunch and dinner menus is cooked to order and will be tailored to special dietary needs. **Open Monday through Saturday for lunch and dinner. Full service, vegan options, fresh juice, BYOB, catering, take-out, $$**

RIDGEWOOD

Nature's Market Place

1 West Ridgewood Ave., Ridgewood, NJ 07450   **(201) 445-9210**
Natural foods. Diners can enjoy a meatless "meatball" sandwich, Bean Burritos, vegetarian tacos or chili, Spinach Lasagna, Falafel, salads, plus much more at Nature's Market Place Deli Cafe. **Open for lunch Monday through Saturday. Closed Sunday. Counter service, vegan options, smoothies, fresh juices, take-out, VISA/MC/AMX, $**

RUNNEMEDE

Li's Peking Chinese Restaurant
Runnemede Plaza, 835 E. Clements Bridge Rd.,
Runnemede, NJ 08078   **(609) 939-4440**
Chinese. Li's has a vegetarian menu with appetizers, many soups, and entrees featuring vegetable, tofu, and mock-meat dishes. There's an excellent vegetarian selection, and foods are low in salt and prepared without MSG. **Open daily. Full service, vegan options, BYOB, take-out, VISA/MC/AMX, $$**

SCOTCH PLAINS

• Udupi Authentic Indian Vegetarian Cuisine
2540 Route 22E, Scotch Plains, NJ 07076   **(908) 233-5511**
Vegetarian/Indian. See entry under Iselin, NJ.

STONE HARBOR

Green Cuisine
302 96th St., Stone Harbor, NJ 08247   **(609) 368-1616**
Natural foods. This restaurant has been serving delicious healthy food for over ten years. Menu selections include gourmet sandwiches, exotic salads, and beautiful fresh fruit selections. Vegetarian items such as Hummus Pita, Tabouli Salad, and veggie burgers are very popular. **Open daily for three meals. Full service, vegetarian options, fresh juice, BYOB, take-out, no credit cards, $$**

TOMS RIVER

Natural Foods Vegetarian Cafe
675 Batchelor St., Toms River, NJ 08753   **(908) 240-0024**
Natural foods. Located inside a natural foods store, this mostly vegetarian cafe features many unique dishes like a vegan German platter, veggie loaf platter, and tempeh and chickpea curry. **Open Monday through Friday for lunch. Limited service, vegan options, take-out, VISA/MC/AMX/DISC, $**

VORHEES

Richard's Natural Foods Restaurant
10 White Horse Rd., Vorhees, NJ 08043   **(609) 627-5057**
Primarily vegetarian/natural foods. Richard's is a restaurant with a natural foods store. It offers many pasta dishes and other vegetarian entrees. The menu is almost entirely vegetarian. Cooking classes are available. **Open Monday through Friday for lunch, and Wednesday through Saturday for dinner. Full service, vegan options, fresh juice, BYOB, take-out, $$**

NEW MEXICO

ALBUQUERQUE

•• Adam's Table
3600 Central and Carlisle, Albuquerque, NM 87106   (505) 266-4214
Vegan. This is Albuquerque's only vegan restaurant serving Southwestern food. You'll find a big salad bar, fresh soups daily, hot buffet lunch, and sugarless desserts. The only non-vegan food is the soy cheese, which contains casein, a milk protein. **Closed Saturday. Full service, fresh juices, catering, take-out, VISA/MC/DISC, $**

Alejandro's New Mexican Restaurant
6416 Zuni SE, Albuquerque, NM 87108   (505) 265-9555

5801 Wyoming NE, Albuquerque, NM 87109   (505) 821-3481
New Mexican. Whether you prefer patio dining at the Zuni location or fireplaces at the Wyoming site, you'll find a vegetarian plate, chili, and other veggie options. Items that can be prepared to meet the dietary standards of the American Heart Association are indicated on the menu. Live guitar music is played on Friday and Saturday nights. **Open daily. Full service, wine/beer, take-out, VISA/MC/AMX/ DISC, $–$$**

Artichoke Cafe
424 Central SE, Albuquerque, NM 87106   (505) 243-0200
International. Stark modern decor, rotating art exhibits, and a dedication to fine food, wine, and service have made the Artichoke Cafe one of Albuquerque's popular dining spots. The food is a mix of French, Italian, and creative American cuisine, and there are limited veggie options. It's pricey. **Closed Sunday. Full service, fresh juices, wine/beer, take-out, VISA/MC/AMX, $$$**

Bangkok Cafe
5901 Central NE, Albuquerque, NM 87108   (505) 255-5036
Thai. An entire vegetarian menu section that includes appetizers, soups, curry dishes, wok fried dishes, rice and noodles, and desserts is included on the Bangkok Cafe menu. All of the foods may be ordered from mild to spicy. Patio dining. **Open daily. Full service, vegan options, wine/beer, take-out, VISA/MC/AMX/ DISC, $$**

Bodhi Tree Restaurant
127 Harvard Dr., SE, Albuquerque, NM 87106   (505) 260-0919
Indian. Vegetarian items are about one-third of the menu, and only vegetable oil is used. There's patio dining with lots of shade. **Open daily. Full service, fresh juices, take-out, $$**

EJ's Cafe
2201 Silver SE, Albuquerque, NM 87106   (505) 268-2233
American/international. Located near the University, EJ's has a menu that includes various vegetarian and non-vegetarian foods for breakfast, lunch, and dinner. Pasta, veggie burgers, stir-fry, and Mexican dishes are offered as is a wide variety of coffees. **Open daily. Full service, vegan options, take-out, VISA/MC, $**

El Patio Restaurant
142 Harvard SE, Albuquerque, NM 87106   **(505) 268-4245**
Mexican. Located near the University, this restaurant has vegetarian green and red chili and usually a veggie special. Savor a vegetarian burrito with fresh avocados, tomatoes, and vegetarian beans. **Open daily. Full service, vegan options, wine/beer, take-out, VISA/MC, $**

• Health Hunters Deli
355 Nara Visa NW, Albuquerque, NM 87107   **(505) 344-8866**
Vegetarian. Salads, sandwiches, hot entrees, specials and desserts make up the menu at Health Hunters. Some examples include Nori Rolls, Chili, and Mexican dishes. There are fresh homemade soups, and selections are mostly dairy-free. Enjoy sunlit atrium dining with local art for sale. **Closed Sunday. Full service, vegan options, fresh juices, limited catering, take-out, VISA/MC, $**

India Kitchen Restaurant
6910 Montgomery NE, Albuquerque, NM 87109   **(505) 884-2333**
Indian. Eleven vegetarian entrees plus soup and appetizers are on the India Kitchen menu. Everything is prepared fresh to order. **Open daily. Full service, vegan options, wine/beer, VISA/MC/AMX/DISC, $**

La Montanita Co-op Supermarket
3500 Central Ave. SE, Albuquerque, NM 87106   **(505) 265-4631**
Health-food-store deli. La Montanita's deli features a wide variety of healthy salads and entrees. Hot soups and sandwiches and vegetarian and vegan foods are also featured. **Open daily. Deli, vegan options, fresh juices, take-out, $**

Oasis Restaurant & Lounge
5400 San Mateo NE, Albuquerque, NM 87109   **(505) 884-2324**
Mediterranean. Oasis features the foods of France, Italy, Greece, and Spain. Vegetarian entrees include Hummus, Falafel, Tabouleh, Moussaka, and pasta dishes. Desserts are homemade. There's live entertainment Wednesday through Saturday evenings. **Open daily for lunch and dinner, Sunday for dinner only. Reservations encouraged. Full service, vegan options, wine/beer/alcohol, take-out, VISA/MC/AMX/DC, $$–$$$**

Shalimar Indian Cuisine
84-5 Montgomery NE, Albuquerque, NM 87111   **(505) 275-7949**
Indian. Vegetarian and non-vegetarian options are available. **Open daily. Full service, wine/beer, take-out, VISA/MC, $$**

LAS CRUCES

• Kalandras Vegetarian Restaurant
1706 South Espina St., Las Cruces, NM 88001   **(505) 525-3384**
Vegetarian. This restaurant opened in 1994 and offers a wide range of vegetarian dishes including salads and soups, veggie burgers, Stuffed Peppers, Mexican Lasagna, Pasta Primavera, Indian Platter, and more. Many dishes have an international flavor and the offerings change each day. **Open for three meals Tuesday**

through Sunday. Closed Monday. Full service, vegan options, take-out, VISA/MC/DISC, $-$$

RIO RANCHO
Fortune Cookie
1011 Rio Rancho Blvd., Rio Rancho, NM 87124   **(505) 892-4500**
Chinese. Full service, wine/beer, take-out, VISA/MC/AMX/DISC, $$

SANTA FE
Baja Tacos
2621 Cerrillos Rd., Santa Fe, NM 87501   **(505) 988-5258**
Mexican. Enjoy fast, healthy and fresh Mexican food with no preservatives or additives. There's a vegetarian menu. **Open for three meals daily. Counter service, vegan options, BYOB, take-out, $**

Cafe Pasqual's
121 Don Gaspar, Santa Fe, NM 87501   **(505) 983-9340**
Natural foods. A Santa Fe classic, Cafe Pasqual's is known for its breakfasts and delicious Southwestern fare that pays particular attention to quality and authenticity. The menu is based on simple ingredients such as red and green chiles, pinto beans, garlic, onions, blue and yellow cornmeal, and white cheese. A lot of the menu items include fish or free-range chicken, but there is a decent selection for vegetarians, and specials are offered. Pasqual's is a place for locals and travelers alike who want innovative meals based on traditional fare. **Open for three meals daily but closed for Wednesday dinner. Full service, fresh juices, wine/beer, take-out, VISA/MC, $$-$$$**

Cloud Cliff Bakery & Restaurant
1805 Second St., Santa Fe, NM 87501   **(505) 983-6254**
Natural foods. Cloud Cliff integrates contemporary arts with fresh foods. The management works closely with local farmers and uses organically grown grains in the European breads and alternative pastries. **Open daily. Full service, fresh juice, wine/beer, take-out, VISA/MC, $$**

• Healthy David's Cafe
418 Cerrillos Rd., Santa Fe, NM 87501   **(505) 982-4147**
Vegetarian. Healthy David's is a Santa Fe classic with a variety of delicious vegetarian entrees, sandwiches, salads, and Middle Eastern foods. **Open daily for lunch and dinner. Full service, vegan options, fresh juices, organic coffee, take-out, $**

🐌 Reviewers' choice   • Vegetarian restaurant   •• Vegan restaurant
$ less than $6 $$ $6-$12 $$$ more than $12
VISA/AMX/MC/DISC/DC—credit cards accepted
Non-alc.—Non-alcoholic   Fresh juices—freshly squeezed

Hunan Chinese Restaurant
2440 Cerrillos Rd., Santa Fe, NM 87501   **(505) 471-6688**
Chinese. If you need a break from Southwestern cuisine, you can find a wide variety
of vegetarian Hunan- and Peking-style Chinese foods at this restaurant. Appetizers, soups, and sixteen vegetarian entrees are offered to delight your taste buds.
**Open daily for lunch and dinner. Full service, vegan options, wine/beer, take-
out, VISA/MC/AMX, $$**

Natural Cafe
1494 Cerrillos Rd., Santa Fe, NM 87501   **(505) 983-1411**
International. Innovative international cuisine features vegetarian and non-vegetarian
dishes. Entrees include East Indian Tempeh Curry, Szechuan Vegetables, and Black
Bean Enchiladas. Whole-wheat French bread and delicous desserts are prepared daily.
Local art decorates the dining room. Garden patio. **Closed Monday. Full service,
vegan options, wine/beer, limited take-out, VISA/MC, $$**

Szechwan Restaurant
1965 Cerrillos Rd., Santa Fe, NM 87501   **(505) 983-1558**
Chinese. Ten vegetable and tofu entrees such as Broccoli with Hot Garlic Sauce
and Sizzling Bean Curd are included on the menu. Appetizers, soup, and daily
vegetarian specials are also offered. **Open daily for lunch and dinner. Full service,
vegan options, wine/beer, take-out, VISA/MC, $$**

Tecolote Cafe
1203 Cerrillos Rd., Santa Fe, NM 87501   **(505) 988-1362**
Mexican/New Mexican. Known for its breakfasts, Tecolote features fresh baked
goods and original atole/pinon hot cakes made with blue cornmeal and roasted
pine nuts. The cafe is also open for lunch and serves various Mexican classics with
a New Mexican twist. Beans and chili sauces are made with pure soy oil and no
lard. The work of local artists is featured on the walls. **Open Tuesday through
Sunday for breakfast and lunch. Full service, fresh juices, wine/beer, take-out,
VISA/MC/AMX/DC, $**

Tomasita's Santa Fe Station
500 S. Guadalupe, Santa Fe, NM 87501   **(505) 983-5721**
New Mexican. Located in a historic red-brick station house, Tomasita's is a distinctive
Northern New Mexican restaurant using recipes that have been handed down for
generations. Vegetarian options are clearly indicated on the menu. Beware, the red
and green chiles do contain beef. **Open Monday through Saturday for lunch and
dinner. Full service, vegan options, take-out, VISA/MC, $$**

Wild Oats Market
1090 St. Francis Dr., Santa Fe, NM 87501   **(505) 983-5333**
Natural foods deli. This deli has vegetarian options and a large selection of breads
and pastries. **Open daily. Deli, fresh juices, take-out, VISA/MC, $**

Apple Tree Restaurant
123 Bent St., Taos, NM 87571 **(505) 758-1900**
Natural foods. Salads, soups, appetizers, and specials all include options for vegetarians. The red and green chile and the beans are vegetarian. Foods are prepared using the freshest ingredients available and reflecting a variety of ethnic persuasions. **Open daily, Sunday brunch. Full service, vegan options, espresso/cappuccino, wine/beer, take-out, VISA/AMX/MC, $–$$$**

The Caffe Tazza
122 Kit Carson Rd., Taos, NM 87571 **(505) 758-8706**
Cafe. An espresso bar with locally made ethnic vegetarian tamales, vegetarian chili plus daily soup specials, and, of course, espresso. There are great magazines and courtyard seating in summer. **Open daily. Limited service, take-out, no credit cards, $**

The Outback
712 Paseo del Pueblo Norte, Taos, NM 87571 **(505) 758-3112**
Pizza. Gourmet pizza with toppings such as dried tomatoes, spinach, artichoke, and pineapple. Pasta and salads also appear on the menu. **Open Monday through Saturday for lunch and dinner, closed Sunday. Full service, espresso/cappuccino, wine/beer, take-out, VISA/MC, $$**

• Wild & Natural Cafe
812B Paseo del Pueblo Norte, Taos, NM 87571 **(505) 751-0480**
Vegetarian. Wild & Natural has a Southwestern-style low-fat, heart-healthy menu. There are non-dairy daily specials, blue corn guacamole enchiladas, tempeh burgers, and veggie burritos. **Open for lunch and dinner Monday through Saturday. Full service, vegan options, fresh juices, espresso/cappuccino, wine/beer, take-out, VISA/MC, $–$$**

NEW YORK

• Dahlia's Vegetarian Bistro
858 Madison Ave., Albany, NY 12208 **(518) 482-0931**
Vegetarian. Dahlia's features international vegetarian cuisine. Every item on the menu is made from scratch. Dinners include Spinach Lasagna, Black Bean Chili, Angel Hair Pasta, and Jamaica Jerk Tempeh. The ice cream bar offers sorbet. **Open for lunch and dinner Sunday through Thursday. Closed November 15 to January 31. Full service, vegan/macrobiotic options, fresh vegetable juice, sorbet-with-7-Up coolers, catering, take-out, VISA/MC, lunch $, dinner $$**

El Loco Mexican Cafe
465 Madison Ave., Albany, NY 12210 **(518) 436-1855**

Mexican. Sample no-lard refried beans, veggie brown Mexican rice, veggie chili and soups, blue cornbread, etc. Most items can be prepared vegetarian. Here you'll find a funky atmosphere, outdoor patio, interesting t-shirts. **Open for lunch and dinner Tuesday through Saturday, Sunday and Monday open later afternoon and dinner time; may begin a Sunday brunch. Full service, wine/ beer/alcohol, catering, take-out, VISA/MC/AMX, $$**

•• Nepenthe Cafe
154 Madison Ave., Albany, NY 12202   **(518) 436-0329**
Vegan. Nepenthe Cafe serves a wide variety of vegetarian food including ethnic dishes, seitan specials, soy-based dishes, steamed vegetables, stir-frys, sea vegetables, and more. **Open for lunch and dinner daily, brunch Saturday. Full service, espresso/cappuccino, fresh juices, smoothies, completely vegan, take-out, VISA/ MC, $$**

ALBERTSON
Vincent's Restaurant & Pizzeria
1004 Willis Ave., Albertson, NY 11507   **(516) 621-7530**
Italian. Offers several vegetarian dishes including a cheeseless potato pizza. **Open daily for lunch and dinner. Full service, take-out, wine/beer, $$**

AMHERST
Pizza Plant
3085 Sheridan Dr., Amherst, NY 14226   **(716) 833-0882**
American with natural food choices. This restaurant offers veggie burgers (vegan), vegetarian chili, burritos, pasta with Pizza Plant's own marinara sauce, vegetarian stew in winter, homemade soups, a large variety of pizzas including soy cheese pizza, and a selection of fresh salads. Over sixty domestic and imported beers are featured. **Open daily. Full service, vegan options, wine/beer, catering, take-out, VISA/MC/AMX/DISC, $$**

AMITYVILLE
• Santosha Vegetarian Dining
40 Merrick Rd, Amityville, NY 11701
(Mailing address: 40 Forrest Place)   **(516) 598-1787**
Vegetarian. Created and owned by an Ashram, Santosha's food is cooked and served by Ashram members. The atmosphere is pleasant and relaxed. Entrees include Tortillas, Tempeh Fillets, Scallops of Tofu, Saffron Couscous African, and more. Desserts include vegan Chocolate Blackout Cake, Banana Berry Parfait, Vegan Berry Pie, and Precious Peach Cake. The in-store bakery will make a carrot wedding cake. **Open for dinner every night except Monday, open for lunch Tuesday through Friday. Full service, vegan options, dairy and non-dairy cappucino, non-alc. beer, catering, take-out, $$$**

ARDSLEY
•• Twilight Cafe
466 Ashford Ave., Ardsley, NY 10502   **(914) 674-0700**

Vegan. Try the lentil millet loaf, barbecued tempeh shishkabob, pad Thai with tempeh, or any of the other creative dishes served at this restaurant located in a greenhouse. **Open daily for lunch and dinner. Full service, fresh juices, espresso/cappuccino, VISA/MC, $–$$$**

BINGHAMTON

Whole in the Wall
43 S. Washington St., Binghamton, NY 13903   **(607) 722-0006**
Natural foods. At Whole in the Wall, bread and bagels are baked fresh every day. Soups are made from scratch; pies are made with fresh fruit and whole-wheat crust. All non-vegetarian items are cooked separately, and the restaurant can accommodate special diets. Tofu, tempeh, and Middle Eastern dishes are served, and live music is featured on Saturday night. **Open Tuesday through Saturday for lunch and dinner. Full service, vegan/macrobiotic options, fresh carrot or grape juices, $$**

BREWSTER

Jaipore
Rt. 22, Brewster, NY 10509   **(914) 277-3549**
Indian. Jaipore is located in an historical Victorian manor and offers more than fifteen vegetarian entrees including rice dishes, freshly baked breads, vegetable curry dishes, plus more. **Open daily for lunch and dinner. Full service, vegan options, catering, beer/wine/alcohol, take-out, VISA/MC/AMX, $$**

BROOKLYN

(For more restaurant listings in the surrounding areas, see New York City.)

The Gourmet Cafe
1622 Coney Island Ave., Brooklyn, NY 11230   **(718) 338-5825**
Kosher/vegetarian (except for some fish)/macrobiotic/ethnic. The fare includes hearty soups such as split pea and mushroom barley, Chopped Vegetarian Liver, Stuffed Cabbage, Veggie Burger, chickenlike schnitzel, Zucchini Muffins, Carrot Cake, and ice cream desserts. Gourmet Cafe retails frozen entrees. **Open Sunday through Thursday for lunch and dinner. Full service, vegan options, catering, take-out, VISA/MC/AMX/DISC, $$**

Healthy Henrietta's
60 Henry St., Brooklyn, NY 11201   **(718) 858-8478**
Mexican/natural foods. Henrietta's has an artsy atmosphere and features great brunches and desserts. Mexican items are offered with tofu sour cream. **Vegan/macrobiotic options, take-out, $–$$.**

Kar Too Restaurant
5908 Ave. N, Brooklyn, NY 11234   **(718) 531-8811**
Chinese. Savor sautéed string beans with pickled cabbage, tangy and spicy tofu, spinach sautéed with Fu-U sauce. Brown rice is available. **Open daily to 10:30 P.M., wine/beer, take-out, VISA/MC/AMX, $$**

• King Vegetarian Restaurant
4705 Church Ave., Brooklyn, NY 11203   **(718) 284-4533**
Vegetarian. This is an East Flatbush restaurant. **Open Monday through Saturday for lunch and dinner. Full service, catering, $**

The Leaf & Bean Cafe
136 Montague St., Brooklyn, NY 11201   **(718) 855-7978**
Natural foods. Located on the parlor floor of a brownstone, the Leaf & Bean Cafe offers a continental menu of salads, omelettes, and items such as Vegetable Lasagna, sandwiches, and desserts. Cakes, tarts, pies, and scones can be ordered to accompany your gourmet coffee or tea selection. Brunch and lunch only. **Open daily. Limited service, gourmet coffee, take-out, VISA/MC/AMX, $$**

Moustache Pizza
405 Atlantic Ave., Brooklyn, NY 11217   **(718) 852-5555**
Middle Eastern. Behind this small neighborhood restaurant is a garden setting with tables and umbrellas. Bread is baked when ordered. **Open daily. Limited service, Turkish coffee, Mideastern citrus drink, mint tea, $**

Mr. Falafel Restaurant
226 Seventh Ave., Brooklyn, NY 11215   **(718) 768-4961**
Egyptian. **Open daily. Full service, Turkish coffee, cappucino, carrot juice, take-out, AMX, $**

Steve and Sons Bakery and Caterers, Inc.
9305 Church Ave., Brooklyn, NY 11212   **(718) 498-5800**
Ethnic/American. This is the home of the vegetarian patties or turnovers. You'll also find vegetarian stew, vegetarian barbecue ribs, vegetable steaks, and gluten in wine sauce. **Open for three meals Sunday through Thursday. Full service, fresh juices, beer, $$**

Taam Eden Restaurant
5001 13th Ave., Brooklyn, NY 11219   **(718) 972-1692**
Kosher. Features French service and a nice dining room. **Open daily for breakfast, lunch, and dinner. Full service and cafeteria style, wine, take-out, $$**

Weiss's Restaurant
1146 Coney Island Ave., Brooklyn, NY 11230   **(718) 421-0164**
Kosher. Kosher dairy cuisine with added vegetarian dishes such as Tofu Primavera, Vegetables & Linguine, and Vegetarian Chopped Liver. **Open Sunday through Thursday from 12 P.M. to 9:30 P.M.; in winter, open Saturday 90 minutes after sundown (after the Sabbath ends). Full service, egg cream, wine/beer/alcohol, catering, take-out, $$**

Who's on Seventh

183 Seventh Ave. (at Second Street), Brooklyn, NY 11215   (718) 765-0597
Natural foods. Enjoy natural sandwiches, soups, entrees, and juices. The restaurant, which also serves fish, is near the Seventh Avenue C/D/Q/F subway stops. **Full service, $$**

BUFFALO

Amy's Place

3234 Main St., Buffalo, NY 14214   (716) 832-6666
Natural foods/American/Middle Eastern. About one-half of the menu is vegetarian. **Open daily for three meals. Full service, take-out, $**

El Charro Mexican Restaurant

3447 Bailey Ave., Buffalo, NY 14215   (716) 837-5300
Mexican. El Charro serves tamales, empanadas, burritos, tacos, tostados. **Open daily. Full service, wine/beer/alcohol, catering, VISA/MC/AMX/DISC, $$$**

CANTON

• Willow Island

1 West Main, Canton, NY 13617   (315) 386-8822
Vegetarian/ethnic. Enjoy eating complete vegetarian cuisine on open or screened decks that overlook the Levasse River. Occasionally, there's live music. All desserts and breads are made on the premises with organic whole-wheat flour and maple syrup or honey. **Open Tuesday through Saturday for lunch and dinner. Closed Thanksgiving week and Christmas week. Full service, vegan options, wine/beer, catering, take-out, VISA/MC/AMX, $$**

GARDEN CITY

Akbar

One Ring Rd. West, Garden City, NY 11530
(On grounds of Roosevelt Field)   (516) 248-5700
Indian. Akbar has a good vegetarian selection with at least four vegan entrees; three others have some dairy. Spicy food is available. **Full service, vegan options, $$**

GREAT NECK

Earth's Harvest

5 Great Neck Rd., Great Neck, NY 11021   (516) 829-8605
Health-food-store counter. **Open daily. Limited service, macrobiotic options, VISA/MC, $**

Garden of Plenty

4 Wellwyn Rd., Great Neck, NY 11021   (516) 482-8868
Ethnic/Chinese. Offers unique vegetarian dishes like Sautéed Chinese Spinach, Snow White Chow Fun Rolls, Fish Fantasy (made out of bean curd), and Enoki Mushrooms. **$$**

U-8-2 Much

1739 Peninsula Blvd., Hewlett, NY 11557   **(516) 569-6888**

Chinese. Located in a shopping center where the towns of Valley Stream, Lynbrook, and Hewlett meet, this restaurant offers a tremendous selection of healthy Chinese dishes. Enjoy creative tofu and gluten dishes, vegetable or noodle entrees, delicious soups, brown rice, plus much more. **Open daily for lunch and dinner. Full service, completely vegan, fresh juices, take-out, VISA/MC/AMX, $$**

Jholla

36 Gerard St., Huntington, NY 1174   **(516) 385-7956**

Indian take-out. Jholla features Northwestern Indian cuisine with the emphasis on vegetarian food. **Open daily. Take-out only, $$**

Tortilla Grill

335 New York Ave., Huntington, NY 11743   **(516) 423-4141**

Mexican. This Mexican restaurant clearly indicates on the menu the dishes suitable for vegetarians. The beans do not contain lard. **Open Tuesday through Sunday for lunch and dinner. Closed Monday. Counter service, $**

ABC Cafe

308 Stewart Ave., Ithaca, NY 14850   **(607) 277-4770**

Natural foods. Also known as the Apple Blossom Cafe, it features free music Tuesday night, Sunday brunch, monthly art shows, seasonal menus. Vegetarian favorites include ABC Burger, Tempeh Reuben, Broccoli Cashew Stir-Fry. **Closed Monday and between Christmas and New Year's. Table service at dinner and brunch only. Counter service other times. Vegan/macrobiotic options, wide selection of coffee and espresso drinks, smoothies, wine/beer, take-out, $–$$**

Moosewood Restaurant ❧

DeWitt Building, Ithaca, NY 14850   **(607) 273-9610**

Natural foods. Moosewood serves gourmet and natural foods cuisine with ethnic specialties on Sunday nights. The cooperatively owned and managed restaurant offers homemade desserts, Bully Hill 100% New York State Grape Juice, and Yuengling beer, ale, and porter. The menu changes daily, rotating through the hundreds of dishes featured in the restaurant's four cookbooks. Friendly ambiance and seasonal outdoor terrace dining. **Open daily, with dinner only on Sunday. Full service, wine/beer, limited catering and take-out, VISA/MC, $$**

Charlies Restaurant

324 Forest Ave., Locust Valley, NY 11560   **(516) 676-6229**

American. Charlies offers pasta dishes, personalized pizzas, and calzones made with a whole-wheat crust, vegetarian sandwiches, and tofu dishes. **Open daily 4 P.M. to midnight. Full service, wine/beer/alcohol, take-out, VISA/MC/AMX/DISC, $$**

LONG ISLAND

For restaurants in this area, see Albertson, Amityville, Garden City, Great Neck, Hewlett, Huntington, Locust Valley, Medford, Merrick, Montauk, Oceanside, Sag Harbor, Seaford, West Hempstead, and Woodmere. For restaurant listings in the surrounding area, see New York City.

MANHATTAN

(For more restaurant listings in the surrounding areas, see New York City.)

Abyssinia Ethiopian Restaurant
35 Grand St., New York, NY 10013　　　　　　**(212) 226-5959**

Ethiopian. The Abyssinia Restaurant has the beguiling air of Ethiopia's 4000-year-old-culture. Its arched vaults and grass-cloth walls are adorned with artifacts from another time, with top African background music and wines. There are no utensils! Vegetarian dishes are eaten with a spongy bread as you sit on hand- carved wooden stools around colorful woven-basket tables called mesobs. All natural ingredients are used in cooking. **Open Monday through Friday for dinner, Saturday and Sunday for lunch and dinner. Full service, vegan options, wine/beer, catering, take-out, AMX, $$**

•• Angelica Kitchen ❧
300 E. 12th St., New York, NY 10003　　　　　　**(212) 228-2909**

Vegan/macrobiotic. This vegan restaurant uses 95 percent organic ingredients. Daily specials are offered along with excellent homemade cornbread and tahini dressing. Angelica's has been rated highly by many New Yorkers. **Open daily. Full service, vegan/macrobiotic options, fresh juices, smoothies,take-out, $$**

Apple Restaurant
17 Waverly Pl., New York, NY 10003　　　　　　**(212) 473-8888**

Ethnic. Lunch, dinner, and brunch are served. This restaurant uses separate cooking equipment when preparing vegetarian foods and features Karaoke sing-a-long. Though Apple serves plenty of meat dishes, there are many interesting natural food choices including Yam Tempura, Watercress Salad, Tempeh Burger, Stir-Fried Cabbage with Soba Noodles, BBQ Seitan, and more. **Open daily for lunch and dinner. Full service, wine/beer/alcohol, catering, take-out, VISA/MC/AMX, $$**

B & H Dairy Restaurant
127 Second Ave., New York, NY 10003   **(212) 505-8065**
Kosher. This vegetarian restaurant does serve fish. Home cooking includes omelettes, baked goods, sandwiches, salads, soups, and hot entrees such as Vegetarian
Stuffed Cabbage and Vegetarian Chili. Sandwiches, salads, and desserts round out
the menu at B & H, which offers daily soup and sandwich specials. **Open daily.**
Limited service, vegan options, fresh juices, take-out, no credit cards, $

•• Bachue
36 W. 21st St., New York, NY 10010   **(212) 229-0870**
Vegan/natural foods. New York City is fortunate to have a new vegan restaurant. Diners
can enjoy vegan breakfasts with items such as waffles, scrambled tofu, and a juice bar
including tropical shakes. Entrees during the day include many international items
such as Chickpea Crêpes, enchiladas, and empanadas. Organic grains and beans as
well as organic produce, when available, are used at this restaurant. Flour is ground
on the premises to make fresh bread. This new restaurant offers a breakfast and lunch
menu that is available until 6 P.M. Future plans include adding on an expanded dinner
menu. **Open Monday through Saturday for breakfast and lunch. Full service, vegan
options, catering, take-out, $$**

Benny's Burritos
93 Avenue A, New York, NY 10009   **(212) 254-3286**

113 Greenwich Ave., New York, NY 10014   **(212) 727-0584**
Mexican. Benny's serves Cal-Mex style cuisine emphasizing fresh vegetarian foods
in a fifties atmosphere. The food contains no preservatives, no lard, and no MSG.
Benny's uses non-dairy tofu sour cream, whole-wheat tortillas, and brown rice.
**Open daily for lunch and dinner. Full service, vegan options, wine/beer/alco-
hol, catering, take-out, $$$**

The Blue Nile Restaurant
103 W. 77th St., New York, NY 10024   **(212) 580-3232**
Ethiopian. This traditional Ethiopian restaurant offers vegetarian entrees and
appetizers. Enjoy its distinct decor of woven-basket-tables and hand-carved stools.
**Open daily for dinner, lunch Friday through Sunday. Full service, vegan options,
wine/beer, catering, take-out, AMX/DISC/DC, $$**

Boostan
85 MacDougal St., New York, NY 10012   **(212) 533-9561**
Natural foods. This restaurant is vegetarian with the exception of one fish dish.
Located in the heart of Greenwich Village, it offers an extensive menu, including
appetizers, soups, salads, sandwiches, pasta dishes, various entrees, and desserts.
Open daily for lunch and dinner. Full service, vegan options, catering, take-out, $$

🍴 Reviewers' choice   • Vegetarian restaurant   •• Vegan restaurant
$ less than $6 $$ $6–$12 $$$ more than $12
VISA/AMX/MC/DISC/DC—credit cards accepted
Non-alc.—Non-alcoholic   Fresh juices—freshly squeezed

• The Candle Cafe
1307 3rd Ave., New York, NY 10021   **(212) 472-0970**
Vegetarian/macrobiotic. You'll find Tofu Salad, watercress, Hummus, Tofu Burger, Spinach Tofu Roll, Broccoli Tofu Knish, daily specials such as Pasta with Peanut Sauce or Tempeh Stew and Stuffed Yam, and a variety of desserts and handmade breads. Sugar-free and dairy-free desserts are available. **Open for three meals Monday through Saturday. Limited service/take-out, vegan/macrobiotic options, VISA/MC, $$**

• Caravan of Dreams
405 E. 6th St., New York, NY 10009
(between First Avenue and Avenue A)   **(212) 254-1613**
Vegetarian/natural foods. This smoke-free restaurant is committed to using only organically grown ingredients whenever available, and to designing balanced dishes for healthful eating. Almost all foods are dairy-free, many are wheat-free, and the water is osmosis-filtered. Caravan offers completely vegetarian foods such as Black Bean Chili, Corn Polenta with Sweet Potato and Leek Sauce, and Grilled Marinated Tofu. It features live music nightly, art gallery, lectures, and various classes. **Open daily to midnight or later. Full service, vegan options, fresh juices, cappuccino/espresso, $-$$**

Good Food Cafe
401 Fifth Ave., New York, NY 10016   **(212) 686-3546**
Natural foods store/cafe and juice bar. This cafe serves healthful foods like Vegetarian Chili, Spinach Pie, Macrobiotic Plate, and Special Brown Rice and Veggies. **Open Monday through Saturday. Limited service, vegan/macrobiotic options, fresh juices, catering, take-out, VISA/MC/AMX, $**

Good Health Cafe
324 E. 86th St., New York, NY 10028   **(212) 439-9680**
Natural foods/ethnic. Foods are mostly dairy-free; some items are made with eggs. Middle Eastern, Mexican, Italian, and Japanese dishes are featured. **Open weekdays for lunch and dinner, weekends for brunch. Full service, fresh juices, non-alc. beer, delivery, take-out, VISA/MC/AMX/DC, $$**

The Great American Health Bar
76 Beaver St., New York, NY   **(212) 344-7522**

2 Park Ave., New York, NY   **(212) 685-7117**

821 Third Ave., New York, NY   **(212) 758-0883**

35 W. 57th St., New York, NY   **(212) 355-5177**
Natural foods/kosher. The Health Bar offers a wide variety of vegetarian entrees such as Eggplant Parmesan, Pizza of the Day, and Pasta of the Day and is know for its fresh-squeezed juices and homemade soups. Sandwiches include Hummus, Falafel, The Garden Patch, and Avocado. **Open daily. Full service, vegan options, fresh juices, catering, take-out, $**

Hana Restaurant
675 Ninth Ave., New York, NY 10036   **(212) 582-9742**

Korean/Japanese. Hana offers a separate vegetarian menu that includes Korean and Japanese specialties. The menu features Jap Cahe (vegetables with rice noodles), Hana Noodle (stir-fried noodles), Woo Dong (soup with noodles and vegetables), and four types of vegetarian sushi. **Open for lunch and dinner Monday through Saturday. Full service, vegan options, carrot juice, sake/plum wine/wine/beer, VISA/MC/AMX, $$**

The Health Nuts

1208 Second Ave., New York, NY 10021   (212) 593-0116

835 Second Ave., New York, NY 10017   (212) 490-2979

2611 Broadway, New York, NY 10025   (212) 678-0054

Natural foods. A natural deli and juice bar are situated inside a large health food store. Freshly prepared gourmet vegetarian salads, pasta, grains, hot foods, pizza, soups, pastries, cakes, and snacks are available. Sometimes a vegan cheese cake is offered! **Open daily. Counter service, vegan options, fresh juices, take-out, VISA/MC/AMX, $**

The Health Pub

371 Second Ave., New York, NY 10010   (212) 529-9200

Natural foods. A spacious dining area and leisurely pace are the hallmarks of this exceptional restaurant. Food is vegan, except for some salmon. Menu items include Marinated Grilled Tofu with Horseradish Dressing, Black Bean Chili with Cilantro and Tofu Sour Cream, Marinated Lima Beans with Fennel and Shallots, delicious desserts such as Lemon Pecan Tart, Hazelnut Carob Torte with Raspberry Sauce, and organic wines. **Open daily. Full service, vegan options, non-alc. beer, organic wine/beer, take-out, AMX, $$–$$$**

• House of Vegetarian

68 Mott St., New York, NY 10013   (212) 226-6572

Vegetarian/Chinese/macrobiotic. House of Vegetarian offers health food and brown rice. There's no meat, chicken, seafood, or MSG. The restaurant serves more than 200 dishes with many different meat imitations. There are assorted mock chicken dishes using pineapple, lemon, mango in season, yams, etc; mock iron steak, imitation fish, vegetarian egg rolls, and more. **Open daily. Full service, vegan/ macrobiotic options, take-out, $–$$**

Indian Delhi

392 Columbus Ave., New York, NY 10024   (212) 570-0962

Indian. Many items are dairy-free; only canola oil is used in cooking. Space is limited. **Open daily. Full service, vegan options, fresh carrot juice, wine/beer, take-out, $$$**

Life Cafe

343 E. 10th St., New York, NY 10009   (212) 477-9001

Natural foods/Cal-Mex. Possibly the hippest restaurant around, Life Cafe has plenty of local color and great food. It's tiny and fills up fast, but the food is worth the crowd. Many offerings are vegetarian or vegan. **Open daily for three meals, brunch on weekends. Full service, vegan options, fresh juice, wine/beer/alcohol, take-out, VISA/MC/DC/Carte Blanche, $$**

Luma

200 Ninth Ave., New York, NY 10011   **(212) 633-8033**

Natural foods/macrobiotic. Luma has an extensive vegetarian menu that uses many organic ingredients. **Open daily for dinner. Full service, catering, take-out, VISA/MC, $$$**

• Madras Mahal

104 Lexington Ave., New York, NY 10016   **(212) 684-4010**

Vegetarian/Indian/kosher. Madras Palace features South Indian kosher vegetarian cooking near Manhattan's Little India section. Dairy products are used but no eggs. **Open daily for lunch and dinner. Full service, vegan options, non-alc. beer, catering, take-out, VISA/MC/AMX/DC, $$**

Mana Restaurant

2444 Broadway, New York, NY 10024
(between 90th and 91st Sts.)   **(212) 787-1110**

Japanese. Mana is vegetarian except for fish and offers Japanese natural and macrobiotic cooking with no sugar, chemicals, preservatives, or dairy products. Filtered water and organic ingredients are used. **Open for lunch and dinner Monday through Saturday. Full service, vegan options, BYOB, take-out, no credit cards, $$**

Mizrachi Kosher Dairy Restaurant

105 Chambers St., New York, NY 10007   **(212) 964-2280**

Kosher/natural foods. Mizrachi provides a fresh salad bar, full breakfast menu, Middle Eastern and vegetarian dishes, different types of pizzas, plus many kinds of sandwiches and homemade soups. **Open for three meals Monday through Thursday, Friday for breakfast and lunch. Cafeteria style, fresh juices, catering, no credit cards, $**

The Natural Food Bar

166 West 72nd St., New York, NY 10023   **(212) 874-1213**

Kosher/natural foods. Vegetarian except for fish, the Natural Food Bar has an extensive vegetarian offering, including Tabouleh Salad, Baba Ghanouj, Veggie-Nut Burgers, and fresh-squeezed juices. It has a small sit-down bar and other limited seating. **Open Monday through Saturday from 8 A.M. to midnight, Sunday from 11 A.M. to 10 P.M. Limited/take-out service, fresh juices, $**

• The Natural Gourmet Cookery School's Friday Night Dinner Club

48 W. 21st St., Second Floor, New York, NY 1001   **(212) 645-5170**

☙ Reviewers' choice   • Vegetarian restaurant   •• Vegan restaurant
$ less than $6 $$ $6–$12 $$$ more than $12
VISA/AMX/MC/DISC/DC—credit cards accepted
Non-alc.–Non-alcoholic   Fresh juices—freshly squeezed

Vegetarian/natural foods. Enjoy a vegetarian meal (including seasonal vegetables) that has been carefully balanced so that it is sugar- and dairy- free, high in fiber and complex carbohydrates, low in fat, and cholesterol-free. **Open Friday only. Reservations required. Closed major holidays. Full service, BYOB, catering, take-out, VISA/MC, $$$**

Naturworks
200 A West 44th St., New York, NY 10036   **(212) 869-8335**
Natural foods. A wide variety of natural food is offered with an emphasis on vegetarian sandwiches, vegetarian soups, and quiche. Baked desserts, frozen yogurt, and non-dairy frozen desserts are available at reasonable prices, and there's a large selection of herbal teas. **Closed Sunday. Cafeteria style, vegan options, fruit juices, take-out, $**

Nawab Restaurant
256 E. 49th St., New York, NY 10017   **(212) 755-9100**
Indian. Serving Northern Indian cuisine, Nawab is open for lunch and dinner and offers a buffet. There's a vegetarian section on the menu and some vegetarian appetizers, soup, salads, and rice items. **Open daily. Full service, vegan options, wine/beer/alcohol, take-out, VISA/MC/AMX, $$–$$$**

Nirvana
30 Central Park South, New York, NY 10019   **(212) 486-5700**
Indian. Near the Fifty-seventh Street N/R and B/Q subway stops, Nirvana has a terrific view north into Central Park. **Formal, full service, $$$**

Nosmo King
54 Varick St., New York, NY 10013   **(212) 966-1239**
Contemporary American. Organically grown food is used, although there are many non-vegetarian dishes. The restaurant uses litttle or no dairy and features such gourmet items as Napolean of Asparagus with Wild Mushrooms. **Open for lunch Monday through Friday, dinner daily. Full service, reservations recommended, fresh juices, wine/beer/alcohol, VISA/MC/AMX, lunch–$$, dinner–$$$**

Nutrisserie
142 W. 72nd St., New York, NY 10023   **(212) 721-3039**
Natural foods. This health food deli and store has an organic juice bar with an extensive vegetarian menu. **Open daily for three meals. Cafeteria style, fresh juices, catering, take-out, VISA/MC/AMX, $**

Ozu Restaurant
566 Amsterdam Ave., New York, NY 10024   **(212) 787-8316**
Macrobiotic. A primarily Japanese menu includes soups, breads, salads, and entrees featuring tofu, grains, noodles, tempura, and vegetables. Fish is also served here as are daily entree and dessert specials. **Open daily. Full service, vegan/macrobiotic options, beer/organic wine, take-out, VISA/MC, $$**

• Plum Tree Vegetarian Restaurant
1501 First Ave., New York, NY 10021   **(212) 734-1412**
Vegetarian/natural foods/macrobiotic. Plum Tree has served vegetarian, macrobiotic,

and vegan cuisine since 1981. The menu includes items such as Azuki and Black Bean Soup, Fire Dragon Chili, Macro-Ratatouille, and Vegetable Crêpes. **Open for lunch and dinner Tuesday through Sunday, closed Monday. Full service, vegan/macrobiotic options, fresh juices, take-out, no credit cards, $$**

Pravine Gourmet Ice Cream
27 St. Marks Pl., New York, NY 10003   **(212) 673-5948**

193 Bleecker St., New York, NY 10012   **(212) 475-1968**

American. If you find yourself in Manhattan searching for a great place to get dessert, try Pravine Gourmet Ice Cream shops. They offer several flavors of Tofutti (vegan ice cream), soy "egg" creams, soy cappuccino, and soy milk shakes. **Open from noon to midnight daily. Counter service, vegan options, take-out, $**

Pumpkin Eater
2452 Broadway, New York, NY 10024   **(212) 877-0132**

Natural foods/juice bar. Located not too far from Columbia University, Pumpkin Eater is usually busy. **Open daily for lunch and dinner. Full service, wine/beer, catering, take-out, AMX, $$**

Quantum Leap
88 W. Third St., New York, NY 10012   **(212) 677-8050**

Natural foods. Many tasty vegan and vegetarian dishes are served in this relaxed and homey atmosphere, natural pies and house dressing, too. **Full service, $$**

Ratner's
138 Delancey St., New York, NY 10002   **(212) 677-5588**

Dairy restaurant. This eatery is near Delancey Street F subway stop and Essex Street J/M subway stop. **Full service, $$**

• Sacred Chow
522 Hudson St., New York, NY 10014   **(212) 337-0863**

Vegetarian. Although pricey, this gourmet foods store is definitely worth checking out. Almost completely vegan, except for the occasional use of honey, gourmet dishes include fennel soysage with roasted garlic tomatoes; dill pickle tempeh with juniper berries and tarragon; and grilled vegetables, seitan robai, and wheat berries with tamarind glaze. Fresh-made juices and milks include orange blossom almond milk and organic orange juice. **Open daily for lunch and dinner. Limited service, vegan options, take-out, VISA/MC/AMX, $$**

The Salad Bowl
A and S Plaza, Floor 7
901 Sixth Ave., New York, NY 10001   **(212) 594-6512**

721 Lexington Ave., New York, NY 10022   **(212) 752-7201**

906 Third Ave., New York, NY 10022   **(212) 644-6767**

South Street Seaport Pier 17, New York, NY 10022   **(212) 693-0590**

Natural foods. Vegetarian sandwiches, soups, and salads are offered at this cafe. All foods are home-cooked. **Open daily. Cafeteria style, fresh juices, catering, take-out, $$**

Scallions
48 Trinity Pl., New York, NY 10006   **(212) 480-9135**
Natural foods/juice bar. Scallions is a health food restaurant specializing in dishes that are low in fat, cholesterol, and sodium. **Open for three meals Monday through Friday from 7:30 A.M. to 7 P.M. Fresh juices, catering, take-out, $**

•• Shojin
23 Commerce St., New York, NY 10014   **(212) 989-3530**
Vegan/Japanese. Known for Tofu Pie, this restaurant serves entrees such as Sweet & Sour Tofu, Tempura, Gluten Cutlet, and Okara Burgers. Absolutely no animal products are used. Malt is used as a sweetener. **Open for dinner Monday through Saturday, closed Sunday. Full service, take-out, $$**

Souen Restaurant
28 E. 13th St., New York, NY 10003   **(212) 627-7150**
Macrobiotic/natural foods. Sample various seitan, tofu, and tempeh entrees, plus appetizers, soups, salads, tempura, and noodle dishes with option of udon or soba noodles. Fish is also served here, and there are indoor and outdoor gardens. **Open daily. Full service, vegan/macrobiotic options, fresh juices, organic coffee, organic wine/beer, take-out, VISA/MC/AMX, $$–$$$**

Spring Street Natural
62 Spring St., New York, NY 10012
(Corner of Lafayette)   **(212) 966-0290**
Natural foods. Enjoy vegetarian soups, salads, entrees, and even some sugar-free and dairy-free desserts. **Open daily. Full service, fresh juices, cappuccino/espresso, catering, take-out, VISA/MC/AMX, $$**

St. Mark's Pizza
23 Third Ave., New York, NY 10003   **(212) 420-9531**
Pizza. In the heart of the East Village, this local corner pizza place has a wide variety of vegetarian pizzas. **Limited service, take-out, $**

Temple in the Village Restaurant
74 W. Third St., New York, NY 10012   **(212) 475-5670**
Natural foods/macrobiotic. This small buffet-style health food restaurant for macrobiotics and vegetarians serves vegetables, noodles, five–seven grain rice, and teas. All foods are prepared on the premises. Seating is limited. **Open for lunch and dinner Monday through Saturday. Cafeteria style, BYOB, catering, take-out, $**

• Vegetarian Heaven
304 W. 58th St., New York, NY 10019
(4 Columbus Circle)   **(212) 956-4678**
Vegetarian/kosher/Chinese. Enjoy vegetarian dishes such as Shredded Beef with Basil, Chicken with Sesame Sauce, or Sweet and Sour Pork, all made from soybean protein, all completely vegetarian. Other dishes include Eggplant in Spicy Sauce, Vegetable Tempura, and Bean Noodle Slice with Vegetables. This restaurant serves numerous vegan dishes as well. It's near the Columbus Circle stop of the

A/B/C/D/1/9 subways. **Open daily for lunch and dinner. Reservations required. Full service, fresh juice, BYOB, catering, take-out, VISA/MC, $$**

• Vegetarian Paradise 3

33–35 Mott St., New York, NY 10013 (212) 406-6988

Vegetarian. Located in the heart of Chinatown, this restaurant is kin to VP2 (see that entry for description).

Village Natural Food Corp.

46 Greenwich Ave., New York, NY 10011 (212) 727-0968

Natural foods. This spacious Greenwich Village restaurant offers whole grains only, and has daily specials. **Full service, take-out, $$**

•• VP2 🐾

144 W. 4th St., New York, NY 10012 (212) 260-7141

Vegan. Extensive menu features exquisite Chinese vegetarian cuisine. The menu includes hot and cold appetizers, salads, desserts, and many entree categories such as bean curd, greens, mock meat, mushroom, wheat gluten, noodle, and rice. Hot clay pots and house specials such as Taro Whole Fish (vegetarian), Stuffed Lotus Leaf, and Spinach Dumpling are featured. It's not to be missed!! You'll find it near the West Fourth Street subway stop on the A/B/C/D/E/F trains. **Open for lunch and dinner daily. Full service, vegan options, fresh juices, catering, take-out, VISA/MC/AMX, $$**

•• VP-2-GO

140 W. 4th St., New York, NY 10012 (212) 260-7049

Vegan take-out. Enjoy outstanding vegetarian fare at excellent prices. The take-out menu lists thirty-five items from Fried Taro Dumplings to Stuffed Lotus Leaf to Lemon Tofu Pudding plus 100-percent vegetarian authentic Dim Sum "like nowhere else in NYC." Wholesale and retail foods are available at this location. **Open daily. Cafeteria style, vegan options, catering, take-out, VISA/MC/AMX, $**

• Whole Earth Bakery and Kitchen

70 Spring St., New York, NY 10012 (212) 226-8280

Vegetarian bakery. Enjoy fresh baked goods that are predominately vegan. Menu includes muffins, cookies, brownies, and much more. Some sandwiches are also offered. **Open daily. Vegan options, take-out, $**

Whole Foods in SoHo

117 Prince St., New York, NY 10012 (212) 673-5388

Health food store and deli. Whole Foods features gourmet natural take-out, deli, and a salad bar. **Open daily. Take-out, VISA/MC/AMX/DISC, $**

🐾 Reviewers' choice   • Vegetarian restaurant   •• Vegan restaurant
$ less than $6 $$ $6–$12 $$$ more than $12
VISA/AMX/MC/DISC/DC—credit cards accepted
Non-alc.—Non-alcoholic   Fresh juices—freshly squeezed

Whole Wheat 'N Wild Berrys
57 W. Tenth St., New York, NY 10011   **(212) 677-3410**
Natural foods. Enjoy items such as Nutburgers, Manicotti, Black Bean Sauté, and
Vegetarian Chili. This small restaurant located near the IND West Fourth Street
station (A/B/C/D/E/F trains) recently celebrated its seventeenth anniversary.
**Open daily for lunch and dinner. Full service, wine/beer/alcohol, catering,
AMX, $$**

Yaffa Cafe
97 Saint Marks Place, New York, NY 10009   **(212) 674-9302**
Natural foods. In this bohemian atmosphere, vegetarian dishes include crêpes, stir
fry, tofu, Baba Ghanouj, salads, and Hummus. There's garden seating during the
summer, as well as a sidewalk cafe. **Open 24 hours daily. Full service, vegan
options, fresh juices, wine/beer, take-out, AMX, $$**

• Zen Palate ✿
663 Ninth Ave., New York, NY 10036 (at 46th street)   **(212) 582-1669**

34 Union Square East, New York, NY 10003   **(212) 614-9345**
Vegetarian/Chinese. Zen Palate offers dishes like Stuffed Cabbage Deluxe, Vegetarian Squid, and Stir-fried Brown Rice with Vegetables. **Open daily for lunch and
dinner. Full service and cafeteria, vegan options, fresh juices, take-out, VISA/
MC/AMX, $–$$**

Zucchini
1336 First Ave., New York, NY 10021   **(212) 249-0559**
Natural foods. The restaurant will cook to order any special dietary requests. Only
olive oil is used in cooking and salads. Items include Baked Stuffed Zucchini,
Four-Bean Vegetarian Chili, and Four-Cheese Zucchini-Spinach Lasagna. **Open
daily for lunch and dinner except in July and August for dinner only. Full service,
catering, take-out, VISA/MC/AMX, $$**

MANLIUS

• Incredible Edibles
209 E. Seneca St., Manlius, NY 13104   **(315) 682-6684**
Vegetarian/natural foods store. This natural-foods-store deli sells all-vegetarian
lunches. Spanikopita, Hummus, hot soups, pasta salad, Tofu Lasagna, egg rolls,
and more are on the menu. There are also cooking classes, massage, and poetry
readings. **Open Tuesday through Saturday. Limited service, vegan options,
macrobiotic options, fresh juices, limited catering, take-out, $**

MEDFORD

Salad Bowl
1699 J Rt. 112, Medford, NY 11763   **(516) 475-1810**
Natural foods. See description under Manhattan.

MERRICK

Tortilla Grill
53 Merrick Ave., Merrick, NY 11566   **(516) 546-4141**
Mexican. See entry under Huntington.

MONTAUK

Naturally Good Foods & Cafe
S. Essex St., Montauk, NY 11954   **(516) 668-9030**
Natural-foods-store cafe. Breakfast, lunch, and dinner are available at this cafe where
you'll also find a deli case, take-out, fresh baked goods daily, fruit smoothies, and
a natural foods store. **Open daily. Limited service, vegan/macrobiotic options,
fresh juices, take-out, AMX, $**

NEW PALTZ

• Wildflower Cafe
18 Church St., New Paltz, NY 12561   **(914) 255-0020**
Vegetarian. Enjoy a nice inside/outside atmosphere with occasional live classical
guitar music while sampling a wide variety of dishes and specials. **Call for hours.
Closed Wednesday. Full service, wine/beer/alcohol, take-out, no credit cards, $$**

NEW YORK CITY

*New York City actually consists of the five boroughs of Manhattan,
Queens, Brooklyn, Bronx, and Staten Island. Most tourists tend to go to
Manhattan, which is generally referred to as New York City. There are
many, many restaurants in Manhattan. If you visit New York, it is easiest
to explore the large variety of restaurants in Manhattan rather than go
off to other areas. You actually can have a fun walk across the Brooklyn
Bridge to Brooklyn, and with a tour guide map find Brooklyn Heights
where there are numerous natural foods restaurants. You can also travel
to other boroughs—except Staten Island—relatively easily by subway. If you
choose to visit other places using mass transit, we would recommend that
you start with Queens and Brooklyn. (Though part of New York City
politically and via mass transit, these boroughs are geographically on
Long Island.)*

*If you have a car, you can visit restaurants on Long Island. This can
end up being a one- to three-hour drive, depending on traffic and how far
out on Long Island you are going. If you are willing to make the trip, see
entries under Albertson, Amityville, Garden City, Great Neck, Hewlett,
Huntington, Locust Valley, Medford, Montauk, Oceanside, Sag Harbor,
Seaford, West Hempstead, and Woodmere.*

*Some New Jersey cities are also within the vicinity of Manhattan. See
entries under Colonia, East Rutherford, Hoboken, Montclair, and New-*

ark. Hoboken and Newark can be reached by "PATH" trains from Manhattan. Buses also go from Manhattan to New Jersey cities.

For detailed listings of restaurants in New York City or the surrounding areas, refer to the individual boroughs or the areas listed above.

NYACK

Harvest Moon Cafe

3 South Broadway, Nyack, NY 10960   **(914) 353-1555**
Natural foods. This smoke-free cafe offers organic items when available, whole-grain dishes, salads, and more. **Open Wednesday through Sunday for lunch and dinner and Tuesday for lunch and dinner during the summer only. Full service, take-out, VISA/MC/AMX, $$**

OCEANSIDE

Prima Pasta

3450 Long Beach Rd, Oceanside, NY 11572   **(516) 536-7660**
Pasta restaurant. This small, cozy pasta restaurant features nineteen entrees, at least six are vegan. Calories, protein, and fat content are listed for Pasta Delites. **Full service, take-out, $$**

OLIREREA

Mountain Gate Indian Restaurant

212 Mc Kinky Hollow Road, Olirerea, NY 12410   **(914) 254-6000**
Ethnic/Indian. Mountain Gate offers a vegetarian buffet and features outdoor dining and hiking trails. **Open daily for lunch and dinner. Full service, wine/ beer/alcohol, take-out, VISA/MC/AMX/DISC/DC, $$**

ONEONTA

The Autumn Cafe

244 Main St., Oneonta, NY 13820   **(607) 432-6845**
Natural foods. This American bistro offers daily specials and uses whole foods. All items are prepared on the premises. **Open daily Tuesday through Saturday from 11 A.M. to 9 P.M.; Sunday brunch, 11 A.M. to 3 P.M. Full service, wine/beer, catering, take-out, VISA/MC/AMX, $—lunch $$—dinner**

QUEENS

(For more restaurant listings in the surrounding areas, see New York City.)

• Annam Brahma Restaurant

84-43 164 St., Jamaica Hills, NY 11432   **(718) 523-2600**
Ethnic/Indian. This completely vegetarian restaurant offers dishes such as Vegetable Kabob, Vegetarian Casserole, and samosas. **Open daily for lunch and dinner. Full service, vegan options, fresh juices, catering, take-out, $–$$**

• Bamboo Garden
41-28 Main St., Flushing, NY 11355 (718) 463-9240

Vegetarian/kosher/Chinese. In the Golden Shopping Mall, Bamboo Garden offers 116 choices served with brown or white rice. Food contains no MSG or dairy. **Open daily. Full service, vegan options, VISA/MC, $–$$**

Hunan Dynasty
271-01 Union Turnpike, New Hyde Park, NY 11040 (718) 962-6868

Ethnic/Hunan. Enjoy such vegetarian options as Moo Shu Vegetables, Eggplant with Garlic Sauce, Bean Curd with Brown Sauce. **Open daily for lunch and dinner. Full service, catering, take-out, VISA/MC/AMX, $$**

India Corner
178-19 Union Turnpike, Flushing, NY 11366 (718) 523-9682

Indian. This restaurant specializes in Northern Indian cuisine. **Open daily except Tuesday. Full service, catering, take-out, VISA/MC/AMX/DISC, $$**

Quantum Leap
65-64 Fresh Meadows Lane, Fresh Meadow, NY 11365 (718) 461-1307

Natural foods/health foods store. See description under Manhattan.

The Salad Bowl
24-20 Jackson Ave., Long Island City, NY 11101 (718) 786-1002

Natural foods. See The Salad Bowl listing under Manhattan.

• Smile of the Beyond
86-14 Parsons Blvd., Jamaica, NY 11432 (718) 739-7453

Vegetarian. Smile of the Beyond started as an ice cream parlor and now sells predominantly traditional American breakfast items plus brown rice veggie salad, mock meats, rice, and salads. **Open daily 7 A.M. to 4 P.M., closed Sunday. Counter service, fresh juices, take-out, $**

ROCHESTER

Aladdin's Natural Eatery
646 Monroe Ave., Rochester, NY 14607 (716) 442-5000

141 State St., Rochester, NY 14614 (716) 546-5000

Natural foods. Aladdin's offers great soups, sandwiches, pasta dishes, salads, and more. **Open for three meals daily. Full service, fresh juices, beer/wine, vegan options, take-out, $–$$**

🕿 Reviewers' choice • Vegetarian restaurant •• Vegan restaurant
$ less than $6 $$ $6–$12 $$$ more than $12
VISA/AMX/MC/DISC/DC—credit cards accepted
Non-alc.—Non-alcoholic Fresh juices—freshly squeezed

Alexi's Restaurant
680 Monroe Ave., Rochester, NY 14607   **(716) 244-1444**
Italian. Vegetarians can dine on a wide variety of gourmet pizzas (whole-wheat crust is available), salads, pasta dishes, Eggplant Parmesan, and Cheese Calzones at Alexi's Restaurant. **Open for lunch and dinner daily. Full service, take-out, $$**

Mamasan's Restaurant
309 University Ave., Rochester, NY 14607   **(716) 262-4580**
Vietnamese. Try vermicelli and noodle salads, vegetable salads, curries, and more at this restaurant. **Open Monday through Saturday for lunch and dinner. Closed Sunday. Full service, take-out, $$**

Shalimar Palace
470 W. Ridge Rd., Rochester, NY 14615   **(716) 621-6900**
Indian. Approximately ten vegetarian dishes are offered at this Indian restaurant. **Open for lunch and dinner daily. Full service, vegan options, take-out, $$**

• Slice of Life Cafe
742 South Ave., Rochester, NY 14620   **(716) 271-8010**
Vegetarian. Munch on an udon-style salad or feast on Bean Burritos, Curried Veggies over rice, scrambled tofu, veggie burgers, Tempeh Ruby, or a Primavera Sub at Slice of Life Cafe. **Open Tuesday through Saturday for three meals. Open for brunch Sunday. Closed Monday. Full service, vegan options, catering, take-out, $**

SAG HARBOR

Provisions of Sag Harbor, Ltd.
Bay & Divisions St., Sag Harbor, NY 11963   **(516) 725-3636**
Natural foods/health-food-store deli. In this homey atomosphere, you'll find a salad bar with organic lettuce, and such natural meals as Scrambled Tofu, Organic Vegetable Pot Pie, and Tempeh Rueben. **Open daily for breakfast, lunch, and early dinner. Full service, vegan options, organic carrot juice, fresh juices, VISA/MC/AMX, $-$$**

SARATOGA SPRINGS

• Four Seasons Natural Foods Cafe
33 Phila St., Saratoga Springs, NY 12866   **(518) 584-4670**
Vegetarian. A wide range of vegetarian and vegan dishes is offered in addition to a salad bar. **Open for lunch and dinner Monday through Saturday. Open for lunch Sunday. Limited service, fresh juices, vegan options, catering, take-out, VISA/MC/DISC, $$**

SCARSDALE

• Mrs. Green's Natural Market
365 Central Park Ave., Scarsdale, NY 10583   **(914) 472-9675**
Vegetarian/health food store/juice bar. **Open daily. Vegan options.**

SEA CLIFF
Ken's Place
64 Roslyn Ave., Sea Cliff, NY 11579 **(516) 674-3752**
California style. Try the vegetable moussaka, vegetarian pizza, or Ken's vegan feast for two—baba ghanouj, taboule potato bread, and organic vegetable salad. **Open Tuesday through Friday for lunch and dinner. Saturday and Sunday dinner only. Full service, vegan options, fresh juices, smoothies, VISA/MC, $$**

SEAFORD
• Earth's Harvest Natural Market
1244 Hicksville Rd., Seaford, NY 11783 **(516) 797-0700**
Vegetarian/health food store. See Earth's Harvest under Great Neck.

STATEN ISLAND

(For more restaurant listings in the surrounding areas, see New York City.)

Dairy Palace
2210 Victory Blvd., Staten Island, NY 10314 **(718) 761-5200**
Kosher/dairy restaurant. This pizza and dairy restaurant features a Chinese menu, mock-meat dishes, and ice cream bar. **Open Sunday through Thursday for lunch and dinner, open Friday from 11 A.M. until sunset, open after sundown Saturday night until 12:30 A.M. Cafeteria style, vegan options, $$**

Taste of India Restaurant
287 New Dorp Lane, Staten Island, NY 10306 **(718) 987-4700**
Indian. Taste of India features Saturday and Sunday buffet with at least two vegetarian options. There are nine vegetarian specials, and coconut soup flavored with almond and pistachio is vegetarian. **Open daily. Full service, wine/beer/alcohol, take-out, VISA/MC/AMX, $$**

SUFFERN
New Harvest Natural Foods
41 Lafayette Ave. (Rt. 59 West), Suffern, NY 10901 **(914) 357-9200**
Natural foods deli and juice bar. With a 1950s diner atmosphere, this establishment offers special vegetarian entrees daily, soups, and baked goods. **Open daily for lunch. Counter service, vegan options, take-out, fresh juices, VISA/MC, $**

SYRACUSE
King David Restaurant
129 Marshall St., Syracuse, NY 13210 **(315) 471-5000**
Middle Eastern. This Middle Eastern style restaurant is in the heart of the Syracuse University area. **Open daily for lunch and dinner, closed one day a week. Full service, wine/beer, VISA/MC/AMX, $$**

UTICA

The Phoenician Restaurant
623 French, Utica, NY 13413   **(315) 733-2709**
Middle Eastern. Vegetarian platters include Falafel, Fattoush, Tabouleh, and other Middle Eastern items. **Closed Sunday. Full service, wine/beer, VISA/MC, take-out, $**

WARWICK

• West St. Whole Foods, Ltd.
80 Ryerson Rd., Warwick, NY 10990   **(914) 986-3669**
Vegetarian/health-food-store deli. You'll find sandwiches and fresh baked goods every day, and fresh bread on Saturday. **Open Monday through Saturday. Limited service, fresh juices, take-out, $**

WEST HEMPSTEAD

Taj Mahal Restaurant
221 Hempstead Turnpike, W. Hempstead, NY 11552   **(516) 565-4607**
Ethnic. **Open daily for dinner, lunch Monday through Saturday. Full service, wine/beer/alcohol, VISA/MC/AMX, $$**

WILLIAMSVILLE

• Earth Spirit
5548 Main St., Williamsville, NY 14221   **(716) 634-5510**
Vegetarian deli and juice bar. A group of ecologists opened this establishment in 1993. Organic produce is used when available. Try one of the veggie burgers, hummus sandwiches, pizzas, or salads. **Open Monday through Saturday for lunch. Limited service, fresh juices, vegan options, $**

Pizza Plant
8020 Transit Rd., Williamsville, NY 14221   **(716) 632-0800**
Pizza/ethnic. Vegetarian items on the menu are indicated by a carrot. Choices include Nachos, Chili, Bread Bowl Stew, and a wide variety of pizzas. Whole-wheat dough and sesame, spinach, or garlic doughs are available. **Open daily. Full service, wine/beer, take-out, VISA/MC/AMX/DISC, $$**

WOODMERE

Earth's Harvest
1002 Broadway, Woodmere, NY 11598   **(516) 295-1505**
Health-food-store counter. See entry under Great Neck.

NORTH CAROLINA

ASHEVILLE

Cafe Max & Rosie's
52 N. Lexington Ave., Asheville, NC 28801   (704) 254-5342
Natural foods. Dine on a number of vegetarian and vegan dishes at Cafe Max & Rosie's including a veggie burger, Tempeh Parmigiana Sub, Fresh Fruit Fantasy, Mideast Bean Pita, Vegan Veggie Pita, Fried Rice, plus much more. **Open for breakfast and lunch Monday through Wednesday. Open for three meals Thursday through Saturday. Closed Sunday. Full service, vegan options, fresh juices, smoothies, take-out, $**

Dinner for the Earth
160 Broadway, Asheville, NC 28801   (704) 253-7656
Natural foods deli. Many vegetarian options are available at this natural foods deli. **Open daily. Counter service, vegan options, take-out, $**

• Laughing Seed Cafe
40 Wall St., Asheville, NC 28801   (704) 252-3445
Vegetarian. Enjoy a wide variety of international vegetarian dishes including a Caribbean Quesadilla, Mid-Eastern Pita Sandwich, Greek Salad, Kung Pao Tofu, Tempeh Fajitas, and more. Indoor and outdoor seating available. **Open for three meals Monday through Saturday and brunch on Sundays. Full service, fresh juices, vegan/macrobiotic options, take-out, VISA/MC/DISC, $$**

CARRBORO

• Govinda's
102 E. Main St., Carrboro, NC 27510   (919) 942-7262
Vegetarian. Enjoy a wide range of international vegetarian dishes and a juice bar at this restaurant. **Open daily for lunch and dinner. Full service, fresh juices, espresso/cappuccino, vegan options, take-out, VISA/MC, $–$$**

CHAPEL HILL

Pyewacket Restaurant 🍜
The Courtyard, 431 W. Franklin St.
Chapel Hill, NC 27516   (919) 929-0297
Natural foods. Vegetarian options are available. **Open daily. Full service, fresh juices, wine/beer/alcohol, take-out, VISA/MC/AMX/DC, $$**

CHARLOTTE

Berrybrook Farm Natural Foods
1257 East Blvd., Charlotte, NC 28203   (704) 334-6528
Natural foods take-out. Homemade soups, salads, and sandwiches are made fresh daily at this natural food grocery and deli. The menu at Berrybrook changes daily

and is primarily vegetarian. **Closed Sunday. Take-out only, vegan options, fresh juices, VISA/MC/DISC, $**

Cafe Verde at Talley's Green Grocery
1408-C East Blvd., Charlotte, NC 28203   **(704) 334-9200**
Natural foods. Ethnic, low-fat vegetarian, vegan, and non-vegetarian dishes are offered in addition to daily soups, a wonderful salad bar, sandwiches, and desserts made without refined sugars. Enjoy the best selection of beers in town. **Open daily. Cafeteria style, vegan options, fresh juices, wine/beer/alcohol, take-out, VISA/MC, $**

Delphi
7211-14 E. Independence Blvd., Charlotte, NC 28227   **(704) 536-9899**
Greek. Vegetarian specialties include spinach puffs, falafel, stuffed grape leaves, and a vegetable pita sandwich. **Open Monday through Saturday for lunch and dinner. Full service, take-out, VISA/MC, $**

Dragon Inn Chinese Restaurant
204A W. Woodlawn Rd., Charlotte, NC 28217   **(704) 503-3900**
Chinese. Dragon Inn features Cantonese-, Hunan-, and Szechuan-style vegetarian options. MSG is omitted upon request. **Open daily. Full service, vegan options, wine/beer, take-out, VISA/MC/AMX/DISC, $$**

House of Chinese Gourmet
5608 Independence Blvd., Charlotte, NC 28212   **(704) 563-8989**
Chinese. Here's a deliciously inviting menu with over twenty vegetarian entrees, plus soups and appetizers. Many tofu dishes are available, and MSG is omitted upon request. **Open daily. Full service, vegan options, wine/beer/alcohol, take-out, VISA/MC/AMX, $$**

India Palace
6140 E. Independence Blvd., Charlotte, NC 28212   **(704) 568-7176**
Indian. Authentic Indian cuisine is offered, and great care is taken in the preparation and use of spices. Nine vegetable entrees are on the menu. **Open daily for dinner. Full service, vegan options, take-out, VISA/MC/AMX, $$**

La Paz Restaurant
523 Frenton Pl., Charlotte, NC 28210   **(704) 372-4168**
Mexican. La Paz does not use lard or meat in the black beans, rice, and refried beans. It offers a variety of vegetarian entrees including Whole Wheat Pesto Tortillas, Whole Wheat Red Chile Tortillas, Veggie Burritos, and Roasted Corn and Zucchini Tamales. **Open daily for dinner. Full service, vegan options, non-alc. beer/wine, beer/wine/alcohol, VISA/MC/AMX/DISC/DC, $$**

People's Natural Food Market Deli
617 S. Sharon Amity Rd., Charlotte, NC 28211 **(704) 364-3891**
Natural-foods-store deli. Located in a natural foods store, this deli offers salads, sandwiches, smoothies, and more. **Open for lunch Monday through Saturday. Closed Sunday. Limited service, fresh juices, vegan options, take-out, non-alc. beer/wine, beer/wine/alcohol, VISA/MC, $**

Pewter Rose
1820 South Blvd. #109, Charlotte, NC 28203 **(704) 332-8149**
Seasonal. Fresh, eclectic cuisine is served in an airy but cozy atmosphere. There are limited vegetarian options, primarily appetizers. **Open daily for lunch and dinner. Full service, wine/beer/alcohol, take-out, VISA/MC/AMX, $$**

Thai Cuisine Restaurant
4800 Central Ave., Charlotte, NC 2820 **(704) 532-7511**
Thai. Tofu is substituted for the meat in any dish to create delicious vegetarian options. There are some vegetarian appetizers, salads, and soup. No MSG or salt is used in the preparation of food. **Open daily. Full service, vegan options, wine/beer/alcohol, take-out, VISA/MC/AMX, $$**

DURHAM

Anotherthyme
109 N. Gregson St., Durham, NC 27701 **(919) 682-5225**
Seasonal. Enjoy gourmet seasonal cuisine with pasta, vegetarian, and non-vegetarian dishes. No red meat is served. **Open daily. Full service, fresh juices, wine/beer/alcohol, take-out, VISA/MC/AMX, $$–$$$**

GREENSBORO

Sunset Cafe
4608 W. Market St., Greensboro, NC 27407 **(919) 855-0349**
Natural foods. A blackboard menu changes daily. At least four of the sixteen entrees are vegetarian and some are vegan. Examples include Russian Cheese Dumplings, Vegetarian Cheese Nut Loaf, Rice and Cheese Croquettes, Grilled Vegetable Kabobs, Vegetarian Lasagna, Spinach Manicotti, and more. **Open daily. Full service, vegan options, wine/beer/alcohol, take-out, VISA/MC, $$**

HILLSBOROUGH

The Regulator Cafe
108 S. Churton St., Hillsborough, NC 27278 **(919) 732-5600**
New American. Located in a restored historic home that George Washington slept in, this cafe serves new American cuisine with a combination of vegetarian and other health-conscious foods. Pasta, tempeh dishes, salads, and appetizers make up the vegetarian selection. **Open daily. Full service, vegan options, wine/beer, take-out, VISA/MC/DISC, $$**

RALEIGH

Irregardless Cafe

901 W. Morgan St., Raleigh, NC 27603   **(919) 833-8898**

Natural foods. A new menu each night features vegetarian, vegan, and non-vegetarian entrees. Fresh baked breads, cookies, and desserts are also available in this totally non-smoking environment. **Open daily, Sunday brunch. Full service, vegan options, espresso/cappuccino, wine/beer/alcohol, take-out, VISA/MC/AMX, $–$$**

WINSTON-SALEM

Rainbow News & Cafe

712 Brookstown Ave., Winston-Salem, NC 27101   **(919) 723-0858**

Cafe. This European-style cafe offers homemade soups, salads, sandwiches, and desserts. **Open for three meals daily. Full service, wine/beer, VISA/MC, $$**

The Rose and Thistle

107 Lockland Ave., Winston-Salem, NC 27103   **(919) 725-6444**

American. The Rose and Thistle features such vegetarian entrees as pizza, Vegetable Medley, eggplant subs, and five salads. **Open daily, dinner served only on Saturday. Full service, fresh juices, non-alc. beer, beer/wine, take-out, $–$$**

NORTH DAKOTA

BISMARCK

Green Earth Cafe

208 E. Broadway, Bismarck, ND 58501   **(701) 223-8646**

Natural foods. Green Earth features daily specials with vegetarian and ethnic options. Co-located with One World Coffeehouse. **Open for coffee and lunch Monday through Saturday, dinner Friday through Saturday. Limited service, catering, take-out, $**

OHIO

AKRON

Mustard Seed Market Cafe

3885 W. Market Street, Akron, OH 44333   **(216) 666-7333**

Natural foods/macrobiotic. Mustard Seed Market is one of the largest natural foods stores in the Midwest. The restaurant located in the store offers great natural foods dishes. There is a strong emphasis on vegetarian dishes including macrobiotic and vegan meals. Some seafood and poultry are also served. Mustard Seed Market emphasizes organic foods and has the best produce department in town. **Open daily for lunch, Tuesday through Saturday for dinner. Full service, vegan options, fresh juice, beer/wine, catering, take-out, VISA/MC, $$**

CALCUTTA

• Ely's Food for Thought
15655 State Rt. 170, Calcutta, OH 43920   **(216) 385-3597**
Vegetarian. Many unique dishes with Vietnamese and American influences are found on Ely's menu. Try the barbecued mock duck salad, vegetable enchiladas, or banh xeo—Vietnamese crepes filled with mung beans, mushroom, and green onion. Several vegan items are clearly marked with a diamond. **Open Monday through Saturday for lunch and dinner. Full service, vegan options, espresso/cappuccino, take-out, VISA/MC/AMX/DISC, $$**

CANTON

Mulligan's
4118 Belden Village St., NW, Canton, OH 44718   **(216) 493-8239**
American. This old-fashioned pub offers a separate vegetarian menu. Enjoy salads, meatless chili, soups, veggie hot dogs, garden burgers, veggie sandwiches, burritos, pasta dishes, and rice and black beans. **Open daily for lunch and dinner. Full service, vegan options, take-out, VISA/MC, AMX, $**

CINCINNATI

Alpha Restaurant
204 W. McMillan St., Cincinnati, OH 45219   **(513) 381-6559**
American. This restaurant features a relaxed and friendly atmosphere. Vegetarian selections are offered for breakfast, lunch, and dinner, and Alpha is willing to accommodate special dietary needs. **Open daily. Full service, vegetarian options, fresh juice, beer/wine/alcohol, take-out, VISA/MC/AMX/DISC, $$**

Arnold's Bar & Grill
210 E. 8th St., Cincinnati, OH 45202   **(513) 421-6234**
American tavern. Arnold's is a unique turn-of-the-century tavern with good food, fresh ingredients, and a strong selection of vegetarian specials and soups. **Open Monday through Friday for lunch and dinner. Full service, vegetarian options, fresh juice, beer/wine/alcohol, take-out, $$**

Cheng-I Cuisine
203 W. McMillan St., Cincinnati, OH 45219   **(513) 723-1999**
Chinese. Cheng-I is a traditional Chinese restaurant with an extensive vegetarian menu. The vegetarian spring rolls were voted best vegetarian appetizer by *Cincinnati Magazine.* **Open Monday through Saturday for lunch and dinner, Sunday for dinner. Full service, vegetarian options, beer/wine/alcohol, catering, take-out, VISA/MC/AMX/DISC/DC, $$**

- ## Clifton Natural Foods Deli & Juice Bar
207 W. McMillan St., Cincinnati, OH 45219   (513) 651-5288
Vegetarian/natural foods. Clifton has an extensive menu of vegetarian salads, entrees, sandwiches, soups, drinks, and desserts. **Open daily. Deli service, vegan options, fresh juice, take-out, $**

Floyd's of Cincinnati, Inc.
129 Calhoun St., Cincinnati, OH 45219   (513) 221-2434
Middle Eastern. Various vegetarian Middle Eastern dishes including Tabouleh, Baba Ghanouj, Hummus, Falafel Sandwich, and salads are offered. **Open daily for lunch and dinner but closed Sunday. Vegan options, take-out, $**

Jerusalem Cafe
235 W. McMillan St., Cincinnati, OH 45219   (513) 241-2323
Ethnic. Enjoy an authentic Middle Eastern dining experience reflective of Mediterranean traditions and culture. All dishes are available without meat, and there is an extensive vegetarian menu. **Open daily for lunch and dinner. Full service, vegan options, BYOB, catering, take-out, VISA/MC, $$**

Mayura Restaurant
3201 Jefferson Ave., Cincinnati, OH 45220   (513) 221-7125
East Indian. This Indian restaurant with its attached bar offers many vegetarian dishes. **Open for lunch and dinner Tuesday through Saturday. Full service, beer/wine/alcohol, catering, take-out, VISA/MC/AMX/DISC, $$**

Myra's Dionysus
121 Calhoun St., Cincinnati, OH 45219   (513) 961-1578
International. An extensive international menu includes Middle Eastern, Chinese, Greek, Brazilian, Mexican, Turkish, Indian, and Italian dishes and features an incredible variety of excellent soups and many vegan selections. Outdoor seating is available. **Open daily for lunch and dinner. Full service, vegan options, wine/ beer, catering, take-out, no credit cards accepted, $**

Red Apple Deli & Cafe
6911 Miami Ave., Cincinnati, OH 45243   (513) 271-6766
Natural foods. The Red Apple Deli & Cafe offers Vegetarian Chili, Veggie Burgers, Barbecue Tofu, Stir-Fry Vegetables with Rice, Veggie Lasagna, various salads, plus much more. **Open daily for lunch and dinner. Counter service, vegan options, fresh juices, take-out, VISA/MC/AMX/DISC, $**

- - ## Ulysses Whole World Foods
350 Ludlow Ave., Cincinnati, OH 45220   (513) 281-5050

🐾 Reviewers' choice   ● Vegetarian restaurant   ●● Vegan restaurant
$ less than $6 $$ $6–$12 $$$ more than $12
VISA/AMX/MC/DISC/DC—credit cards accepted
Non-alc.—Non-alcoholic   Fresh juices—freshly squeezed

Vegan/international. Ulysses offers the finest in vegetarian cuisine, including an array of fresh, homemade soups, sandwiches, salads, chili, entrees, and desserts. All food is prepared without milk, butter, cheese, eggs, meat, chicken, or fish. **Open Tuesday through Saturday for lunch and dinner. Full service, vegan options, limited catering, take-out, VISA/MC, $–$$**

CLEVELAND

(For more restaurant listings in the surrounding areas, see Cleveland Heights.)

Ali Baba Restaurant
12021 Lorain Rd., Cleveland, OH 44111   (216) 251-2040
Middle Eastern. Ali Baba has delicious Middle Eastern specialities and a vegetarian section on the menu. The recipes used are those of the owner's grandmother. Falafel, Hummus, and Baba Ghanouj are outstanding. Brown rice, whole-wheat pita, and all other foods are prepared without MSG, artificial flavorings, or preservatives. The hosts are friendly, cheerful, and accommodating. **Open Tuesday through Friday for lunch and dinner, dinner only on Saturday. Full service, catering, take-out, $$**

Parma Pierogies Restaurant
5580 Ridge Rd., Cleveland, OH 44129   (216) 888-1200
Polish/ethnic. This no-smoking restaurant offers fifteen varieties of vegetarian pierogies. The dough has no preservatives. **Limited service. Open daily, vegan options, non-alc. beer/wine, take-out, $**

CLEVELAND HEIGHTS

Taj Mahal Restaurant
1763 Coventry Rd. at Mayfield Road
Cleveland Heights, OH 44118   (216) 321-0511
Indian. Savor very good vegetarian curry selections. Meals include pure vegetarian lentil/pea soup and basmati rice pilaf with raisins and nuts. Many vegetarian appetizers and main entrees are available. **Open daily for dinner, Sunday brunch. Full service, vegan options, beer/wine/alcohol, catering, take-out, VISA/MC/ AMX, $$**

Tommy's
1820 Coventry Rd., Cleveland Heights, OH 44118   (216) 321-7757
Greek. Cleveland Heights natives have told us this is the place to go. Taped music is played, and Falafel, Hummus, Spinach Pies, Tempeh Burgers, and fruit freezes are offered. **Open daily. Full service and counter service, vegan options, fresh juices, take-out, $$**

Yaakov's Kosher Restaurant
13969 Cedar Rd., Cleveland Heights, OH 44118   (216) 932-8848
Kosher. Excellent pizza, Falafel, and Eggplant Parmesan. **Cafeteria style, vegan options, take-out, $**

CLIFTON

(For restaurant listings in the surrounding areas, see Dayton.)

COLUMBUS

Estrada's Restaurant
240 King Ave., Columbus, OH 43201   **(614) 294-0808**
Mexican. Very inexpensive, fresh, and good Mexican food—the best Mexican food in town—is featured. There are many vegetarian and a few vegan options. Lard is not used in the preparation of the food. **Open Monday through Saturday for lunch and dinner. Full service, vegan options, catering, take-out, DISC, $**

• King Avenue Coffeehouse
247 King Ave., Columbus, OH 43201   **(614) 294-8287**
Vegetarian/ethnic. The coffeehouse features daily menu additions, vegan options, and organic ingredients whenever possible. A non-smoking environment and art exhibits are also featured. Made-to-order brunch is available on Sunday. **Open Tuesday through Sunday for lunch and dinner. Full service, vegan options, fresh juice, take-out, VISA/MC/AMX/DISC, $-$$**

Nong's Hunan Express
1634 Northwest Blvd., Columbus, OH 43212   **(614) 486-6630**
Thai/Oriental. Nong's offers a huge variety of vegetarian dishes, including soups and egg rolls. The atmosphere is casual. **Full service, vegetarian options, take-out, $$**

Rigsby's Cuisine Volatile
698 North High St., Columbus, OH 43215   **(614) 461-7888**
American. This formal restaurant offers several vegetarian and a few vegan selections. **Full service, vegan options, $$**

• Whole World Bakery
3269 N. High St., Columbus, OH 43202   **(614) 268-5751**
Vegetarian/American. Whole World offers baked goods made without sugar, whole-wheat pizza, tofu sloppy Joes, veggie burgers, and great vegetarian soups. A wide variety of entrees is offered. **Closed Monday. Full service, vegan options, BYOB, catering, take-out, $-$$**

DAYTON

(For more restaurant listings in the surrounding areas, see Fairborn, Kettering, and Yellow Springs.)

Euro Bistro
5524 Airway Rd., Dayton, OH 45431   **(513) 256-3444**
Natural foods/bistro. This smoke-free bistro offers freshly baked breads, specialty sandwiches, homemade salads, soups and quiche, incredible cookies and cheesecakes. Outdoor seating available. **Closed Sunday. Limited service, catering, take-out, $**

Euro Bistro

1328 Kauffman Ave., Fairborn, OH 45324   **(513) 878-1989**

Natural foods/bistro. See entry under Dayton, OH.

The Zephyr

106 W. Main, Kent, OH 44240   **(216) 678-4848**

Natural foods. This restaurant is vegetarian with the exception of some fish dishes. The menu features Middle Eastern appetizers, salads, veggie stir fry, Potato Pancakes, veggie burger, Falafel, plus much more. Desserts are baked fresh daily. **Open Tuesday through Sunday for breakfast, lunch, and dinner. Full service, catering, take-out, $**

• Kettering Medical Center Cafeteria

3535 Southern Blvd., Kettering, OH 45429   **(513) 296-7262**

Vegetarian. The menu has a twenty-eight-day cycle. Most items have dairy and eggs. **Open daily for three meals. Cafeteria style, vegan options, $**

• Sycamore Hospital Cafeteria

2150 Leiter Rd., Miamisburg, OH 45342   **(513) 866-0551**

Vegetarian. This smoke-free establishment offers vegetarian and vegan entrees, a salad bar, freshly baked breads, and desserts. **Open daily for three meals. Cafeteria-style service, $**

Jalmers Health Foods

1488 Sylvania Ave., Toledo, OH 43612   **(419) 476-7918**

Health-food-store deli/juice bar. **Open Monday through Saturday. Limited service/deli, fresh juice, take-out, VISA/MC, $**

Carol's Kitchen

101 Corry St., Yellow Springs, OH 45387   **(513) 767-7959**

🍴 Reviewers' choice   ● Vegetarian restaurant   ●● Vegan restaurant
$ less than $6 $$ $6–$12 $$$ more than $12
VISA/AMX/MC/DISC/DC—credit cards accepted
Non-alc.—Non-alcoholic   Fresh juices—freshly squeezed

American. This smoke-free establishment offers a sandwich, soup, and fruit bar. Other options include fresh breads, croissants, muffins, and pastries, and there are many vegetarian selections. **Cafeteria service, $$**

Ha Ha Pizza
108 Xenia Ave., Yellow Springs, OH 45387   (513) 767-1261
Pizza. Ha Ha features homemade white or whole-wheat dough, sauce, and fresh vegetables. Several meat alternatives are offered. Soy cheese is available for the pizzas. **Lunch and dinner daily, dinner only on Sunday. Full service, catering, take-out, $**

• Organic Grocery
225 Xenia Ave., Yellow Springs, OH 45387   (513) 767-7215
Vegetarian deli. This smoke-free deli offers vegetarian chili, sandwiches, thick fruit drinks, Hummus, and more. **Full counter, vegan options, fresh juice, $**

Sunrise Cafe
259 Xenia Ave., Yellow Springs, OH 45387   (513) 767-1065 or -7211
Natural/ethnic foods. This charming restored 1940's diner uses fresh ingredients, and everything is made from scratch. The smoke-free diner continues to expand its vegetarian offerings. **Open daily. Full service, vegan options, catering, take-out, VISA/MC, $**

Winds Cafe And Bakery
215 Xenia Ave., Yellow Springs, OH 45387   (513) 767-1144
Natural foods. Specialities include fresh baked breads and pastries, scrambled tofu, and a constantly changing menu that always includes several vegetarian selections. **Open Monday through Saturday for lunch and dinner, brunch on Sunday. Full service, vegan options, fresh juice, beer/wine/alcohol, take-out, VISA/MC/ AMX/DISC, $$–$$$**

Oklahoma

NORMAN

The Earth Natural Foods & Deli
309 S. Flood St., Norman, OK 73069   (405) 364-3551
Natural foods store/deli. This deli offers sandwiches, salads, and drinks to go. Seating is not available. **Open daily. Deli/counter service only, vegetarian options, fresh juice, catering, take-out, VISA/MC/AMX, $**

Love Light Restaurant
529 Buchanan St., Norman, OK 73069   (405) 364-2073
American/ethnic. In a bright airy atmosphere with patio dining, you'll find a "sandwich factory" where you choose your own ingredients for sandwiches and

salads. Homemade whole-grain bread and bakery items are also offered. Love Light offers the best vegetarian selection in Norman. **Open daily. Counter service, vegan options, fresh juice, beer, take-out, VISA/MC, $**

OKLAHOMA CITY

The Earth Natural Foods & Deli
1101 NW 49th St., Oklahoma City, OK 73118 (405) 840-0502
Natural foods. This natural foods restaurant and store offers a menu with many vegetarian selections. Limited service is available only in the evenings. **Open daily. Limited deli service, fresh juice, catering, take-out, VISA/MC/AMX, $**

OREGON

ASHLAND

Ashland Bakery & Cafe
38 E. Main St., Ashland, OR 97520 (503) 482-9463
Cafe/bakery. This restaurant offers an extensive vegetarian menu, including vegetarian chili and soups, and fresh baked goods. **Open daily. Full service, wine/ beer, take-out, VISA/MC, $–$$**

Geppetto's
345 E. Main St., Ashland, OR 97520 (503) 482-1138
Italian. Enjoy a wide selection of vegetarian meals, including great Eggplant Burgers. **Open daily. Full service, vegetarian options, fresh juice, beer/wine/alcohol, take-out, VISA/MC, $–$$$**

House Of Thai Cuisine
1667 Siskiyou Blvd., Ashland, OR 97520 (503) 488-2583
Thai. This family-owned-and-operated restaurant offers a separate vegetarian menu. It was voted best Oriental restaurant in Ashland in 1992. **Open for lunch Monday through Saturday, open daily for dinner. Full service, beer/wine, catering, take-out, VISA/MC, $$**

• North Light Vegetarian Restaurant
120 E. Main St., Ashland, OR 97520 (503) 482-9463
Vegetarian. North Light is a cooperatively managed restaurant with a great regular menu and daily specials. Organic ingredients are used whenever possible. **Open daily. Full service with buffet, vegan options, fresh juice, beer/wine/alcohol, catering, take-out, VISA/MC, $$**

ASTORIA

The Columbia Cafe
1114 Marine Dr., Astoria, OR 97103 (503) 325-2233
Natural foods. Here you'll find lots of delicious vegetarian and vegan options including rice and veggie dishes, bean burritos, homemade pasta, and other

international options. The owner is the cook and is very hospitable. Salsas are made out of all types of fruits and vegetables. Crêpes are a speciality. **Open daily. Full service, vegan options, fresh juices, non-alc. beer, wine/beer, $$**

BEAVERTON

McMenamins Pub
2927 SW Cedar Hills Blvd., Beaverton, OR 97005   **(503) 641-0151**
Tavern. Enjoy a pub atmosphere featuring an extensive vegetarian menu. **Open daily for lunch and dinner. Full service, vegetarian options, beer/wine, catering, take-out, VISA/MC, $**

BEND

Cafe Sante
718 NW Franklin St., Bend, OR 97701   **(503) 383-3530**
American. This cafe-style restaurant has an almost exclusively vegetarian menu and is a local favorite. Organic ingredients are used whenever possible. **Open daily for breakfast and lunch. Full service, vegan options, fresh juice, espresso, beer/ wine, non-alc. beer/wine, take-out, VISA/MC, $–$$**

CLACKAMAS

• New Earth Vegetarian Restaurant and Bake Shop
15571 SE 82nd Dr., Clackamas, OR 97015   **(503) 657-7148**
Vegetarian. Enjoy delicious soups and main dishes made from scratch, as well as delicious baked goods. **Open Sunday through Thursday for lunch and dinner. Open for lunch Friday. Closed Saturday. Full service, fresh juices, vegan options, take-out, $**

CORVALLIS

The Beanery
500 SW 2nd St., Corvallis, OR 97333   **(503) 753-7442**

2541 NW Monroe St., Corvallis, OR 97330   **(503) 757-0828**
Coffeehouse. The Beanery features Vegetarian Lasagna, burritos, soups, salads, espresso, cappuccino, and desserts. **Open late daily. Counter service, espresso/ cappuccino, take-out, VISA/MC/DISC, $$**

Bob's Burger Express
360 NW 5th, Corvallis, OR 97330   **(503) 754-1583**
Fast food. A mainstream, fast-food joint, Bob's also sells an inexpensive vegetarian burger, yogurt, and soups. **Open daily. Counter service, take-out, $**

**⌘ Reviewers' choice   • Vegetarian restaurant   •• Vegan restaurant
$ less than $6 $$ $6–$12 $$$ more than $12
VISA/AMX/MC/DISC/DC—credit cards accepted
Non-alc.—Non-alcoholic   Fresh juices—freshly squeezed**

China Blue
2307 NW 9th St., Corvallis, OR 97330 **(503) 757-8088**
Chinese. China Blue has a large vegetarian selection including sweet and sour tofu and other tofu dishes. **Full service, vegan options, take-out, $–$$**

• Nearly Normal's Gonzo Cuisine
109 NW 15 St., Corvallis, OR 97330 **(503) 753-0791**
Vegetarian. This very local, finely crafted restaurant has an extensive and diverse vegetarian menu. Great salads with seasoned tofu and homemade dressings and homemade desserts are featured. There are farm-fresh specials from the family farm in the summertime. All visitors should have a Nearly Normal's experience while in the area! **Open Monday through Saturday, Sunday brunch in the spring and summer. Limited service, vegan options, fresh juice, beer/wine/alcohol, catering, take-out, $–$$**

EUGENE

(For more restaurant listings in the surrounding areas, see Springfield.)

Anitolio's
992 Willamette, Eugene, OR 97401 **(503) 343-9661**
Natural foods/Mediterranean. This restaurant offers a wide variety of Mediterranean vegetarian dishes including an eggplant and chickpea stew, several curries, soups, and salads. **Open Monday through Saturday for lunch and dinner; Sunday, dinner only. Full service, non-alc. beer, wine/beer, take-out, VISA/MC, $$**

The Beanery
152 W. 5th St., Eugene, OR 97401 **(503) 342-3378**

2465 Hilyard St., Eugene, OR 97405 **(503) 344-0221**
Coffeehouse. See entry under Corvallis, OR.

Bob's Burger Express
620 West 6th St., Eugene, OR 97402 **(503) 342-3121**

296 Coburg Road, Eugene, OR 97401 **(503) 485-4332**

1990 West 11th St., Eugene, OR 97405 **(503) 686-9313**
Fast food. See listing under Corvallis, OR.

Casablanca
Fifth St. Market, Eugene, OR 97401 **(503) 342-3885**
Middle Eastern. Enjoy a good selection of vegetarian foods. **Cafeteria style, vegan options, take-out, $**

The Glenwood Restaurants
1346 Alder St., Eugene, OR 97401 **(503) 343-8303**

2588 Willamette St., Eugene, OR 97405 **(503) 687-8201**
American/Californian. Enjoy a wide variety of vegetarian options—quiche, Tofu Burrito, Spicy Tofu Stir-Fry, Cabbage Rolls, Fried Rice Mandarin, Kima, and

others. **Alder Street location open 24 hours daily; Willamette open daily 6:30 A.M. to 9 P.M. Vegan options, wine/beer, take-out, VISA/MC/AMX/DISC, $**

• Govinda's Vegetarian Buffet
270 W. 8th Street, Eugene, OR 97401   **(503) 686-3531**
Vegetarian/natural foods. Self-serve buffet offers all-you-can-eat salad bar and ten hot entrees including such items as curried vegetables, lasagna, enchiladas, and tofu dishes. Other options are also available. **Open Monday through Friday for lunch and dinner. Limited buffet-style service, vegan options, take-out, $–$$**

Keystone Cafe
395 W. 5th Ave., Eugene, OR 97401   **(503) 342-2075**
American. Breakfast is served all day. Plate-sized pancakes are a specialty, including oatmeal/sesame, whole-wheat, corn/rice, and buckwheat barley varieties. **Open daily 7 A.M. to 3 P.M. Full service, vegan options, fresh juice, very limited catering, take-out, $**

Mekala's Thai Restaurant
296 E. 5th Ave., Eugene, OR 97401   **(503) 342-4872**
Thai/ethnic. Experience outstanding Thai vegetarian dishes containing no MSG. Only canola oil is used. Located in the Fifth Street Public Market, the restaurant has a very nice atmosphere. **Open daily for lunch and dinner. Full service, vegan options, fresh juice, beer/wine, catering, take-out, VISA/MC, $–$$**

• Rainy Day Cafe
50 E. 11th Ave., Eugene, OR 97401   **(503) 343-8108**
Vegetarian. This cafe is mostly vegan with the exception of a few dishes made with cheese. Choose from a wide selection of appetizers, salads, soups, entrees, and desserts. **Open daily for lunch and dinner. Full service, smoothies, $–$$**

GRANTS PASS

Sunshine Natural Food Cafe
128 SW H St., Grants Pass, OR 97526   **(503) 474-5044**
Natural foods. Enjoy Sunshine's organic salad bar, and a buffet Tuesday through Friday. **Closed Sunday. Full service and buffet, vegan options, fresh juice, beer/wine, take-out, $**

HOOD RIVER

Big City Chicks
1302 13th St., Hood River, OR 97031   **(503) 387-3811**
Multi-ethnic. Vegetarian dishes "inspired by many regional cuisines" include rasta pasta, herbed polenta cakes, curried risotto, and bean curd pad Thai. Dishes prepared without dairy are marked with an asterisk. **Open daily for dinner. Full service, vegan options, espresso/cappuccino, wine/beer/alcohol, VISA/MC, $$**

ॐ Reviewers' choice   • Vegetarian restaurant   •• Vegan restaurant
$ less than $6 $$ $6–$12 $$$ more than $12
VISA/AMX/MC/DISC/DC—credit cards accepted
Non-alc.—Non-alcoholic   Fresh juices—freshly squeezed

JUNCTION CITY

Bob's Burger Express
890 Ivy St., Junction City, OR 97448   **(503) 998-3264**
Fast food. See listing under Corvallis.

PORTLAND

(For more restaurant listings in the surrounding areas, see Beaverton and Troutdale.)

• The Daily Grind Restaurant
4026 SE Hawthorne Blvd., Portland, OR 97214   **(503) 233-5521**
Vegetarian. This eatery offers a steam table that is dairy- and egg-free with soup, three entrees, vegetables, mashed potatoes, and gravy. There's also a large salad bar. Menu items include vegetarian sandwiches and burgers, and other items. **Open daily for lunch and dinner. Limited service/cafeteria, vegan options, fresh juice, take-out, VISA/MC, $**

• Garden Cafe
Portland Adventist Medical Center
10123 SE Market St., Portland, OR 97216   **(503) 251-6125**
Vegetarian/natural foods. This is a full-service cafeteria offering vegetarian entrees, salad bar, fresh fruit bar, and a fast-food grill featuring fifteen vegetarian sandwiches. Over 1000 meals are served daily. Vegetarian meals have been served here for over 100 years. Enjoy a wide variety of foods in a comfortable dining area with indoor and outdoor seating just six blocks off Interstate 205. **Closed Saturday and Sunday. Cafeteria-style service, vegan options, catering, take-out, $**

• Healthway Food Center
524 SW 5th, Portland, OR 97204   **(503) 226-2941**
Health-food-store deli. The Healthway deli features fresh juice, soups, and salads. **Open weekdays for lunch. Counter service, take-out, $**

Old Wives Tales
1300 E. Burnside, Portland, OR 97214   **(503) 238-0470**
Ethnic. Enjoy a soup and salad bar, soy products, rice noodles, black bean stew, Mexican dishes, an Egyptian loaf, plus much more. **Open daily for three meals. Full service, fresh juices, non-alc. beer/wine, wine/beer, take-out, VISA/MC/ DISC, $$**

Plainfield Mayur ॐ
852 SW 21st St., Portland, OR 97205   **(503) 223-2995**
Indian. Probably one of the most elegant Indian restaurants you'll find, Plainfield Mayur is located in one of Portland's landmark homes with table settings of fine European crystal, china, and full silver service. The menu includes a vegetarian section with delicious, original entrees, appetizers, and soup. The Tandoor Show Kitchen is the only one in Oregon, and private dining rooms are available for

business meetings or private gatherings. **Reservations recommended. Full service, vegan options, wine/beer/alcohol, take-out, VISA/MC/AMX/DISC, $$**

• Song of the Rose Cafe
1310 NW 23rd, Portland, OR 97210   **(503) 224-0863**
Vegetarian. Located next door to a bookstore, this vegetarian restaurant uses organic ingredients when available. Try Black Bean Burritos, quiche, various soups and salads, veggie burgers, Mushroom Tofu Stroganoff, plus much more. **Open for lunch and dinner Monday through Saturday. Full service, vegan options, espresso/cappuccino, fresh juices, smoothies, take-out, VISA/MC/AMX/DISC, $$**

Thanh Thao Restaurant
4005 SE Hawthorne, Portland, OR 97214   **(503) 238-6232**
Ethnic. Thanh Thao has recently expanded its vegetarian options and now offers a wide selection of tofu, vegetable, eggplant, and mock-meat entrees. Appetizers, soup, and noodle dishes are also available. **Open for lunch and dinner every day except Tuesday. Full service, vegan options, take-out, $–$$**

REDMOND
Bob's Burger Express
433 W. Antler St., Redmond, OR 97756   **(503) 548-1405**
Fast food. See entry under Corvallis, OR.

SALEM
Bob's Burger Express
1415 Capitol St., NE, Salem, OR 97303   **(503) 363-8983**

3999 Commercial St., Southeast Salem, OR 97302   **(503) 364-5798**

5130 River Rd., North Salem, OR 97303   **(503) 393-1072**

890 Lancester Dr., Northeast Salem, OR 97301   **(503) 399-8383**

831 Lancaster Dr., Northeast Salem, OR 97301   **(503) 399-7710**

710 Wallace Rd., Northwest, Salem, OR 97304   **(503) 399-7933**
Fast food. See entry under Corvallis, OR.

SPRINGFIELD
Bob's Burger Express
5803 Main Street, Springfield, OR 97477   **(503) 747-5544**

720 South 8th St., Springfield, OR 97477   **(503) 747-3421**
Fast food. See listing under Corvallis, OR.

Kuraya's Thai Cuisine
1410 Mohawk Blvd., Springfield, OR 97477   **(503) 746-2951**
Thai/ethnic. Kuraya's is a full-service traditional Thai restaurant offering many wonderful vegetarian selections. **Open daily. Dinner only on Sunday. Full service, vegan options, beer/wine, catering, take-out, VISA/MC, $**

TROUTDALE

Multnomah Falls Lodge Restaurant
Hwy. 30 at Multnomah Falls, Troutdale, OR 97060   (503) 695-2376
American. This is a standard American restaurant that has a Garden Burger on the menu. **Open daily. Full service, non-alc. beer, wine/beer/alcohol, VISA/MC/ AMX, $$**

PENNSYLVANIA

ANNVILLE

Great Life Cafe
29 E. Main St. (Rt. 422), Annville, PA 17003   (717) 867-5565
Natural foods. Enjoy organic whole-wheat crust pizzas, Tempeh Burgers, Seitan Melt Sandwiches, Falafel, Vegetarian Lasagna, blue corn tamales, and a Macrobiotic Platter at the Great Life Cafe. Organic ingredients are used when available. **Open for breakfast and lunch Wednesday and Thursday. Open for three meals Friday and Saturday. Full service, vegan options, take-out, $–$$**

ARDMORE

Saladalley
Suburban Square, Coulter Ave. and Saint James St.
Ardmore, PA 19003   (215) 642-0453
American. This is the main office for a chain of franchised restaurants around Philadelphia. Call for the location near you. Saladalley features an extensive salad bar with a wide variety of vegetarian salads, soups, and entrees. Every unit has non-smoking sections and easy access for the handicapped. Some units have live entertainment, happy hour specials, and displays of local artists' work. **Full service, non-alc. beer, wine/beer/alcohol, take-out, $$**

BALA CYNWYD

The Carrot Bunch
51 E. City Line Ave, Bala Cynwyd, PA 19004   (215) 664-5231
Natural foods. **Open Monday through Saturday for lunch and dinner. Full service. Fresh juices, take-out, VISA/MC, $**

🐾 Reviewers' choice   • Vegetarian restaurant   •• Vegan restaurant
$ less than $6 $$ $6–$12 $$$ more than $12
VISA/AMX/MC/DISC/DC—credit cards accepted
Non-alc.—Non-alcoholic   Fresh juices—freshly squeezed

EAST STROUDSBURG

Chang's Garden
Pocono Plaza, Lincoln Ave., K Mart Shopping Center
E. Stroudsburg, PA 18301   **(717) 424-8655**
Chinese. The menu's vegetable section includes tofu and vegetable dishes, an eggplant dish, and Vegetable Egg Foo Young. **Open daily. Full service, VISA/ MC/AMX/DC, $$**

HARRISBURG

Passage to India
525 S. Front St., Harrisburg, PA 17104   **(717) 233-1202**
Indian. Sample from a large selection of vegetarian options like chana masala (chickpeas cooked with onions, tomatoes, and spices) and aloo methi (potatoes cooked with mustard seed, fenugreek, and other spices) at this restaurant over-looking the Susquehanna River. **Open daily for three meals. Full service, vegan options, catering, take-out, VISA/MC, $$**

·HONESDALE

Nature's Grace Health Foods and Deli
947 Main St., Honesdale, PA 18431   **(717) 253-3469**
Health-food-store deli. Soft-serve frozen yogurt is available seasonally. Homemade soups, enchiladas, salads, baked goods, hoagies, and other entrees are available daily. **Open Monday through Saturday, 10 A.M. to 5 P.M. Counter service, fresh juices, take-out, $**

LANCASTER

Asian Restaurant
553 North Pine St., Lancaster, PA 17603   **(717) 397-7095**
International. The Asian Restaurant has eight options in the vegetable section of the menu plus chow mein and lo mein dishes. **Closed Monday. Open Tuesday through Sunday for lunch and dinner. Full service, vegan options, VISA/MC/ DC, $–$$**

Lanvina
1762 Columbia Ave., Lancaster, PA 17603   **(717) 393-7748**

1651 Lincoln Hwy. E., Lancaster, PA 17602   **(717) 399-0199**
Vietnamese. When you visit the Amish area in Lancaster, Pennsylvania, stop by Lanvina restaurants. They offer a huge separate vegetarian menu including Spring Rolls, Tomato and Bean Curd Soup, Vegetable Chow Mein and Lo Mein, Rice Noodles, Fried Rice, curry dishes, and much more. **Open for lunch Monday through Friday and for dinner daily. Full service, vegan options, take-out, $**

LITITZ

• Meadows Natural Foods
10 E. Front St., Lititz, PA 17543   **(717) 626-7374**
Vegetarian/macrobiotic. **Open Monday and Wednesday at 5 P.M. for take-out, Friday at 6 P.M. for eat-in or take-out. Reservations required by noon, $$**

MARSHALL'S CREEK

Naturally Rite Restaurant and Natural Foods Market
Route 209, Marshall's Creek, PA 18335   **(717) 223-1133**

Natural foods. It's a pleasure to find this restaurant among the Pocono vacation spots. Among the wide variety of menu selections are Garden Burgers, Millet Croquettes, Pasta and Broccoli, and Fettucini Pomadora. Vegetarian and non-dairy soy products are available. Desserts can be served with non-dairy ice cream. A health-food store and clinic are connected to the restaurant; however, you do not feel as if you are in a store as the restaurant has its own atmosphere. Informal, outdoor patio. **Open daily except Tuesday. Breakfast is available on weekends.** Full service, fresh juices, take-out, VISA/MC, $$

NARBERTH

Garden of Eatin'
231 Haverford Ave., Narberth, PA 19072   **(215) 667-7634**

Natural foods. This restaurant is in the rear of Narberth Natural Foods. **Open Monday through Saturday for lunch.** Full service, fresh juices, take-out, VISA/MC, $

NEW CUMBERLAND

• Avatar's Golden Nectar
321 Bridge St., New Cumberland, PA 17070   **(717) 774-7215**

Vegetarian. Daily specials and smoothies are available. **Open daily except Sunday.** Full service, fresh juices, take-out, VISA/MC, $

NEWFOUNDLAND

• White Cloud
RD 1, Box 215, Newfoundland, PA 18445   **(717) 676-3162**

Vegetarian. Nestled in the Pocono Mountains, White Cloud is a casual vegetarian and natural foods restaurant and inn. A good selection of vegetarian foods is offered, and organic foods are served when available. **Open for three meals daily during the summer, only on weekends the rest of the year. Reservations are required.** Full service, fresh juices, take-out, VISA/MC/DISC, $$

OXFORD

Taco Shell's
15 N. Third St., Oxford, PA 19363   **(215) 932-9445**

ಶಾ Reviewers' choice   • Vegetarian restaurant   •• Vegan restaurant
$ less than $6 $$ $6–$12 $$$ more than $12
VISA/AMX/MC/DISC/DC—credit cards accepted
Non-alc.—Non-alcoholic   Fresh juices—freshly squeezed

Mexican. Restaurants are limited as it is in this area of southeastern PA so finding Taco Shell's, which has excellent homemade Mexican food in a small-town restaurant atmosphere, is a real treat. The rice and homemade salsa are delicious, and you can always get a filling vegetarian burrito or enchilada. **Open Tuesday through Friday for lunch and dinner. Full service, limited vegan options, BYOB, take-out, $**

PENNS CREEK

Walnut Acres Organic Farm
Walnut Acres Rd., Penns Creek, PA 17862   **(717) 837-5095**
Natural foods. Walnut Acres is an organic farm with a lunch counter. **Open Monday through Saturday for lunch. Limited service, VISA/MC/DISC, $**

PHILADELPHIA

(For more restaurant listings in the surrounding areas, see Ardmore, Bala Cynwyd, and Narberth. Springfield, Wayne, and Willow Grove are farther away.)

•• A-free-ya's
6108 Germantown Ave., Philadelphia, PA 19144   **(215) 848-5006**
Vegan. A-free-ya's offers an exciting new concept in healthy foods with its extensive menu of interesting and creative raw foods dishes. Some stir-fries and soups are available during the winter. **Open Tuesday through Friday, 11 A.M. to 2 P.M. for take-out only. Open at other times Tuesday through Saturday for sit-down. Full service, fresh juices, fresh-pressed solar wines, catering, take-out, VISA/MC, $$**

• The Basic Four Vegetarian Juice Bar
Reading Terminal Market, 12th and Filbert Sts.
Philadelphia, PA 19107   **(215) 440-0991**
Vegetarian. Located in the heart of Philadelphia, this is a food-stand in Reading Terminal. Savor fast-food vegetarian style, including sandwiches, salads, veggie steaks, veggie burgers, mock chicken and tuna salad. **Open Monday through Saturday, 11:30 A.M. to 4:30 P.M. Cafeteria style, fresh juices, take-out, $**

Ben's Restaurant
The Franklin Institute, 20th and the Parkway
Philadelphia, PA 19103   **(215) 448-1355**
American. Ben's claims "An All-American menu with a nutritional twist." **Open daily for breakfast and lunch. Cafeteria style, take-out, $**

• Center Foods Natural Grocer
337 S. Broad St., Philadelphia, PA 19107   **(215) 735-5673**
Vegetarian. Center Foods features a completely organic take-out counter with macrobiotic options. **Open Monday through Saturday. Take-out only, macrobiotic options, $**

Charles Plaza
234-236 N. 10th St., Philadelphia, PA 19107   **(215) 829-4383**
Chinese. This formal restaurant features a vegetarian menu including soups, appetizers, and mock meat entrees made of bean curd, carrot, and seitan, or wheat gluten. **Open daily for lunch and dinner. Full service, reservations required, fresh juices, VISA/MC/AMEX/DISC, $$**

•• Cherry Street Chinese Vegetarian Restaurant ❧
1010 Cherry St., Philadelphia, PA 19107   **(215) 923-3663**
Vegan/Chinese. This smoke-free Chinese restaurant has an extensive menu, featuring vegetable, tofu, and mock-meat dishes. Sample Sesame Lemon Beef, Watercress with Tofu Soup, Eggplant in Black Bean Sauce, and more. An upstairs banquet room is available. **Open for lunch and dinner daily. Full service, vegan/macrobiotic options, take-out, VISA/MC/AMX/DISC, $$**

The Dining Car
8826 Frankford Ave., Philadelphia, PA 19136   **(215) 338-5113**
American. This diner offers some vegetarian meals. **Open 24 hours daily. Full service, alcohol, take-out, $**

Essene Cafe
719 South 4th St., Philadelphia, PA 19147   **(215) 928-3722**
Natural foods. Located next door to a very large natural foods store, Essene Cafe offers a wide variety of vegetarian dishes including soups, salads, Gingered Tofu and Grilled Vegetables, Tempeh Burgers, Sautéed Tofu-Teriyaki Burger, Vegetable Lasagna, and a Macrobiotic Plate. **Open for lunch and dinner Wednesday through Monday. Open only for dinner on Tuesday. Full service, fresh juices, vegan options, take-out, VISA/MC, $$–$$$**

Golden Empress Garden
610 S. 5th St., Philadelphia, PA 19147   **(215) 627-7666**
Chinese. A separate menu lists vegetarian options. No MSG is used. **Open daily. Full service, vegan options, take-out, $–$$.**

Golden Pond Chinese Restaurant
1006 Race St., Philadelphia, PA 19107   **(215) 923-0303**
Chinese. Golden Pond has an extensive vegetarian menu. **Open daily for lunch and dinner. Full service, take-out, VISA/MC, $$**

•• Harmony Vegetarian Restaurant ❧
135 N. 9th St., Philadelphia, PA 19107   **(215) 627-4520**
Vegan/Chinese. Any vegetarian who visits Philadelphia will undoubtedly hear "make sure you visit Harmony!" from friends familiar with this Philadelphia treasure. Harmony is a highly rated, completely vegan Chinese restaurant with a very extensive menu. Many delicious soups, appetizers, and countless vegetable, tofu, and mock-meat dishes are featured. The service is friendly and the atmosphere is pleasant. Weekends are usually very busy. Non-smoking. **Open Monday through Saturday for lunch and dinner. Full service, completely vegan, BYOB, take-out, VISA/MC, $$**

Jumby Bay Juice Bar Cafe
250 South St., Philadelphia, PA 19148   (215) 625-2596
Juice Bar. A wide variety of fresh juices is available. **Open daily. Counter service, take-out, $**

Kawabata
110 Chestnut St., Philadelphia, PA 19106   (215) 928-9564

2455 Grant Ave., Philadelphia, PA 19114   (215) 969-8225
Japanese. Dishes include vegetarian sushi and sukiyaki. **Open daily. Full service, vegetarian/macrobiotic options, take-out, VISA/MC/AMX, $$$**

Keyflower Dining Room
20 S. 36 St., Philadelphia, PA 19104   (215) 386-2207
Natural foods. **Open Monday through Friday for lunch and dinner. Non-smoking, cafeteria style, take-out, $**

Lemon Grass Thai Restaurant
3626-30 Lancaster Ave., Philadelphia, PA 19104   (215) 222-8042
Thai. Request the vegetarian menu. **Open daily for lunch and dinner. Full service, take-out, VISA/MC/AMX/DISC, $$**

Mary's Restaurant
400 Roxborough Ave., Philadelphia, PA 19128   (215) 487-2249
Natural foods. This mostly vegan restaurant offers freshly baked breads and desserts. **Open for dinner Tuesday through Sunday. Sunday Brunch. Full service, vegan/macrobiotic options, take-out, VISA/MC/AMX/DISC, $$**

Middle East Restaurant
126 Chestnut St., Philadelphia, PA 19106   (215) 922-1003
Middle Eastern. This restaurant offers several vegetarian dishes. **Open 5 P.M. to midnight. Full service, vegan options, wine/beer/alcohol, take-out, VISA/MC/ AMX/DISC, $**

Saladalley
Temple University Campus, 1926 Park Mall
Philadelphia, PA 19122   (215) 787-5151
American. See entry under Ardmore, PA, for description.

•• Singapore Vegetarian Restaurant ?❧
1029 Race St., Philadelphia, PA 19107   (215) 922-3288

❧ Reviewers' choice   • Vegetarian restaurant   •• Vegan restaurant
$ less than $6 $$ $6–$12 $$$ more than $12
VISA/AMX/MC/DISC/DC—credit cards accepted
Non-alc.—Non-alcoholic   Fresh juices—freshly squeezed

Vegan/Chinese. This new vegan restaurant is located in Philadelphia's Chinatown. Both the food and service are outstanding. **Open daily for lunch and dinner. Full service, vegan options, fresh juices, take-out, VISA/MC, $$**

South East Restaurant
1000 Arch St., Philadelphia, PA 19107 (215) 629-1888
Chinese. South East has a good selection of vegetarian dishes. **Open daily for lunch and dinner. Full service, vegan/macrobiotic/Pritikin options, take-out, VISA/MC/AMX/DISC, $$**

Szechuan Empire
1699 Grant Ave., Philadelphia, PA 19115 (215) 676-6220
Chinese. Szechuan Empire features an extensive vegan menu. **Open daily, only for dinner on Sunday. Full service, alcohol, take-out, VISA/MC/AMX, $$**

Tang Yean
220 N. 10th St., Philadelphia, PA 19107 (215) 925-3993
Chinese. Here you'll find a great vegetarian menu with vegan options. **Open daily 3 P.M. to midnight. Full service, vegan options, take-out, VISA/MC/AMX, $$**

Taste of India
4015 Chestnut St., Philadelphia, PA 19104 (215) 662-1777
Indian. Savor vegetarian options and a buffet lunch daily. **Open daily for lunch and dinner. Full service, take-out, VISA/MC/AMX/DISC, $$**

Tel Aviva Restaurant and Pizzaria
6724 Castor Ave., Philadelphia, PA 19149 (215) 722-7877
Middle Eastern/pizza. Vegetarian Middle Eastern dishes and veggie pizzas are featured here. **Open daily for lunch and dinner. Full service, vegan options, wine/beer/alcohol, take-out, $$**

Thai Royal
123 S. 23rd St., Philadelphia, PA 19103 (215) 567-2542
Thai. Several vegetarian dishes are offered. **Open daily, only for dinner on weekends. Full service, take-out, wine/beer/alcohol, VISA/MC/AMX, $**

•• Uhuru's Place
4900 Chestnut St., Philadelphia, PA 19139 (215) 474-0226
Vegan. The menu changes daily and includes homemade desserts. **Open Monday through Saturday for lunch and dinner. Full service, vegan options, take-out, $**

Ziggy's
1210 Walnut St., Philadelphia, PA 19107 (215) 985-1838
Japanese. Ziggy's offers some vegetarian dishes. **Open daily for dinner. Full service, take-out, VISA/MC/AMX, $$**

PHOENIXVILLE

Taste of India
450 W. Bridge St., Phoenixville, PA 19460   **(215) 935-3663**
Indian. Taste of India offers a buffet lunch daily. Menu items include pakoras, samosas, and entrees such as eggplant, chickpea, spinach, and potato dishes. **Open daily 11:30 A.M. to 2:30 P.M. and 4:30 P.M. to 10:00 P.M. Full service, take-out, VISA/MC/AMX/DISC, $$**

PINE FORGE

Gracie's New Age Eatery and 21st Century Cafe
Manatawny Rd., Pine Forge, PA 19548   **(215) 323-4004**
Natural foods. The atmosphere has a Southwestern flavor with an outdoor dining terrace. Gracie's goal is to provide a place where both vegetarians and non-vegetarians can be comfortable and share a delicious meal. Foods served include Black Bean Chili, Middle Eastern Sampler, Saffron Curry, and Broccoli with Ravioli. **Open Wednesday through Saturday for dinner, Friday for lunch also. Reservations appreciated. Full service, fresh juices, non-alc. beer, wine/beer/alcohol, take-out, AMX, $$$**

PITTSBURGH

Ali Baba Restaurant
404 S. Craig St., Pittsburgh, PA 15213   **(412) 682-2829**
Middle Eastern. Located in the Oakland section, Ali Baba offers a variety of vegetarian Middle Eastern dishes including a noteworthy couscous dish. **Open Monday through Friday for lunch and daily from 4 P.M. to 10 P.M. Full service, vegan options, beer, take-out, VISA/MC/AMX/DISC, $$**

Star of India
412 S. Craig St., Pittsburgh, PA 15213   **(412) 681-5700**
Indian. There are several vegan dishes plus many other selections using dairy. Open Monday through Friday for lunch, daily for dinner. **Full service, vegan options, dairy or non-dairy mango shake, non-alc. beverages, VISA/MC/AMX, $$**

PORT TREVERTON

• Somewhere in Time
Routes 11 and 15, RD 1, Box 901
Port Treverton, PA 17864   **(717) 374-2202**
Vegetarian. Homemade baked goods are available. **Open Monday through Saturday for three meals. Full service, take-out, VISA/MC, $**

READING

Nature's Garden Natural Foods
Reading Mall, Reading, PA 19606   **(215) 779-3000**
Natural-foods-store deli. Sample Tofu Hogi (tofu, sprouts, and more in whole-wheat

pita), Brown Rice Burgers, and Banana Whirl Blender Treat. **Open Monday through Saturday. Limited service, fresh juices, macrobiotic options, take-out, VISA/MC, $**

Someplace Special
1401 Lancaster Ave., Reading, PA 19607 **(215) 777-2516**
Natural foods/American/herbal store. This store sells herbal plants and herbal seasonings, and uses herbs from its own garden in its prepared foods. You can try Vegetarian Chili with Tempeh over Basmati Rice, Hot Seitan Mock Beef on Pita, and other interesting dishes. The owners prefer that you call ahead for the vegetarian options. There is in-store seating, but it's 99 percent take-out. Cooking classes are offered. **Open Thursday through Sunday for lunch, Tuesday through Sunday for dinner. Take-out, vegan options, usually macrobiotic options, $**

SCRANTON

Siam Restaurant
345 Adams Ave., Scranton, PA 18503 **(717) 963-0303**
Thai. This small Thai restaurant located in downtown Scranton offers several vegetarian dishes including Broccoli and Bean Sprouts, Mixed Vegetables, and Stir-Fried Rice Noodles. **Open for lunch and dinner Tuesday through Friday. Full service, take-out, $**

SPRINGFIELD

Saladalley
1001 Baltimore Pike, Springfield Square
Springfield, PA 19064 **(215) 328-5880**
American. See entry under Ardmore, PA, for description.

STROUDSBURG

• Earthlight Supply
Quaker Plaza, Stroudsburg, PA 18360 **(717) 424-6760**
Vegetarian/health-food-store deli. Snack-bar lunches, soups, casseroles, and sandwiches are served. **Open Monday through Saturday for lunch. Counter service, fresh juices, take-out, $**

Everybody's Cafe
905 Main St., Stroudsburg, PA 18360 **(717) 424-0896**
Natural foods/European. Polish and Italian dishes and other European-style fare include such dishes as Mushroom Picata and many creative entrees. **Open daily for lunch and dinner. Full service, take-out, AMX, $**

🐾 Reviewers' choice   • Vegetarian restaurant   •• Vegan restaurant
$ less than $6 $$ $6–$12 $$$ more than $12
VISA/AMX/MC/DISC/DC—credit cards accepted
Non-alc.—Non-alcoholic   Fresh juices—freshly squeezed

Great Pumpkin Market and Deli
607 E. Market St., Market St. Plaza
West Chester, PA 19380   **(215) 696-0741**
Natural foods deli. The deli moved in 1992 and expanded significantly, adding an organic produce section and nice deli counter. Vegetarian Chili, Tofu Meatball Sandwich, Falafel, a mini salad bar and daily macro platter, daily specials such as Lasagna, baked goods, and two soups are served. **Open daily. Deli, vegan/macrobiotic options, non-alc. beer, take-out, VISA/MC, $**

Hunan Chinese Restaurant
1103 West Chester Pike,
Town and Country Shopping Center
West Chester, PA 19382   **(215) 429-9999**
Chinese. Hunan added a very extensive vegetarian menu in 1992 with numerous appetizers, soups, and entrees, including a large selection of tofu dishes and mock meats. The food is excellent and the staff is very friendly. This is a real treasure for vegetarians, especially for those living in southeastern PA! **Open daily for lunch and dinner. Full service, take-out, VISA/MC/AMX/DISC, $–$$**

Star of India
155 W. Gay St., West Chester, PA 19380   **(215) 429-0125**
Indian. Star of India opened in 1992 and is West Chester's only Indian restaurant. It is located in quaint downtown West Chester and has many vegetarian options. **Full service, take-out, $$**

Nature's Harvest Cafe and Natural Foods Market
101 C E. Moreland Rd., Willow Grove, PA 19090   **(215) 659-7705**
Natural foods. Sandwiches, salads, hot entrees, and Middle Eastern selections are available. **Open Monday through Saturday, 10 A.M. to 8 P.M., Sunday from noon to 4 P.M. Limited service, fresh juices, take-out, VISA/MC/AMX/DISC, $**

PUERTO RICO

Nutrilife
Calle Miguels Casillas #9
Humacao, Puerto Rico 00791   **(809) 852-5068**
Natural foods. This health food store and vegetarian restaurant offers fruit shakes. **Closed Sunday. Cafeteria style, fresh juices, beer, take-out, catering, $**

MAYAGUEZ

• # Bella Vista Hospital Cafeteria
Bella Vista Hospital
Mayaguez, Puerto Rico 00681   **(809) 834-2350**
Vegetarian. This cafeteria serves only vegetarian food. **Open daily for three meals. Cafeteria style, take-out, $**

RHODE ISLAND

BLOCK ISLAND

• # Froozies
PO Box 372 Dodge St., Block Island, RI 02807   **(401) 466-2230**
Vegetarian juice bar. Froozies is not open during the winter; the rest of the year, it offers fresh juices, smoothies, veggie sandwiches on organic bread, and more. This smoke-free establishment has both indoor and outdoor seating. **Open for lunch and dinner daily (closed during the winter). Limited service, fresh juices, vegan options, take-out, $**

EAST PROVIDENCE

Curry in a Hurry
1235 Wampanoag Trail, E. Providence, RI 02915   **(401) 433-4449**
Indian. See description under Providence, RI.

NEWPORT

Harvest Natural Foods & Catering
1 Casino Terr., Newport, RI 02840   **(401) 846-8137**
Health-food-store deli. This deli offers a veggie-pocket bar, fresh salad bar, homemade muffins, hearty soups and stews, sandwiches, oriental stir-fries, and pastas. **Closed Sunday. Limited service, vegan options, take-out, VISA/MC/AMX, $**

PROVIDENCE

Bread & Circus Whole Foods Market
261 Waterman St., Providence, RI 02906   **(401) 272-1690**
Natural foods deli. Enjoy a wide variety of vegetarian and vegan options offered in Bread & Circus's deli and bakery. **Open daily for lunch and dinner. Counter service, macrobiotic/vegan options, espresso/cappuccino, take-out, VISA/MC, $**

Curry In A Hurry
272 Thayer St., Providence, RI 02906   **(401) 453-2424**

Indian. Diners must place their orders at a counter upon arriving at this restaurant; however, your meal is then brought to your table. Several vegetarian curries are available. **Open daily for lunch and dinner. Counter service, take-out, $**

Taj Mahal Restaurant
230 Wickendon St., Providence, RI 02903   **(401) 331-2442**
Indian. Nine options are included on the vegetarian menu, plus some appetizers and soups. **Open Monday through Saturday for lunch and dinner, Sunday for dinner only. Full service, vegan options, take-out, VISA/MC/AMX/DISC, $$**

Taste of India
221 Wickendon St., Providence, RI 02903   **(401) 421-4355**
Indian. A vegetarian section on the menu lists several options. **Full service, vegan options, take-out, $$**

SOUTH CAROLINA

Angel Fish
520 Folly Rd., Merchant Village Center
Charleston, SC 29412   **(803) 762-4722**
Natural foods. Everything is fresh at Angel Fish, and there are daily specials in addition to the regular menu, which lists soups, salads, and pasta dishes with vegetarian options. No meat base is used in soups. **Closed Monday. Full service, vegan options, fresh juices, wine/beer/alcohol, take-out, VISA/MC/AMX, $$**

Doe's Pita Plus
334 E. Bay St., Charleston, SC 29401   **(803) 577-3179**
Middle Eastern. Sandwiches are made with freshly baked pita bread and a variety of fillings. Salads, Stuffed Grape Leaves, Hummus, and other Middle Eastern foods are served. Everything is made on the premises with only the freshest ingredients. **Open daily. Counter service, vegan options, take-out, $**

Annabelle's of Columbia
Dutch Square Mall, Columbia, SC 29210   **(803) 772-5586**

🐌 Reviewers' choice   • Vegetarian restaurant   •• Vegan restaurant
$ less than $6 $$ $6–$12 $$$ more than $12
VISA/AMX/MC/DISC/DC—credit cards accepted
Non-alc.—Non-alcoholic   Fresh juices—freshly squeezed

Family restaurant. This is a regular family restaurant, but a local vegetarian recommends the Stir-Fry Vegetable Platter, and says the chef is willing to create various veggie dishes. **Open daily. Full service, vegan option, wine/beer/alcohol, take-out, VISA/MC/AMX, $$**

The Basil Pot
928 Main St., Columbia, SC 29201-3964   **(803) 799-0928**
Natural foods/macrobiotic. This is the home of the kitchen of the original Southern Vegetarian Hunting Lodge. Here you will find the elusive pinto bean and the more common but equally succulent tofu loaf. Soups and salads, Chili, Tofu Burger, Pizza, sandwiches, daily specials, and a breakfast menu are featured. Primarily vegetarian, Basil Pot serves chicken, turkey, and tuna. **No dinner served on Sunday. Full service, vegan options, fresh juices, non-alc. beer, take-out, VISA/MC, $–$$**

Nice-N-Natural
1217 College St., Columbia, SC 29201   **(803) 799-3471**
Natural foods. Nice-N-Natural specializes in sandwiches and salads, with soups and some side orders to round out the menu. Numerous fresh fruit salads are available. **Open Monday through Friday. Limited service, vegan options, fresh juices, take-out, no credit cards, $**

GREENVILLE
Annie's Cafe
121 S. Main St., Greenville, SC 29601   **(803) 271-4872**
Natural foods. This natural foods restaurant offers some Mexican and other ethnic options. Vegetarian, low-sugar, and low-salt dishes are available. No preservatives are used. Bread is baked fresh daily. **Open daily. Full service, wine/beer, take-out, VISA/MC/AMX, $$**

SOUTH DAKOTA

YANKTON
Body Guard
2101 Broadway Mall, Yankton, SD 57078   **(605) 665-3482**
Natural foods. Experience a natural foods bakery with a lot of specialty and non-allergenic baked goods. **Open daily. Limited service, take-out, $**

TENNESSEE

•• Country Life Buffet
3748 Ringgold Rd., Chattanooga, TN 37412   **(615) 622-2451**
Vegan. Enjoy an all-you-can-eat vegan buffet with different entrees each day, brown rice, beans, cornmeal rolls, and a salad bar. **Open Sunday through Thursday for lunch only. Buffet, take-out, VISA/MC, $–$$**

•• Foods for Life
3220 Brainerd Rd., Chattanooga, TN 37411   **(615) 624-2829**
Vegan. Foods for Life offers vegan entrees made of grains, wheat gluten, tofu, and legumes. Whole-grain breads and a salad bar are also available. **Open Monday through Friday for lunch and dinner. Self service, fresh juices, limited catering, take-out, VISA/MC/DISC, $**

Choices
108 4th Ave. So., Franklin, TN 37064   **(615) 791-0001**
American. Located in an old hardware store, Choices is an eclectic restaurant offering a wide variety of food. Live jazz can be heard some evenings. Vegetarian dishes include a Vegan Lentil-Pea Soup, pasta, Veggie Burritos, Puff Pastry Ravioli, and a Vegetable Platter. **Open daily for lunch and dinner. Full service, beer/ wine/alcohol, VISA/MC/AMX, $$**

El Charro
6701 Kingston Pike, Knoxville, TN 37919   **(615) 584-9807**
Mexican. The veggie burritos, enchiladas, tacos, and rice and beans are prepared without lard. **Open daily. Full service, non alc. beer/wine, wine/beer/alcohol, take-out, VISA/MC/AMX, $–$$**

Falafel Hut
601 15th St., Knoxville, TN 37916   **(615) 522-4963**
Middle Eastern. Falafel Hut offers Hummus, Tabouleh, lentil soups, and salads. **Open daily for breakfast, lunch, and dinner. Full service, non-alc. beer, take-out, VISA/MC/AMX, $–$$**

Hawkeye's Corner
1717 White Ave., Knoxville, TN 37916   **(615) 524-5326**
American/continental. You'll find a wide range of homemade foods with some vegetarian options, and the management is willing to accommodate special requests. Try the Vegetarian Alfredo, Vegetarian Pita, and the salads. There are live concerts Thursdays and Fridays and no cover charge. **Open daily until midnight. Full service, non-alc. beer, wine/beer/alcohol, take-out, VISA/MC/AMX/DISC/ DC, $$**

La Paz

8025 Kingston Pike, Knoxville, TN 37919 **(615) 670-5250**

Mexican. This restaurant and bar combo serves no meat or meat stock in beans or sauces. You can get Vegetarian Chili, and Mexican dishes with spinach fillings. Inquire about the rice as it contained chicken stock at the time of this writing. **Open Tuesday through Sunday for dinner. Full service, non-alc. beer, wine/ beer/alcohol, VISA/MC/AMX, $$**

Mexicali Rose

6500 Kingston Pike, Knoxville, TN 37919 **(615) 588-9191**

Mexican. Beans are made without lard, and there are three types of enchiladas and burritos. **Open Tuesday through Saturday. Full service, non-alc. beverages, beer, $$**

Silver Spoon Cafe

7250 Kingston Pike, Knoxville, TN 37919 **(615) 584-1066**

American cafe. The cafe offers Italian specialties with vegetarian options, including three to four strict vegetarian entrees. Pasta salads and whole-wheat breads are available. **Open daily. Full service, non-alc. beer/wine, wine/beer/alcohol, take-out, VISA/MC/AMX/DISC/DC, $–$$**

The Tomato Head

12 Market Square, Knoxville, TN 37902 **(615) 637-4067**

Italian. Gourmet pizzas, vegetarian and vegan sandwiches, a hummus pita, and tofu enchiladas are all served in a dining room that doubles as an art gallery. **Open Monday through Friday for lunch, Thursday through Saturday for dinner. Full service for dinner, limited service at lunch, vegan options, VISA/MC/AMX, $**

Wang's Place

4009 Chapman Hwy., Knoxville, TN 37920 **(615) 573-4580**

Chinese. The menu lists five vegetarian entrees, a vegetables and tofu dish, and two vegetarian soups. Wang's Place will accommodate vegetarians. **Open daily. Full service, non-alc. beer, wine/beer/alcohol, take-out, VISA/MC/AMX/ DISC/DC, $**

MADISON

Sitar

116 21st Ave. N., Madison, TN 37115 **(615) 321-8888**

Indian. Enjoy several vegetarian entrees at this Indian restaurant including vegetable curries, freshly baked breads, soup, and more. **Open daily for lunch and dinner. Full service, take-out, $$**

• Tennessee Christian Medical Center Cafeteria

500 Hospital Dr., Madison, TN 37115 **(615) 865-37115**

🐾 Reviewers' choice • Vegetarian restaurant •• Vegan restaurant
$ less than $6 $$ $6–$12 $$$ more than $12
VISA/AMX/MC/DISC/DC—credit cards accepted
Non-alc.—Non-alcoholic Fresh juices—freshly squeezed

Vegetarian. This Seventh-day-Adventist-run cafeteria serves only vegetarian food including options such as Cheese Manicotti, burritos, Cashew Casserole, and quiche. There's also a great salad bar. **Open daily. No breakfast on weekends. Cafeteria style, limited take-out, $**

MEMPHIS

La Montagne Restaurant
3550 Park Ave., Memphis, TN 38111   **(901) 458-1060**
Natural foods. This restaurant offers several vegetarian options including daily specials such as veggie burgers, Vegetables Alfredo, pizza, and burritos. **Open for lunch and dinner daily. Full service, espresso/cappuccino, take-out, VISA/MC, $$**

Squash Blossom
5101 Sanderlin #124, Memphis, TN 38117   **(901) 685-2293**

1720 Poplar, Memphis, TN 38104   **(901) 725-4823**
Natural foods. Enjoy a Tofu and Tempeh Vegetable Stir-Fry, Oat Burgers, Linguine Marinara, and other dishes at this smoke-free restaurant. **Open daily. Cafeteria style, vegan options, fresh juices, smoothies, espresso/cappuccino, take-out, VISA/MC/AMX/DISC, $–$$**

NASHVILLE

• Country Life
1917 Division St., Nashville, TN 37203   **(615) 327-3695**
Vegetarian. Country Life features fresh fruit and fresh vegetable salad bars, soups, and hot entrees. **Closed Saturday and Sunday. Cafeteria/buffet style, vegan options, take-out, $**

Garden Allegro
1805 Church St., Nashville, TN 37203   **(615) 327-3834**
Natural foods. This informal, primarily vegetarian restaurant offers Tofu Sloppy Joes, Veggie Reuben Sandwich, Tempeh Burgers, burritos, Vegetarian Curry, Lasagna, Chili Rellenos, Baked Potatoes, plus more. **Open Monday through Saturday for three meals. Full service, vegan options, smoothies, take-out, VISA/MC/AMX, $–$$**

Las Brisas
27 Arcade, Nashville, TN 37219   **(615) 255-6343**
Mexican. Vegetarian options at this restaurant include burritos, Spinach Enchiladas, Veggie Fajita Roll, Chalupas, and more. **Open for lunch Monday through Friday. Counter service, vegan options, take-out, $**

Slice of Life Restaurant and Bakery ❧
1811 Division St., Nashville, TN 37203   **(615) 329-2525**
Natural foods. The emphasis here is on healthy and delicious entrees including Spinach Lasagna, and Black Bean Cakes with Artichoke Stuffing. All items are free of sugar and preservatives. **Open daily. Full service, vegan/macrobiotic options, wine/beer, take-out, VISA/MC/AMX/DISC, $$**

Sunshine Grocery
3201 Belmont Blvd., Nashville, TN 37212 **(615) 297-5100**
Natural-food-store deli. Buy various ethnic vegetarian dishes at this deli counter located in a natural foods store. **Open for three meals Monday through Saturday. Closed Sunday. Take-out only, fresh juices, smoothies, VISA/MC, $**

Windows on the Cumberland
112 2nd Ave. North, Nashville, TN 37201 **(615) 244-7944**
Natural foods. This almost completely vegetarian restaurant offers "lunch and dinner with a view," and live entertainment. **Cafeteria service for lunch, full service for dinner, $**

SAVANNAH

• Gina's Country Health and Vegan Shoppe
1315 Wayne Rd., Savannah, TN 38372 **(901) 925-7220**
Vegetarian. The food served here is vegan. There is honey in some dishes. **Open weekdays. Limited service, vegan options, take-out, $**

TEXAS

AMARILLO

Back to Eden Snack Bar and Deli
2425 I-40 W., Amarillo, TX 79109 **(806) 353-7476**
Natural foods. Described as the healthiest place to eat in Amarillo, this restaurant features fresh baked goods and salads, homemade salad dressings, and fresh soups made without MSG. **Closed Sunday. Limited service, catering, take-out, VISA/ MC/AMX/DISC, $–$$**

AUSTIN

El Mercado
1302 South 1, Austin, TX 78724 **(512) 447-7445**
Mexican. You'll find some vegetarian and some vegan items here. **Full service, take-out, $$**

Martin Bros. Cafe
914 N. Lamar, Austin, TX 78703 **(512) 476-7601**

2815 Guadalupe St., Austin, TX 78705 **(512) 478-9001**
Natural foods. Martin Bros. is a good place to people-watch—artists, musicians, professionals, and politicians. Enjoy Chalupas with Beans and Cheese, soft whole-wheat tacos with black beans or hummus, Nachos, Vegetarian Tamale and Brown Rice Dinner. Frozen desserts include ice cream, yogurt, and sorbet. **Open daily for three meals. Counter service, vegan options, fresh juices, smoothies, take-out, $**

Mother's Cafe and Garden
4215 Duval, Austin, TX 78751   **(512) 451-3994**
Vegetarian. International vegetarian food includes Enchiladas, Stir-Fry, Veggie Burger, Lasagna, soups, salads, and desserts. **Open daily for lunch and dinner. Full service, vegan options, fresh juices, wine/beer, take-out, VISA/MC/DC, $$**

• Mr. Natural
1901 E. First St., Austin, TX 78702   **(512) 477-5228**
Vegetarian. Mr. Natural features Mexican vegetarian food—Vegetarian Fajitas, Veggie Burgers, Veggie Ceviche, Veggie Tamales, Breakfast Tacos with Veggie Chorizo (sausage)— a whole-wheat bakery, and a juice bar. **Open daily 7 A.M. to 8 P.M. Cafeteria style, fresh juices, take-out, $**

• West Lynn Cafe
1110 W. Lynn, Austin, TX 78703   **(512) 482-0950**
Vegetarian. Enjoy a delicious selection of various vegetarian foods from a variety of countries. Soups, sandwiches, light fare, pasta, Southwestern, Mexican, Indian and other international specialties are offered in an eclectic, historic neighborhood close to downtown. **Open daily for lunch and dinner. Weekend brunch. Full service, vegan options, fresh juices, espresso/cappuccino, wine/beer, take-out, VISA/MC/AMX, $–$$**

DALLAS

(For more restaurant listings in the surrounding areas, see Denton, Richardson, and Waxahachie.)

Francis Simun's
1507 N. Garret Ave., Dallas, TX 75206   **(214) 824-4910**
Vegetarian. This vegetarian establishment serves international cuisine including Mexican and Italian food. **Open daily for lunch and dinner. Full service, fresh juices, wine/beer, catering, take-out, AMX/DISC/DC, $–$$$**

H and M Natural Foods Grocery
9191 Forest Lane, Dallas, TX 75243   **(214) 231-6083**
Natural foods. Enjoy the salad bar and entrees such as vegetable burger, vegetarian soup, Tabouleh, Hummus, Avocado Sandwich, Nachos. **Open Monday through Saturday in the afternoon. Limited service, vegan options, fresh juices, VISA/MC/AMX, $**

• Kalachandji's Restaurant and Palace
5430 Gurley Ave., Dallas, TX 75223   **(214) 821-1048**

🍴 Reviewers' choice   • Vegetarian restaurant   •• Vegan restaurant
$ less than $6 $$ $6–$12 $$$ more than $12
VISA/AMX/MC/DISC/DC—credit cards accepted
Non-alc.—Non-alcoholic   Fresh juices—freshly squeezed

Vegetarian/natural foods. No preservatives or refined sweeteners are used. A House Tamarind Tea and fresh homemade breads are served. There's an Indian gift shop and indoor or outdoor dining. **Open Tuesday through Sunday. Self-service buffet, VISA, $$**

Macro Gourmet
850 S. Greenville Ave., Suite 110, Dallas, TX 75081   (214) 669-8328
Macrobiotic. Soups, entrees, desserts, and sandwiches feature organic whole-cereal grains and vegetables. Foods are prepared without dairy, sugar, or preservatives. **Open Monday through Saturday for breakfast and lunch. Dinner is served Thursday through Saturday. Limited service, vegan/macrobiotic options, catering, VISA/MC, $$**

Phil's Natural Eats Cafe
2815 Elm, Dallas, TX 75226   (214) 761-8400
Natural foods. Several years ago, The Vegetarian Resource Group sponsored a restaurant gathering at Phil's Natural Eats Cafe. The food was absolutely delicious. Diners should certainly try the Tex-Mex dishes including Gregg's Tofu Nachos, Guac Tacos, Tamale Plate, enchiladas, and Mushroom Spinach Quesadillas. **Open daily for lunch and dinner. Counter service, vegan options, fresh juices, take-out, $$**

Roy's Nutrition Center
130 Preston Shopping, Dallas, TX 75230   (214) 987-0213
Health-food-store deli/juice bar. Roy's is a deli, bakery, and juice bar cafe offering salads, sandwiches, and entrees such as Lasagna, Brown Rice and Stir-Fry Vegetables, and calzones. **Open Sunday through Friday morning and afternoon. Closes early on Friday in the winter. Juice bar, fresh juices, take-out, VISA/MC/AMX/DISC, $**

Thai Lotus Kitchen
3851 D Cedar Springs, Dallas, TX 75219   (214) 520-9385
Thai. Thai cooking classes are offered in this smoke-free restaurant. **Open Friday and Saturday for lunch and dinner. Full service, take-out, VISA/MC/AMX, $–$$**

DENTON

Mr. Chopsticks
1120 W. Hickory, Denton, TX 76201   (817) 382-5437
Thai. The Denton Area Vegetarian Organization said Mr. Chopsticks' owner has been wonderful about accommodating vegetarians and will make special items. **Open daily. Limited service, take-out, VISA/MC, $**

EL PASO

Body Matter Juice Cafe
4224 N. Mesa, El Paso, TX 79902   (915) 533-5433
Natural foods. In addition to delicious drinks and shakes, enjoy soups, salads, sandwiches, burritos, spinach lasagna, enchiladas, whole-wheat pizza, and more. **Open for three meals Monday through Saturday. Closed Sunday. Full service, fresh juices, vegan options, take-out, $**

Eating With Grace
6110 N. Mesa, El Paso, TX 79912   **(915) 585-9099**
Natural foods. Eating With Grace offers daily specials including soups, salads, veggie burgers, stir-frys, and casseroles. **Open for three meals Monday through Saturday. Closed Sunday. Full service, vegan options, catering, take-out, VISA/ MC, $**

FORT WORTH

(For more restaurant listings in the surrounding area, see Waxahachie.)

The Back Porch
3400-B Camp Bowie, Ft. Worth, TX 76107   **(817) 332-1422**
Sandwich and salad shop. Located across the street from the museums and Omni theater, The Back Porch offers a salad bar (items sold by weight), vegetarian sandwiches and burgers, and low-fat ice cream. **$**

HOUSTON

Asian Restaurant
3701 Weslayan, Houston, TX 77027   **(713) 850-0450**
Chinese/Vietnamese. A separate vegetarian menu includes such items as Mongolian Vegetable Clay Pot, Charlie's Sizzling Plate, Lemon Grass Tofu, and more. Management claims to have the best macrobiotic food in town. **Open Monday through Saturday. Full service, vegan/macrobiotic options, wine/beer, catering, take-out, VISA/MC/AMX/DISC/DC, $**

Bombay Palace
3901 Westheimer, Houston, TX 77027   **(713) 960-8472**
Indian. Bombay Palace is a member of a worldwide chain of Indian restaurants. The daily luncheon buffet includes vegetarian options. **Open daily for lunch and dinner. Full service, wine/beer/alcohol, catering, take-out, VISA/MC/AMX, $$**

Guilin Chinese Cafe
4005 H Bellaire, Houston, TX 77025   **(713) 661-1963**
Chinese. Some vegan entrees are available. **Counter service, $**

• Happy Vegetarian Mart
6131 Wilcrest, Houston, TX 77072   **(713) 879-8989**
Vegetarian. This vegetarian Chinese restaurant offers a large number of appetizers, soups, and main dishes some of which include tofu or mock meats made of soy or gluten. **Open Thursday through Tuesday for lunch and dinner. Closed Wednesday. Full service, vegan options, take-out, $–$$**

Healthy Food Express
4400 Memorial Dr. (at the Bayou Park Club)
Houston, TX 77007   **(713) 861-2800**

1319 Twinbrooke
Houston, TX 77088

Natural foods/macrobiotic. Healthy Food Express is a food delivery business, supplying the client with a week's worth of food, split into two deliveries. Vegetarian, macrobiotic, and Mexican/American foods contain no eggs, dairy, or white sugar. Pasta dishes, whole grains, vegetables, salads, fruit-juice-sweetened desserts, and more are available. **Macrobiotic options, delivery, wine/beer/alcohol, take-out, VISA/MC/DISC, $$**

A Moveable Feast
2202 West Alabama, Houston, TX 77098   (713) 528-3585
Natural foods. Several people recommended this restaurant, which offers blackboard specials and at least one macrobiotic plate daily. The wide selection of vegetarian food includes Chili Tempeh Burgers, Blue Corn Enchiladas with Black Beans, Cheeseless Florentine Lasagna, Vegetarian Barbecue (made with seitan), Vegan Spinach Enchiladas, Vegetarian Chicken Fried Steak with Roasted Potato Sticks, Meatless Happy Burgers, Vegetarian Fajitas, Pita Pizzas, and more. Breakfast is served on weekends. **Open daily 9 A.M. to 10 P.M. Limited service, vegan/ macrobiotic options, fresh juices, organic coffee, take-out, catering, VISA/MC/ AMX/DISC, $–$$**

On the Border
9705 Westheimer, Houston, TX 77042   (713) 977-9955

4608 Westheimer, Houston, TX 77027   (713) 961-4494
Mexican. A *Vegetarian Journal* reader wrote to tell us that this is "Not a vegetarian restaurant, but the only Mexican restaurant in town that I know of that serves Grilled Vegetable Fajitas. Great!!" **Full service, $$**

Red Pepper Restaurant
5626 Westheimer, Houston, TX 77056 (713) 622-7800
Chinese. Savor such unique selections as Vegetarian Peking Duck, Vegetable Dumplings, Spinach Bean Curd Soup, Shredded Dry Bean Curd, Vegetarian Fish (made from black mushrooms wrapped in bean curd skin), Spinach in Light Fresh Garlic Sauce, Red Pepper's Bean Curd, and much more. The restaurant is somewhat formal, but you can dress casually. **Open daily. Full service, wine/beer/alcohol, catering, take-out, VISA/MC/AMX/DC, $$**

Seekers Natural Foods and Vitamins
4004 Bellaire, Houston, TX 77025   (713) 665-2595
Natural foods. This restaurant inside a health food store uses no salt or white sugar. As much organic produce as possible is served at the ninety-item salad bar. Menu includes Rice-N-Veggies, Whole-Wheat Noodle Lasagna, Tofu Spring Rolls, Veggie Cheese Burger, and other items. **Open daily. Full service, vegan/macrobiotic options, fresh juices, smoothies, wine/beer, take-out, VISA/MC/AMX, $**

🐾 Reviewers' choice   • Vegetarian restaurant   •• Vegan restaurant
$ less than $6 $$ $6–$12 $$$ more than $12
VISA/AMX/MC/DISC/DC—credit cards accepted
Non-alc.—Non-alcoholic   Fresh juices—freshly squeezed

Thai Pepper
2049 W. Alabama, Houston, TX 77098   **(713) 520-8225**
Thai. We've been told that the staff is accommodating, the cooks are willing to turn meat entrees into veggie entrees, and it's the best Thai food in Houston. **Full service, $$**

•• Wonderful Vegetarian Restaurant
7549 Westheimer, Houston, TX 77063   **(713) 977-3137**
Vegan/Chinese/kosher. More than 100 dishes are vegan, and there's a special "all-you-can-eat" buffet lunch. You'll find seven wheat-gluten dishes, ten soybean gluten platters, eight marinated mushroom plates, nine types of imitation seafood, and other selections. **Open Tuesday through Sunday. Full service, vegan options, wine/beer, VISA/MC/AMX/DC, $**

RICHARDSON

Macro Gourmet Restaurant
850 S. Greenville #110, Richardson, TX 75081   **(214) 669-8328**
Macrobiotic/natural foods. Food served at the Macro Gourmet Restaurant is primarily vegan and macrobiotic, except fish is served occasionally. Entrees are served with soup, brown rice, blanched vegetables with a tofu dressing, and a salad. Organic ingredients are used whenever possible. **Open for three meals Monday through Saturday. Closed Sunday. Counter service, vegan options, VISA/MC, $–$$**

SAN ANTONIO

Fiesta Patio Cafe
1421 Pat Booker, San Antonio, TX 78148   **(512) 658-5110**
Mexican/natural foods. Whole-grain brown rice is prepared Spanish style. No lard is used; foods are made with peanut oil. Foods are prepared without preservatives, MSG, or other artificial ingredients. Alfalfa sprouts and natural cheese are available. **Open daily except Monday. Full service, wine/beer, VISA/MC/AMX, $**

Gini's Home Cooking and Bakery
7214 Blanco, San Antonio, TX 78216   **(512) 342-2768**
American/natural foods. Good old-fashioned foods are prepared a healthy way and served in a totally smoke-free atmosphere. A *Vegetarian Journal* reader called the fresh baked breads, pies, and cookies "scrumpdilliicious!!" Pritikin-style meals and baked goods are available. Menu choices for vegetarians include seasonal fresh fruit and whole-wheat pancakes. **Open daily. Full service, fresh juices, wine/beer, VISA/MC/AMX, $$**

Thai Kitchen
445 McCarty, San Antonio, TX 78216   **(512) 344-8366**
Thai/Chinese. Enjoy nine vegetarian entrees plus soups and appetizers including Spring Rolls, Hot and Sour Soup, Bean Curd with Hot Pepper, and Noodles with Vegetable Gravy. **Open Monday through Saturday for lunch and dinner. Full service, wine/beer, VISA/MC/AMX/DISC/DC, $$**

Twin Sisters Bakery and Cafe
6322 N. New Braunfels, San Antonio, TX 78209 **(512) 822-0761**
Natural foods/American/Mexican. The owners call this an "herbally influenced restaurant." Whole-wheat Chalupas and Quesadillas are samples of the natural choices. Oatmeal Special and Tacos are included on the breakfast menu. **Open for breakfast daily. Lunch and dinner served Tuesday through Saturday. Closed Sunday. Full service, vegan/macrobiotic options, fresh juice, wine/beer, $–$$**

Zuni Grill
511 Riverwalk, San Antonio, TX 78205 **(512) 227-0864**
Southwestern. This relatively new restaurant is located one block from the San Antonio Convention Center. In the heart of the Riverwalk tourist district, it has both indoor and outdoor seating. Zuni Grill offers vegetarian and vegan soups and three vegetarian entrees. Vegans may request that dishes be prepared without cheese. **Open daily for breakfast, lunch, and dinner. Full service, vegan options, catering, take-out, VISA/MC/AMX/DISC/DC, $$**

WACO

Joe's Sandwich Shop
1900 S. 12th St., Waco, TX 76706 **(817) 756-5151**
International/American. Close to Baylor University, this shop features Veggie Sandwich (pita stuffed with vegetables), Falafel, Thyme Pizza, Labneh Sandwich (Middle Eastern cheese spread with tomatoes and dried mint), and Tabouleh. **Open daily except Sunday; in the summer, lunch hours only. Cafeteria style, catering, take-out, $**

Waco Natural Foods
1424 Lake Air Dr., Waco, TX 76710 **(817) 772-5743**
Natural foods. You'll find a vegetarian menu; vegan food is available. **Hours vary. Full service, vegan options, take-out, $**

WAXAHACHIE

Kirkpatrick's Natural Foods
207 S. College, Waxahachie, TX 75165 **(214) 937-0010**
Natural foods. Lunches include homemade soups, soy burgers, and homemade pastas. Dinner is new-American-cuisine style served by candlelight. **Open for lunch Monday through Friday. Open for dinner Thursday through Saturday. Full service, catering, take-out, VISA/MC/AMX, $–$$$**

WESLACO

Pelly Health Ranch
1616 S. Bridge Ave., Weslaco, TX 78596 **(512) 968-5343**
Natural foods. Pelly specializes in raw food dishes. **Open daily. Full service, take-out, $**

U.S. Virgin Islands

• ## The Garden of Luscious Licks
Cruz Bay, St. Johns, U.S. Virgin Islands   (809) 693-8400
Vegetarian. This restaurant, located across from the National Park Services, offers Whole Wheat/Oatmeal Pancakes, Falafel Sandwiches, various soups, pizza, veggie burgers, salads, and soy shakes. **Open Monday through Saturday for three meals. Closed Sunday. Full service, fresh juices, espresso/cappuccino, vegan options, take-out, $**

ST. THOMAS

• ## Akasha Sweet Life
Smith Bay, St. Thomas, U.S. Virgin Islands   (809) 775-2650
Vegetarian. This is a small vegetarian cafe. **Open for lunch and dinner daily. Full service, VISA/MC, $$**

Wok and Roll
Red Hook, St. Thomas, U.S. Virgin Islands   (809) 775-6246
Chinese. This take-out restaurant offers four vegetarian entrees including Curry Tofu and Buddha's Delight. It is located across the street from the ferry dock. **Open daily for lunch and dinner. Take-out only, $$**

Zorba's
Charlotte Amalie, St. Thomas, U.S. Virgin Islands   (809) 776-0444
Greek/Mediterranean. This restaurant offers several vegetarian and vegan options. **Open Monday through Saturday for lunch and dinner. Full service, vegan options, take-out, VISA/MC/AMX, $-$$**

Utah

BOULDER

Pole's Place
465 N. Highway 12, Boulder, UT 84716   (801) 335-7422
American. This restaurant is located across the street from Anasazi State Park. It offers a veggie burger and salads. **Open daily. Counter service, $**

HURRICANE

New Garden Cafe
130 S. Main , Hurricane, UT 84737   (801) 635-9825
Natural foods. Outdoor seating is available next to a garden—a wonderful setting

for a meal. Fresh dessert specials and cappuccino are featured. **Closed Sunday. Self-serve counter, espresso/cappuccino, $**

MOAB

Honest Ozzie's Cafe and Desert Oasis
60 N. 100 W., Moab, UT 84532 (801) 259-8442

Natural foods. Moab's only natural foods restaurant and bakery, Honest Ozzie's features garden seating and displays of local artwork. This nearly vegetarian restaurant serves whole grains for breakfast, and tempting appetizers, salads, and entrees for lunch and dinner. **Open daily. Closed in December and January. Full service, vegan options, carrot juice, organic coffee and tea, fruit smoothies, wine/beer, $-$$**

OGDEN

Bright Day Natural Lunches
952 28th St., Ogden, UT 84403 (801) 394-7503

Natural foods. Bright Day features soups made from fresh vegetables, sandwiches on seven-grain bread, fruit shakes, and baked goods. **Closed Sunday, open for lunch Monday through Saturday. Counter service, vegan options, fresh juices, take-out, $**

Harvest Restaurant
341 27th St., Ogden, UT 84401 (801) 621-1627

Natural foods. Enjoy a wide variety of sandwiches, soups, and salads at Harvest Restaurant. **Open Monday through Saturday for three meals. Full service, fresh juices, smoothies, catering, take-out, VISA/MC/AMX, $**

The Mexican Place - Senior Frogs
455 25th St., Ogden, UT 84405 (801) 394-2323

Mexican. Only vegetable oil is used, and many entrees can be made without cheese. **Open daily. Full service, vegan options, wine/beer/alcohol, take-out, VISA/MC, $-$$**

PROVO

Good Earth Cafe
384 West Center, Provo, UT 84601 (801) 377-7447

Natural foods. Located in a natural foods store, this cafe offers a wide variety of salads, sandwiches, tofu hot dogs, and more. **Open Monday through Saturday for three meals. Counter service, vegan options, take-out, $**

🕏 Reviewers' choice • Vegetarian restaurant •• Vegan restaurant
$ less than $6 $$ $6–$12 $$$ more than $12
VISA/AMX/MC/DISC/DC—credit cards accepted
Non-alc.—Non-alcoholic Fresh juices—freshly squeezed

Bangkok Thai
1400 Foothill Dr., #210, Salt Lake City, UT 84108   (801) 582-8424
Thai. Enjoy vegetarian "palace-style cuisine" like pad tofu sauteed with chilies, garlic, broccoli, peppers, and basil; or woon sen kai, which is glass noodles sauteed with bamboo shoots, egg, bean sprouts, onions, and Thai seasonings. Vegetable stock is used in all vegetarian dishes. According to the menu, most dishes can be ordered vegetarian upon request. Indicate to your server if you want your meal prepared vegan. **Open daily for dinner, Monday through Friday for lunch. Full service, vegan options, take-out, VISA/MC/AMX, $$**

Deloretto's
2939 E. 3300 So., Salt Lake City, UT 84109   (801) 485-4534
Italian. Some vegetarian options are available here. **Open daily. Full service, beer, take-out, $**

New Frontiers Natural Foods
2454 S. 700 East, Salt Lake City, UT 84106   (801) 359-7913

802 E. 200 South, Salt Lake City, UT 84102   (801) 355-7401
Natural foods. This natural bakery and deli features items made to order from scratch and excellent desserts. **Open daily. Counter service, fresh juices, catering, VISA/MC/AMX/DISC, $**

• Park Ivy Garden Cafe
878 S. 900 East, Salt Lake City, UT 84102   (801) 328-1313
Vegetarian. This restaurant views vegetarianism as "a global ecological neccessity," and works towards educating its patrons. Specialties include freshly baked breads, "Save the Chicken" Salad, and homemade soups. Dinner specials change nightly. **Closed Sunday. Limited service, vegan options, catering, VISA/MC, $$**

Panda Garden
8805 Zion Park Blvd., Springdale, UT 84676   (801) 772-3535
Chinese. Panda Garden is located near Zion National Park. It offers eight vegetarian Chinese dishes, including several with tofu. **Open daily for lunch and dinner. Full service, vegan options, take-out, $$**

Zion Pizza & Noodle Company
Zion National Park
Town Center, Springdale, UT 84767   (801) 772-3815
Pizzeria. Enjoy several different types of veggie pizza, as well as a veggie stir-fry with pasta, and other dishes. **Open daily for dinner. Full service, take-out, $$**

Capitol Reef Cafe
360 West Main St., Torrey, UT 84775   (801) 425-3271

Natural foods. This cafe is located next to an inn a few miles from Capitol Reef National Park and offers a wide variety of vegetarian dishes including salads, sandwiches, stir-fry vegetables, Fettuccine Primavera, Mushroom Lasagna, and more. **Hours vary according to season; call ahead. Full service, fresh juices, espresso/cappuccino, take-out, $$**

VERMONT

BRATTLEBORO

Common Ground
25 Elliot St., Brattleboro, VT 05301   **(802) 257-0855**
Natural foods. A community-based worker-owned cooperative, Common Ground emphasizes the use of local and organic foods. The restaurant strives to maintain a balance between business needs and social and environmental concerns. Fish is served on weekends only, and stir-fry and seitan dishes are always served. **Closed Tuesday. Vegan options, take-out, fresh juices, wine/beer, no credit cards, $**

BURLINGTON

• Origanum Natural Foods Cafe
227 Main St., Burlington, VT 05401   **(802) 863-6103**
Vegetarian deli. This deli offers an excellent selection of hot dishes, soups, veggie burgers, sandwiches, salads, beverages, and an extensive salad bar with many organic ingredients. Various ethnic foods are featured as well. Eggs are not used. **Open daily. Cafeteria style, vegan options, fresh juices, take-out, VISA/MC, $**

MANCHESTER CENTER

Bagel Works
Routes 11 & 30, Manchester Center, VT 05255   **(802) 362-5082**
Bagel deli. More than sixteen varieties of bagels are available with various topping options including cream cheeses, tofutti spreads, salads, and vegetarian combinations. Ingredients are all natural and prepared without preservatives. Bagel Works is environmentally conscious and socially active in the community. **Open daily. Counter service, vegan options, fresh juices, take-out, $**

MONTPELIER

• Horn of the Moon Cafe
8 Langdon St., Montpelier, VT 05602   **(802) 223-2895**
Vegetarian. Established in 1977, the Horn of the Moon is the oldest vegetarian restaurant in New England. The menu lists salads, sandwiches, soups, homemade breads, and daily specials. Vegan and heart-healthy dishes are clearly indicated on the menu, and local organic produce and ingredients are used when possible. The walls of the cafe are decorated with the work of local artists in a rotating exhibit. **Open Tuesday through Sunday for three meals; Monday for breakfast and lunch. Full service, vegan options, fresh juices, wine/beer, catering, take-out, no credit cards, $**

State Street Market Grocery and Deli
20 State St., Montpelier, VT 05602   **(802) 229-9353**
Natural foods. Homemade natural foods include soups, sandwiches, deli salads, and hot entrees. **Closed Sunday. Cafeteria style, take-out, $**

NEWPORT
• ## Newport Natural Foods Bakery & Cafe
66 Main St., Newport, VT 05855   **(802) 334-2626**
Vegetarian. Several hot soups and entrees are offered daily plus sandwiches, salads, desserts, and fresh baked goods. A chalkboard menu changes daily. **Closed Sunday. Cafeteria style, take-out, $**

VIRGINIA

ALEXANDRIA
Bombay Curry Company
3102 Mt. Vernon Ave., Alexandria, VA 22305   **(703) 836-6363**
Indian. Try the vegetarian curry, vegetarian thali, or vegetable biryani. **Open daily for lunch and dinner. Full service, VISA/MC/DISC/DC, $$**

Mediterranean Bakery and Cafe
352 S. Pickett St., Alexandria, VA 22304   **(703) 751-1702**
Natural foods/Middle Eastern. Mediterranean decor— including arches, columns, and a terra cotta canopy—is found in this wonderful cafe. Dine on Middle Eastern vegetarian delicacies including Falafel, Hummus, Baba Ghanouj, Stuffed Grape Leaves, various salads, spinach pies, and casseroles. All baked goods are prepared fresh on the premises. A grocery store offering Middle Eastern, Italian, and Greek items is also located here. **Open daily for breakfast, lunch, and dinner. Limited service, take-out, $–$$**

ARLINGTON
Adulis Restaurant
2325 Eads St., Arlington, VA 22202   **(703) 920-3188**
Ethiopian. Eight vegetarian specials plus appetizers are available at Adulis. **Full service, vegan options, espresso/cappuccino, wine/beer, $–$$**

Bardo Rodeo
2000 Wilson Blvd., Arlington, VA 22201   **(703) 527-9399**
Pub. This pub, seating 600 indoors and 400 on the outdoor patio, serves no red meat and offers many vegetarian dishes (some of which require your specifying that the chicken or fish be omitted) including Indonesian Sauté, Hummus, an Indian platter, Salsa, Guacamole, Grilled Vegetable Lasagna, tostadas, burritos,

salads, and sandwiches. The menu changes regularly. **Open daily. Full service, vegan options, wine/beer, VISA/MC, $–$$**

Bombay Curry House
2529 Wilson Blvd., Arlington, VA 22201 (703) 528-0849

Indian. Bombay Curry House has several options for vegetarians. **Open daily. Full service, wine/beer, take-out, VISA/MC/AMX, $–$$**

Chesapeake Seafood & Crab House
3607 Wilson Blvd., Arlington, VA 22201 (703) 528-8888

International. A pleasant surprise for any vegetarian who might find himself here, the Chesapeake House has a wide selection of unique and creative vegetarian appetizers, soups, and gourmet specialties. Examples include Lemon Grass Tofu, Mongolian Vegetable Clay Pot, and Cantonese Chow Mein. **Open daily. Full service, vegan options, wine/beer, take-out, VISA/MC/AMX/DISC, $–$$**

China Gourmet Cafe
2154 Crystal Plaza Arcade, Arlington, VA 22202 (703) 415-0300

Chinese. Located underground in Crystal City, China Gourmet offers low-priced lunch and dinner combination specials featuring many meatless dishes. China Gourmet is willing to accommodate special requests. **Closed Sunday. Limited service, vegan options, wine/beer, take-out, $**

Kabul Caravan Restaurant
1725 Wilson Blvd., Arlington, VA 22209 (703) 522-8394

International. Authentic international foods are prepared fresh daily. There is a vegetarian menu section with four options plus side dishes. **Open daily. Full service, vegan options, wine/beer/alcohol, take-out, VISA/MC/AMX, $$**

• Madhu Ban
3217 N. Washington Blvd., Arlington, VA 22201 (703) 528-7184

Vegetarian/Indian. This new vegetarian restaurant is located in the Virginia suburbs of Washington, D.C. It offers a wide variety of Indian breads, soups, salads, and entrees including curry and rice, masala dosas, and more. **Open daily for lunch and dinner. Full service, non-alc. beer/wine, catering, take-out, VISA/ MC, $$**

Pamir Afghan Restaurant
561 S. 23rd St., Arlington, VA 22204 (703) 979-0777

Afghan. Three vegetarian entrees plus appetizers make up the veggie selections at Pamir. **Closed Sunday. Full service, vegan options, wine/beer/alcohol, take-out, VISA/MC/AMX, $$**

ಿ Reviewers' choice   • Vegetarian restaurant   •• Vegan restaurant
$ less than $6 $$ $6–$12 $$$ more than $12
VISA/AMX/MC/DISC/DC–credit cards accepted
Non-alc.–Non-alcoholic   Fresh juices–freshly squeezed

BLACKSBURG
South Main Cafe
117 S. Main St., Blacksburg, VA 24060   **(703) 552-3622**
Ethnic foods. A variety of delicious-sounding, international vegetarian entrees includes Lemon Grilled Tempeh Filet, Thai Eggplant, and Tofu and Pad Thai. Chicken and fish are also served. **Open for lunch and dinner. Closed Sunday. Full service, vegan options, fresh juice, wine/beer/alcohol, take-out, $–$$**

CENTREVILLE
• Herb Garden Express
5705 Regimental Court, Centreville, VA 22020   **(703) 818-8477**
Vegetarian. Herb Garden Express is a catering service that offers vegetarian, vegan, and macrobiotic meals with an international flavor. Herb Garden caters weddings and other parties, and also delivers to homes. **Catering, $$**

CHARLOTTESVILLE
Integral Yoga Natural Foods
923 Preston Ave., Charlottesville, VA 22901   **(804) 293-4111**
Vegetarian. This self-serve restaurant offers deli food by the pound, sandwiches, baked goods, knishes, Lasagna, Hummus, pasta dishes, Indian and Mexican foods. **Open daily. Self-serve, vegan options, non-alc. beer/wine, take-out, VISA/MC, $**

Ming Dynasty
1417 Emmet St., Charlottesville, VA 22901   **(804) 979-0909**
Chinese. This Chinese restaurant offers a huge vegetarian selection. Dine on mock meat, fish, and poultry dishes. Enjoy Mixed Vegetables, Fried Rice, Spring Rolls, Steamed Dumplings, Rice Noodles, bean curd dishes, and more. **Open for lunch and dinner daily. Full service, take-out, VISA/MC/AMX, $$**

FALLS CHURCH
Panjshir Restaurant
924 West Broad St., Falls Church, VA 22046   **(703) 536-4566**
Afghan. Panjshir features vegetarian eggplant, pumpkin, and spinach dishes. **Open daily. Full service, wine/beer/alcohol, take-out, VISA/MC/AMX, $$**

FREDERICKSBURG
Sammy T's Light Food and Ale
801 Caroline St., Fredericksburg, VA 22401   **(703) 371-2008**
Natural foods. Foods are made fresh to order with vegan and vegetarian options, some Middle Eastern and Mexican dishes, and a wide selection of beer. **Open for three meals daily. Full service, vegan options, wine/beer, take-out, VISA/MC/ DISC, $–$$**

HERNDON

Ariana Afghan Restaurant

283 Sunset Park Dr., Herndon, VA 22070   **(703) 435-0151**

International. One of the few restaurants offering Afghan cuisine, Ariana special-izes in kabobs, low-cholesterol, low-fat, and vegetarian dishes. Indian and Middle Eastern specialities are also offered. The vegetable dishes include eggplant, spin-ach, pumpkin, leek, cauliflower, and lentils. No MSG is used. **Closed Sunday. Full service, vegan options, non-alc. beer, wine/beer, take-out, VISA/MC, $$**

A Little Place Called Siam

328 Elden St., Herndon, VA 22070   **(703) 742-8881**

Asian. An extensive vegetarian selection distinguishes the Thai and Southeast Asian cuisine here. Many tofu, eggplant, and vegetable entrees are available as are appetizers and soup. **Full service, vegan options, wine/beer/alcohol, take-out, VISA/MC/AMX, $$**

LEESBURG

Andy's Pizza & Subs

9F Catoctin Circle SW, Leesburg, VA 22075   **(703) 771-0277**

Deli. Many Middle Eastern favorites such as Falafel, Hummus, Baba Ghanouj, and Stuffed Grape Leaves are offered. Andy will make Lemon-Tahini Sauce for the Falafel for vegans. **Full service, vegan options, $**

LURAY

Mindi's Mexican Restaurant

Rt. 211 West, Luray, VA 22835   **(703) 743-7550**

Mexican. Enjoy several vegetarian Mexican dishes including tacos, burritos, enchi-ladas, and more. Kids are especially welcomed! **Open for lunch and dinner Tuesday through Sunday. Full service, vegan options, non-alc. beer, beer/wine, $**

RICHMOND

• Grace Place

826 W. Grace St., Richmond, VA 23220   **(804) 353-3680**

Vegetarian. This twenty-year-old vegetarian restaurant specializes in international cuisine. Grace Place, with its rotating art show on the walls, is a sanctuary to artists, musicians, the sensitive, and well-informed. **Closed Sunday. Full service, vegan options, fresh juices, organic coffee, wine/beer/alcohol, take-out, VISA/MC $$**

ROANOKE

•• The Eden Way Place

307 Market St., SE, Roanoke, VA 24011   **(703) 344-3336**

Vegan. Located in the historic market district of downtown Roanoke, Eden Way offers a low-fat vegan menu with entrees, soups, burgers, and Falafel. Whole-grain breads and desserts are baked fresh in the restaurant's bakery, and there's a natural foods store in the same location. **Closed Saturday. Full service, vegan, take-out, $**

VIENNA

Panjshir II Restaurant
224 W. Maple Ave., Vienna, VA 22180   **(703) 281-4183**
Afghan. See listing under Falls Church.

VIRGINIA BEACH

The Cool Breeze Cafe
1102 Atlantic Ave., Virginia Beach, VA 23451   **(804) 437-9433**
American. The Cool Breeze Cafe is open during the summer season only. It offers vegetarian options including salads and veggie pita sandwiches. **Open for three meals daily Memorial Day through Labor Day only. Full service, vegan options, take-out, $**

Fresh Market Deli, Inc.
550 First Colonial Rd., Hilltop Square Shopping Center
Virginia Beach, VA 23451   **(804) 425-5383**
Natural foods. Unique and creative vegetarian food. **Open Monday through Saturday. Full service, fresh juices, smoothies, take-out, $**

The Heritage Cafe
314 Laskin Rd., Virginia Beach, VA 23451   **(804) 428-0500**
Natural foods. Many of the entrees, sandwiches, soups, and fresh baked desserts are prepared free of wheat, dairy, sugar, and animal ingredients. **Open daily for three meals. Limited service, vegan options, fresh juices, smoothies, take-out, VISA/MC/AMX/DISC, $**

India Restaurant
5760 Northampton Blvd., Virginia Beach, VA 23455   **(804) 460-2100**
Indian. Vegetarian items offered at India Restaurant include curry dishes, vegetable biryani, freshly baked Indian breads, plus more. **Open daily for lunch and dinner. Full service, vegan options, take-out, $$**

WILLIAMSBURG

Chez Trinh
Williamsburg Shopping Center
Monticello Ave. at Richmond Rd.
Williamsburg, VA 23185   **(804) 253-1888**
Vietnamese. All dishes are prepared fresh and cooked to order; service can, therefore, be slow at times. Vegetarian dishes include Bean Curd with Vegetables, Vegetarian Noodles, Tofu Cutlets and Peanut Sauce served with Rice Paper, and Sautéed String Beans. **Open daily for lunch and dinner. Full service, take-out, $$**

WASHINGTON

Natural Gourmet
Harold's Square, Bainbridge Island, WA 98110   **(206) 842-2759**
Natural foods. Vegetarian dishes include fresh salads, entrees, soups, and sandwiches. **Closed Sunday. Limited service, vegan options, fresh juices, espresso, take-out, VISA/MC, $**

BELLEVUE

Thai Chef
1645 140th Ave., NE, Bellevue, WA 98005   **(206) 562-7955**
Thai. A wide selection of Thai foods includes vegetarian appetizer, soup, and entree specialties. **Open daily. Full service, vegan options, wine/beer, take-out, VISA/MC/AMX, $$**

Twelve Baskets Restaurant & Catering
825-116th Ave., Bellevue, WA 98004   **(206) 455-3684**
Natural foods. All seating is non-smoking in this country cottage atmosphere. Enjoy vegetarian entrees, excellent homemade soups, sandwiches, salads, pasta, and desserts. Christian music, drama, and entertainment are featured on weekends. **Closed Sunday. Full service, vegan options, fresh juices, espresso, take-out, VISA/MC/AMX/DISC, $$**

BELLINGHAM

Bangkok House Restaurant
2500 Meridan, Bellingham, WA 98225   **(206) 733-3322**
Thai. Many tofu dishes are offered. **Closed Sunday. Full service, vegan options, non-alc. beer, wine/beer, take-out, VISA/MC, $$**

Old Town Cafe
316 W. Holly St., Bellingham, WA 98225   **(206) 671-4431**
Natural foods. The Old Town Cafe has a special philosophy regarding its staff: "The people who work here are a team. All jobs are equally important and all tips are shared equally by the cooks, dishwashers, and waitpersons." This social consciousness extends to recycling everything possible, reducing use of non-recyclables, and supporting local food suppliers. Sandwiches, salads, soups, and vegetarian specials are offered. **Open daily for breakfast and lunch. No smoking. Full service, vegan options, fresh juices, espresso, $**

🍴 Reviewers' choice   ● Vegetarian restaurant   ●● Vegan restaurant
$ less than $6 $$ $6–$12 $$$ more than $12
VISA/AMX/MC/DISC/DC—credit cards accepted
Non-alc.—Non-alcoholic   Fresh juices—freshly squeezed

Taste of India
3930 Meridan St., #J, Bellingham, WA 98226   **(206) 647-1589**
Indian. Many vegetarian specialties are prepared to order. The breads are delicious. **Open daily for lunch and dinner. Full service, vegan options, wine/beer, $$**

Thai House
3930 Meridan St., Bellingham, WA 98226   **(206) 734-5111**
Thai. Vegetarian offerings include rice and noodle dishes, and spring rolls. **Take-out, $–$$**

COLLEGE PLACE

• Walla Walla College Cafeteria
32 SE Ash, College Place, WA 99324   **(509) 527-2732**
Vegetarian. Sample meat analogues, Mexican food bar, and "Nature's Inn" bar without eggs or dairy. Desserts are sweetened with dates. **Open daily during school year. Limited hours in summer. Cafeteria service, vegan options, take-out, $**

ELLENSBURG

Valley Cafe & Takeout
105 W. 3rd, Ellensburg, WA 98926   **(509) 925-3050**
Northwest cuisine. Pacific Northwest cuisine is featured in an original art deco facility. There are some vegetarian options, and all dishes are prepared fresh using only the best ingredients. **Open 11 A.M. to 9 P.M. Monday through Friday, 7:30 A.M. to 10 P.M. Saturday and Sunday. MC/VISA/AMX/DISC**

FEDERAL WAY

Marlene's Market & Deli
31839 Gateway Center Blvd., S.
Federal Way, WA 98003   **(206) 839-0933**
Natural foods. This clean and inviting deli/restaurant has an adjoining espresso bar serving only organically grown coffee. There's easy access next to Interstate 5. **Open daily. Limited service, fresh juices, take-out, VISA/MC, $**

MT. VERNON

The Deli Next Door
202 S. First St., Mt. Vernon, WA 98723   **(206) 336-3886**
Natural foods. Enjoy wholesome sandwiches, salads, specialties, hot entrees, deli salads, and kids' plates. **Open daily. Limited service, fresh juices, espresso, $**

OLGA

Doe Bay Cafe
Star Route 86, Olga, WA 98279   **(206) 376-2291**
Natural foods. Doe Bay Cafe is situated in a turn-of-the-century building overlooking Otter Cove at the historic Doe Bay Village Resort and Retreat on Orcas Island. Serving dishes with an international flavor, Doe Bay has a casual and social setting.

Mineral spring hot tubs, cedar sauna, massage, and a daily guided kayak-trip help build appetites worthy of the meals at Doe Bay Cafe. Indoor and outdoor seating. **Open daily in summer, only weekends and holidays after September. Full service, wine/beer, $$**

OLYMPIA

Red Apple Natural Foods
400 Cooper Point Rd., Olympia, WA 98502   **(206) 357-8779**
Health-food-store deli. This deli offers soups, veggie burgers, sandwiches, Chili, and vegan espresso in case you need a little boost! **Closed Sunday. Counter service, vegan options, fresh juices, organic coffee, espresso, take-out, VISA/MC, $**

The Urban Onion
116 Legion Way, Olympia, WA 98501   **(206) 943-9242**
Health-conscious cuisine. The Urban Onion is located in the Hotel Olympian across from Sylvester Park. Vegetarian health-conscious cuisine is featured along with espresso and delicious desserts. **Open daily. Full service, fresh juices, espresso, wine/beer, take-out, VISA/MC/AMX, $$**

PORT ANGELES

Cafe Garden
1506 E. First St., Port Angeles, WA 98362   **(206) 457-4611**
Ethnic. Breakfast items are served all day, and there are creative salads, pasta, and Szechuan stir-fries. **Open daily. Vegan options, wine/beer, $$**

ROCKPORT

Cascadian Farm Organic Market
5375 Hwy 20, Rockport, WA 98283   **(206) 853-8629**
Juice bar. This organic farm offers juices, espresso, freshly baked goods, and sorbet. There's a picnic area, and self-guided tours are permitted. **Open until dusk from May until October. Counter service, fresh juices, espresso, VISA/MC, $**

SAN JUAN ISLAND

Springtree Cafe
310 Spring St., Friday Harbor
San Juan Island, WA 98250   **(206) 378-4848**
Cafe. Innovative and tasty vegetarian entrees are served every night. **$$**

SEATTLE

(For additional restaurant listings, see Bellevue and Federal Way.)

•• Araya's Vegetarian Place
4732 University Way NE, Seattle, WA 98105   **(206) 524-4332**
Vegan. Enjoy 50 vegan Thai dishes at this Seattle restaurant that opened in 1994. Don't miss the all-you-can-eat buffet lunch on Saturdays, which is fantastic. **Open**

for lunch and dinner Monday through Saturday, and only for dinner on Sunday. Full service, completely vegan, take-out, VISA/MC/AMX, $–$$

Bagel Express
205 1st Ave., So., Seattle, WA 98104   **(206) 682-7202**
Sandwich shop. "Handcrafted" soups are the specialty here; 80 percent of them are vegetarian. Lunch special is a bagel sandwich with a cup of soup. Vegetarian sandwiches are also on the menu. **Open Monday through Friday, also Saturday in July and August only. Counter service, vegan options, fresh juices, take-out, $**

Bahn Thai Restaurant
409 Roy St., Seattle, WA 98109   **(206) 283-0444**
Thai. Thirteen vegetarian entrees, appetizers, and rice and noodle dishes are included on this Thai menu. **Open daily. Full service, vegan options, wine/beer, take-out, VISA/MC/AMX/DISC, $**

•• Bamboo Garden
364 Roy St., Seattle, WA 98109   **(206) 282-6616**
Vegan/Chinese. The extensive vegetarian menu features delicious vegan Chinese cuisine. Don't be confused when you see turkey and chicken; they're all made from vegetable protein. Eggs and dairy products are not used. **Open for lunch and dinner daily. Reservations accepted. Full service, completely vegan, wine/beer/alcohol, take-out, VISA/MC/AMX, $$**

Bangkok Hut
2126-3rd Ave. & Blanchard, Seattle, WA 98121   **(206) 441-4425**
Thai. Eleven vegetarian options, appetizers, and salad are offered. **Open daily. Full service, vegan options, wine/beer, take-out, VISA/MC/AMX, $–$$**

• Black Cat Cafe
4110 Roosevelt Way, Seattle, WA 98105   **(206) 547-3887**
Vegetarian. Nearly vegan, this restaurant uses no eggs and offers such dishes as Tofu Rancheros and Blue Corn Pancakes for brunch. Soups, salads, and sandwiches are also available. **Open Tuesday through Sunday. Closed Monday. Full service, catering, vegan options, take-out, $**

• The Blue Planet Cafe
2208 N. 45th St., Seattle, WA 98103   **(206) 632-0750**
Vegetarian. Almost everthing served at this cafe is organically grown. Tofu Nut Burgers, lasagna, pasta, salads, and vegan pastries are featured. **Open daily. Full service, vegan options, fresh juices, organic coffee, take-out (in your own container), VISA/MC, $$**

🐾 Reviewers' choice   • Vegetarian restaurant   •• Vegan restaurant
$ less than $6 $$ $6–$12 $$$ more than $12
VISA/AMX/MC/DISC/DC—credit cards accepted
Non-alc.—Non-alcoholic   Fresh juices—freshly squeezed

Cafe Counter Intelligence
94 Pike Suite 32, Seattle, WA 98101   **(206) 622-6979**
Natural foods. Egg dishes, soups, and salads are served here. **Open Monday through Wednesday for breakfast and lunch. Full service, wine/beer, take-out, $**

• Cafe Flora
2901 E. Madison, Seattle, WA 98112   **(206) 325-9100**
International vegetarian. Savor fine international vegetarian food featuring the flavors of Mexico, Japan, and India. The many creative dishes include Sage Pappardelle with Wild Mushrooms, Grilled Nutburger, Oaxaca Tacos, and Indian Chickpea Stew. **Closed Monday. Full service, vegan options, fresh juices, non-alc. beer, take-out, VISA/MC, $$**

Cafe Loc
407 Broad St., Seattle, WA 98109   **(206) 441-6883**
Cafe. Cafe Loc offers family-style cooking with vegetarian options. **Open daily. Full service, beer, take-out, $**

Cause Celeb
524 15th Ave. E., Seattle, WA 98112   **(206) 323-1888**
Natural Foods. Enjoy Spinach Nut Burgers, and stir-fries. **Open daily. Full service, catering, wine/beer, take-out, $**

Cyclops Cafe
2416 Western Ave., Seattle, WA 98121   **(206) 441-1677**
Cafe. Vegetarian fare is offered in a fun, eclectic setting. **Open daily. Weekend breakfasts. Full service, espresso, wine/beer, take-out, VISA/MC, $$**

Elliot Bay Cafe
101 S. Main St., Seattle, WA 98104   **(206) 686-6664**
Cafe. In a cozy cafe under a bookstore in a historic area of Seattle, a chalkboard menu features some vegetarian options. **Open daily. Cafeteria style, wine/beer, take-out, no credit cards, $**

•• Five Loaves Deli & Bakery
2719 E. Madison, Seattle, WA 98112   **(206) 726-7989**
Vegan. The bakery and deli feature freshly baked whole-grain bread and muffins made without refined oils, sugars, or animal products. Sandwiches, burgers, soups, salads, desserts, and fruit shakes are offered for lunch. **Open for three meals every day except Saturday, buffet brunch on Sunday. Limited service, vegan options, fresh juices, take-out, VISA/MC, $**

•• The Globe Cafe & Bakery
1531 14th Ave., Seattle, WA 98122   **(206) 324-8815**
Vegan. This funky coffeehouse has monthly art shows, occasional acoustic music, poetry readings, good food and baked goods, breakfast and brunch menu. **Closed**

Monday. **Limited service, completely vegan, fresh juices, espresso, soy latte, take-out, no credit cards, $**

• Grand Illusion Vegetarian Cafe
1405 NE 50th, Seattle, WA 98105   **(206) 525-9573**
Vegetarian. Sample granola, baked goods, soups, salads, and quiches. **Open daily, counter service, take-out, $**

Gravity Bar
113 Virginia, Seattle, WA 98101   **(206) 448-8826**

415 Broadway E., Seattle, WA 98102   **(206) 325-7186**
Natural foods. Modern food is offered in a high tech but very human atmosphere. The extensive menu (with raw to macrobiotic choices and a breakfast menu) and the decor are creative and out of this world! **Open for three meals daily. Full/limited service, vegan/macrobiotic options, fresh juices, take-out, no credit cards, $–$$**

The Hi Spot Cafe
1410 34th Ave., E., Seattle, WA 98122   **(206) 325-7905**
Natural foods. Situated in a Victorian house, Hi Spot Cafe has a bakery featuring low-salt, low-sugar, and whole-grain pastries. Sweets and decadent desserts are also offered. The menu includes various sandwiches, soups, salads, and beverages for vegetarians and non-vegetarians alike. No smoking and no cellular phones are allowed inside! **Open daily except Tuesday for breakfast and lunch. Full service, vegan options, fresh juices, wine/beer, take-out, VISA/MC as a last resort, $**

• Honey Bear Bakery
2106 N. 55th, Seattle, WA 98103   **(206) 545-7296**
Vegetarian. A Seattle institution, Honey Bear specializes in whole, organic baked goods and pastries, and offers Black Bean Chili, soups, salads, and more in a homey and fun atmosphere. **Open daily 6 A.M. to 11 P.M. Self service, vegan options, fresh juices, espresso, no credit cards, $**

India House
4737 Roosevelt Way, NE, Seattle, WA 98105   **(206) 632-5072**
Indian. Authentic Indian cuisine includes an extensive vegetarian menu. The Indian decor is elegant with many paintings and artifacts. **Open daily. Full service, vegan options, wine/beer/alcohol, take-out, VISA/MC/AMX, $$**

Kokeb Restaurant
926 12th Ave., Seattle, WA 98122   **(206) 322-0485**
Ethiopian. Eight to ten vegetarian options are offered. **Open daily. Full service, wine/beer/alcohol, take-out, VISA/MC/AMX/DISC, $–$$**

New Orleans Creole Restaurant
114 First Ave. S., Seattle, WA 98104   **(206) 622-2563**
Creole/Cajun. The menu features a vegetarian section. Very little salt, animal fats, or stocks are used. Located in historic Pioneer Square, this restaurant offers live

jazz and blues every evening. **Open daily for lunch and dinner. Full service, vegan options, wine/beer/alcohol, take-out, VISA/MC/AMX/DC, $$**

Ranee Thai Restaurant
121 Prefontaine Pl. S., Seattle, WA 98104   (206) 223-9456
Thai. Several vegetarian options include Tofu Hot and Sour Soup, curries, Vegetable Pot Pie, and other vegetable dishes. **Open for lunch. Closed Sunday. Full service, vegan options, beer, take-out, $–$$**

• Silence-Heart-Nest Restaurant
5247 University NE, Seattle, WA 98105   (206) 524-4008
Vegetarian/Indian. Sample Western-style Indian cooking with a menu to please vegans and vegetarians alike—from burgers and "Neatloaf" to curries, samosas, and finger-licking chutneys to fresh salads! Prices are affordable and the atmosphere is peaceful, enlightening, and uplifting. **Closed Sunday and Wednesday. Full service, vegan options, take-out, $**

Sound View Cafe
1501 Pike Place #501, Seattle, WA 98101   (206) 623-5700
Natural foods. This health-minded restaurant has an unusual variety of vegetarian specialties. **Open daily. Cafeteria style, wine/beer, take-out, $**

• Sunlight Cafe
6403 Roosevelt Way, NE, Seattle, WA 98115   (206) 522-9060
Vegetarian. Known for its eggless waffles and pastries, Sunlight offers many vegan options including desserts, sautéed vegetables, and much more. **Open daily for three meals. Full service, vegan options, fresh juices, organic espresso, wine/beer, take-out, $$**

• SunSpot
2510 NE Blakeley, Seattle, WA 98105   (206) 527-2831
1123 Post Alley, Seattle, WA 98101   (206) 682-2236
Vegetarian. Many organic ingredients are used at this all-vegetarian fast-food restaurant. Try a "house special" rollup made with ethnic fillings, including Indian and Thai, in organic whole wheat chapatis. There are also salads, soups, and noodle dishes. SunSpot has a comprehensive recycling program inside the restaurant—and outside where food waste is composted. **Open daily for three meals. Limited service, vegan options, VISA/MC, $**

Thai Palace
2224 8th Ave. and Blanchard, Seattle, WA 98121   (206) 343-7846
Thai. No MSG is used in the preparation of foods, and vegetarian options are available. **Open daily. Full service, vegan options, wine/beer/alcohol, take-out, VISA/MC/AMX, $**

🌢 Reviewers' choice   • Vegetarian restaurant   •• Vegan restaurant
$ less than $6 $$ $6–$12 $$$ more than $12
VISA/AMX/MC/DISC/DC—credit cards accepted
Non-alc.—Non-alcoholic   Fresh juices—freshly squeezed

Viet My
129 Prefontaine Pl. S., Seattle, WA 98104   **(206) 382-9923**
Vietnamese. Viet My offers lots of vegetarian dishes including appetizers, veggie rolls, curry, Tofu Peanut Sauce, and other tofu dishes. **Open Monday through Friday. Full service, vegan options, take-out, $**

SPOKANE

China Best
West 223 Riverside, Spokane, WA 99201   **(509) 455-9042**
Chinese. In addition to twenty-two vegetarian menu items with excellent tofu dishes, China Best is willing to accommodate special diets. Every dish is freshly prepared to order. **Open daily. Full service, vegan options, wine/beer/alcohol, take-out, VISA/MC/AMX/DISC, $$**

• Eat Rite Vegetarian Restaurant
W. 314 Sprague, Spokane, WA 99204   **(509) 838-0382**
Vegetarian. The menu is free of saturated fats, cholesterol, and sugar. Main entrees change daily and feature various ethnic dishes. There's also a fourteen-foot-long salad bar, bread, soups, and desserts. **Closed Saturday. Cafeteria style, vegan options, fresh juices, take-out, $**

Niko's
W. 725 Riverside, Spokane, WA 99201   **(509) 624-7444**

S. 321 Dishman Mica Rd., Spokane, WA 99206   **(509) 928-9590**
Greek/Middle Eastern. Niko's offers many vegetarian items and an all-you-can-eat lunch bar. **Full service, $$**

STANWOOD

Cookie Mill
9808 SR 532, Stanwood, WA 98292   **(206) 629-2362**
Natural foods. This deli offers baked goods, a gift shop, and a blackboard menu. **Open daily. Cafeteria style, take-out, no credit cards, $**

VASHON ISLAND

Dog Days Cafe
17530 Vashon Highway, SW, Vashon, WA 98070   **(206) 463-6404**
Juice bar. Daily vegetarian specials are fresh, and homemade desserts are complemented by a full juice bar and extensive coffee menu. **Open daily except Monday. Full service, fresh juices, beer/wine, $**

Sound Food
20312 Vashon Highway, SW, Vashon, WA 98070   **(206) 463-3565**
Natural foods. Enjoy tofu and vegetable dishes, fresh baked breads, organic produce when available, sandwiches, and salads. **Open daily. Full service, non-alc. beer, beer/wine, VISA/MC/AMX, $$–$$$**

WEST VIRGINIA

• Mountain People's Kitchen
1400 University Ave., Morgantown, WV, 26505   (304) 291-6131
Vegetarian. This vegetarian restaurant attached to a natural foods co-op offers sandwiches, dairy and non-dairy entrees, and Sunday brunch. The casual and funky atmosphere is conducive to finding out what is going on in town, music, etc. **Open daily. Cafeteria style, take-out, VISA/MC, $**

• Palace of Gold Restaurant
RD 1 NBU #24, Moundsville, WV 26041   (304) 843-1812
Vegetarian/Indian. Authentic Indian cuisine includes vegetarian options. **Open daily. Full service, take-out, VISA/MC, $$**

WISCONSIN

Los Banditos
2335 W. Mason St., Green Bay, WI 54303   (414) 494-4505

1258 Main St., Green Bay, WI 54302   (414) 432-9462
Mexican. Authentic Mexican food features vegetable or quacamole fillings. Beans contain a ham-soup base. **Open daily for lunch and dinner, Sunday for dinner only. Full service, wine/beer/alcohol, take-out, VISA/MC/AMX, $–$$**

Zimmani's
333 Main St., Green Bay, WI 54301   (414) 436-2340
Italian. Fresh pasta specials and homemade pasta salads are highlighted at this up-scale restaurant with a full bar and complete deli/bakery. At least one vegetarian special is offered each day, and the staff is willing to accommodate special orders. **Closed Sunday. Full service, wine/beer/alcohol, take-out, VISA/MC/AMX, $–$$**

ᴥ Reviewers' choice   • Vegetarian restaurant   •• Vegan restaurant
$ less than $6 $$ $6–$12 $$$ more than $12
VISA/AMX/MC/DISC/DC—credit cards accepted
Non-alc.–Non-alcoholic   Fresh juices–freshly squeezed

MADISON

• Country Life
2465 Perry St., Madison, WI 53713   **(608) 257-3286**
Vegetarian. The primarily vegan menu is complemented by a great salad bar and many imitation meat products. **Closed Saturday. Full service, vegan/macrobiotic options, $–$$**

Himal Chuli
318 State St., Madison, WI 53705   **(608) 251-9225**
Nepalese. Authentic Nepalese cuisine is featured on a menu divided into vegetarian and non-vegetarian dishes. Seven vegetarian entrees feature various vegetable stews and dumplings. **Open daily. Limited service, beer, take-out, $–$$**

Husnu's
547 State St., Madison, WI 53703   **(608) 256-0900**
Turkish/Italian. Sample Hummus, Falafel, eggplant, and vegetable couscous. **Open daily for breakfast, lunch, and dinner. Full service, non-alc. beer, take-out, VISA/MC, $$**

Mt. Everest Restaurant
1851 Monroe St., Madison, WI 53711   **(608) 255-1704**
Indian. Mt. Everest offers exotic vegetarian and non-vegetarian Indian cuisine. **Closed Sunday. Reservations recommended Friday through Saturday. Full service, wine/beer/alcohol, take-out, VISA/MC/AMX, $$**

Ovens of Brittany
305 State St., Madison, WI 53703   **(608) 257-7000**

3244 University Ave., Madison, WI 53705   **(608) 233-7710**
1831 Monroe St., Madison, WI 53711   **(608) 251-2119**

1718 Fordem Ave., Madison, WI 53704   **(608) 241-7779**
American. On a menu that ranges from simple to fancy, there's stir-fry and occasional vegetarian specials such as Quiche with Goat Cheese, and Spinach Gateau. An excellent bakery and desserts are also available. **Open daily. Full service, non-alc. beer, beer/wine/alcohol, take-out, $$**

Rocky Rocco
Main Office   **(608) 271-6411**

1618 W. Beltline Hwy., Madison, WI 53713   **(608) 251-0304**

411 W. Gilman St., Madison, WI 53703   **(608) 256-0600**

3001 N. Sherman Ave., Madison, WI 53704   **(608) 241-4423**

651 State St., Madison, WI 53703   **(608) 255-6888**

3730 University Ave., Madison, WI 53705   **(608) 238-3558**

4002 E. Washington Ave., Madison, WI 53704   **(608) 241-8001**

4 West Towne Mall, Madison, WI 53562   **(608) 829-2901**

694 S. Whitney Way, Madison, WI 53711   **(608) 273-1223**
Pizza chain. Enjoy whole-wheat-crust pizza by the slice, an excellent salad bar, and
pasta dishes in a family atmosphere. **Open daily for lunch and dinner. Counter
service, vegan options, non-alc. beer, beer, take-out, VISA/MC, $**

Sunprint Cafe & Gallery
638 State St., Madison, WI 53703   **(608) 255-1555**
Ethnic. Several international vegetarian dishes and gourmet desserts are available at
this European-style cafe and art gallery on the university campus. **Open daily. Full
service, fresh juices, espresso/cappuccino, wine/beer/alcohol, take-out, VISA/MC, $$**

MIDDLETON

Rocky Rocco
2620 Allen Blvd., Middleton, WI 53562   **(608) 836-5444**
Pizza chain. See entry under Madison, WI. **Delivery only.**

MILWAUKEE

Abu's Restaurant
1978 N. Farwell Ave., Milwaukee, WI 53202   **(414) 277-0485**
Middle Eastern. Sample spinach pies, Hummus, Eggplant Casserole, lentils, egg-
plant, Baba Ghanouj, Egyptian Chili, and many more interesting dishes. **Open
daily. Full service, take-out, $**

Au Bon Appetit
1016 E. Brady St., Milwaukee, WI 53202   **(414) 278-1233**
Lebanese. This family-owned and operated restaurant offers many Lebanese vege-
tarian dishes including Hummus, Baba Ghanouj, Spinach Pie, Falafel, Carrot
Soup, Lentil Soup, Tabouli, Couscous Ratatouille, and more. **Open for lunch and
dinner Monday through Saturday. Closed Sunday. Full service, fresh juices,
wine, Lebanese coffee, vegan options, catering, take-out, VISA/MC, $$**

Beans & Barley
1901 E. North Ave., Milwaukee, WI 53202   **(414) 278-7878**
Natural foods. Vegetarian, Mexican, and Middle Eastern specialties include homemade soups, salads, sandwiches, burritos, and stir-fry. All foods are prepared using
the freshest ingredients possible. **Open daily for lunch and dinner. Full service,
vegan options, fresh juices, wine/beer, take-out, VISA/MC, $$**

OSCEOLA

Organica Restaurant
Aveda Spa Osceola
1015 N. Cascade St., Osceola, WI 54020   **(800) 283-3202**
Natural foods. Located in a spa near the St. Croix River, this restaurant offers
vegetarian and vegan dishes using local organic produce whenever possible. The
menu changes daily. **Open daily for lunch and dinner. Full service, fresh juices,
reservations required, vegan options, take-out, $$**

RACINE

Old Country Buffet

Westgate Mall, 4901 Washington Ave., Racine, WI 53406   (414) 634-5122
American. This large restaurant with a wide selection of vegetarian items, vegetables, and desserts features an all-you-can-eat buffet. **Cafeteria style, vegan options, $$**

WYOMING

CASPER

Peking Chinese Restaurant

333 E. A, Casper, WY 82601   (307) 266-2207
Chinese. Vegetarian menu includes six entrees as well as soups. **Open daily for lunch and dinner. Full service, wine/beer, take-out, VISA/MC, $**

CHEYENNE

Twin Dragons

1809 Carey Ave., Cheyenne, WY 82007   (307) 637-6622
Chinese. This Mandarin Chinese restaurant offers ten vegetarian entrees including tofu dishes, Broccoli and Garlic Sauce, Vegetable Lo Mein, Chow Mein, and Veggie Egg Rolls. **Open daily for lunch and dinner. Full service, wine/beer/alcohol, take-out, VISA/MC/AMX, $**

CODY

The Hong Kong Restaurant

1244 Sheridan Ave., Cody, WY 82414   (307) 527-6420
Chinese. Enjoy vegetable and bean curd dishes. **Open for lunch and dinner daily during the summer, Tuesday through Sunday during the winter. Full service, wine/beer/alcohol, take-out, VISA/MC, $-$$**

LANDER

China Garden

140 N. 7th St., Lander, WY 82520   (307) 332-7666
Chinese. Several vegetarian dishes including Tofu and Mixed Vegetables, Noodles and Vegetables, and Stir-Fry Broccoli are offered at this Chinese establishment. **Open daily. Full service, BYOB, take-out, $$**

RIVERTON

The Golden Coral

400 N. Federal, Riverton, WY 82501   (307) 856-1152
Steak house. Although this is a family-style steak house, there is a huge salad bar with baked potatoes. **Open daily. Sunday breakfast buffet. Full service, VISA/MC, $-$$**

CANADA

ALBERTA

Michael's Cafe
415 Banff Ave., Banff, AB T0L 0C0   **(403) 762-9339**
Natural foods. Vegetarian dishes include Hearty Lentil Soup, Hummus, Curried Tofu Veggie Crêpe, Whole-Wheat Spaghetti, Totini with Pesto, and Tamari Ginger Tofu Stir-Fry. Menu items do not contain MSG or refined sugar. Organically grown short-grain brown rice is used and, when available, organically grown produce. The restaurant does serve non-vegetarian items. **Open for three meals daily. Full service, vegan options, non-alc. beer, take-out, wine/beer/alcohol, VISA/MC/AMX, $$**

Cedars Restaurant
1009A 1st St., SW, Calgary, AB T2R 0T8   **(403) 264-2532**

Eau Claire Market
2nd St. and 2nd Ave., SW, Calgary, AB T2P 4R5   **(403) 263-0285**
Lebanese. Vegetarian and vegan options are available. The owner is the author of several cookbooks. **Open Monday through Saturday. Full service, vegan options, wine/beer, take-out, VISA/MC/AMX, $$**

The King and I Thai Cuisine
822 11th Ave., SW, Calgary, AB T2R 0E5   **(403) 264-7241**
Thai. Enjoy the contemporary decor with soft jazz background music. Vegetarian selections include Chili Club Tofu made with Japanese eggplant. **Open daily. Full service, wine/beer/alcohol, take-out, VISA/MC/AMX, $$**

Meelen Restaurant, Ltd.
118 32nd Ave., NE, Calgary, AB T2E 7C8   **(403) 291-3188**
East Indian. This restaurant features traditional family recipes. **Open daily for lunch and dinner. Full service, reservations required, wine/beer/alcohol, take-out, VISA/MC/AMX/DISC, $$**

Thai sa-on
351 10th Ave., SW, Calgary, AB T2R 0A5   **(403) 264-3526**
Thai. Authentic Thai cuisine is featured here, including homemade curries, sauces, and desserts. **Open for lunch and dinner Monday through Friday, and only for dinner on Sunday. Full service, catering, beer/wine/alcohol, $$**

ABC Health Shoppe
10550 82nd Ave., Edmonton, AB T6E 1Z9   **(403) 432-7885**
Natural foods. Soups, burgers, and salads are joined by a daily vegetarian special. **Open daily except Sunday. Counter service, fresh juices, non-alc. beer, take-out, $**

High Level Diner
10912 88 Ave., Edmonton, AB T6B 0V6   **(403) 433-0993**
Natural foods. The High Level Diner is an environmentally responsible natural foods eatery furnished with antiques and decorated with local artwork. **Open 9 A.M. to midnight Tuesday through Saturday, to 11 P.M. Sunday and Monday. Full service, wine/beer/alcohol, take-out, VISA/MC/AMX, $$**

• High Level Natural Foods and Cafe
10313 82 Ave., N.W., Edmonton, AB T6E 1Z9   **(403) 433-6807**
Vegetarian. You'll enjoy great veggie burgers and wheat-free baked foods in a casual atmosphere. **Open daily until 5:30 P.M. Full service, vegan options, fresh juices, catering, take-out, VISA/AMX, $**

The King and I Thai Cuisine
10160 82nd Ave., Edmonton, AB T6E 1Z4   **(403) 433-2222**
Thai. The owners emphasize healthy cooking, and special requests will be cooked to order. The Vegetarian Bird's Nest is a must! **Open for lunch Monday through Friday, and dinner Monday through Saturday. Full service, wine/beer/alcohol, take-out, VISA/MC/AMX, $$**

New Asian Village Restaurant
8230 103 Street, NW, Edmonton, AB T6E 4B2   **(403) 433-3804**
Indian. In an atmosphere of Indian decor and music, vegetarian options are provided by a friendly staff. **Open daily. Full service, wine/beer/alcoholic/non-alc. beverages, take-out, catering, VISA/MC/AMX, $$**

Sidney's Deli and Pizza
10416 118 Ave., Edmonton, AB T5X 0P7   **(403) 471-1560**
Ethnic/mixed. Enjoy homemade foods at this family restaurant offering fifteen vegetarian dishes. **Open daily. Full service, wine/beer/alcohol, take-out, VISA/MC/AMX**

• Veggies
10331 82nd Ave., Edmonton, AB T6E 1Z9   **(403) 432-7560**
Vegetarian. Enjoy many vegetarian dishes such as veggie burgers, whole-wheat pizza, and various ethnic entrees in a homey and smoke-free atmosphere. **Open daily except Monday. Full service, vegan options, wine/beer, catering, take-out, VISA/MC/AMX, $$**

BRITISH COLUMBIA

BURNABY

• Govinda's
5462 SE Marine Dr., Burnaby, B.C. V5J 3G8   (604) 433-2454
Vegetarian. Enjoy dining in a relaxed atmosphere with a spiritual theme where you can take a stroll before or after diner in the park-like grounds. **Open daily except Sunday. Cafeteria style, take-out, catering, $$**

COURTENAY

• Bar None Cafe
244 4th St., Box 3093, Courtenay, B.C. V9N 5N3   (604) 334-3112
Vegetarian. A vegetarian buffet features fresh juices and an espresso bar. **Open daily except Sunday. Cafeteria style, fresh juices, espresso, take-out, catering, $–$$**

NELSON

• The Alleyway Cafe'
620 Herridge Lane, Nelson, B.C. V1L 6A7   (604) 352-5200
Vegetarian. Enjoy a variety of vegetarian Mexican, American, and Italian dishes. **Open daily except Sunday. Full service, vegan options, take-out, catering, MC, $–$$**

NORTH VANCOUVER

• Woodlands Natural Food Restaurant
93 Lonsdale Ave., N. Vancouver, B.C. V7M 2E5   (604) 985-9328
Vegetarian. Menu includes sandwiches, burgers, salads, soups, and breakfast items. **Open daily except Sunday. Cafeteria style, take-out, catering, VISA, $**

VANCOUVER

(For additional restaurants in the surrounding areas, see Burnaby, North Vancouver, and West Vancouver.)

Afghan Horsemen Restaurant
445 W. Broadway, Vancouver, B.C. V5Y 1R4   (604) 873-5923
Afghani. Enjoy Afghan soups, salads, and entrees such as Hummus, Badenjan Borani (baked eggplant), and Dahl (lentil stew). **Open daily except Sunday. Full service, wine/beer/alcohol, take-out, VISA/MC/AMX, $$**

ᏒᎧ Reviewers' choice   • Vegetarian restaurant   •• Vegan restaurant
$ less than $6 $$ $6–$12 $$$ more than $12
VISA/AMX/MC/DISC/DC—credit cards accepted
Non-alc.–Non-alcoholic   Fresh juices—freshly squeezed

• Bodai Vegetarian Restaurant
337 E. Hastings St., Vancouver, B.C. V6A 1P3   **(604) 682-2666**
Vegetarian/ethnic. Pure vegetarian food is provided in a smoke-free environment. Entrees include Colorful Bamboo Shoots, Celery with Mushrooms, and Chili Bean Curd with Sesame Seed Oil. **Open daily. Full service, take-out, VISA/MC, $$**

• Bo-Jik Vegetarian Restaurant
820 W. Broadway, Vancouver, B.C. V5Z 1J8   **(604) 872-5556**
Vegetarian/Asian. Enjoy pure Buddhist vegetarian cuisine. **Open daily. Full service, take-out, VISA/MC, $$**

•• Circling Dawn
1045 Commercial Dr., Vancouver, B.C. V5L 3X1   **(604) 255-2326**
Vegan/organic food store. This vegan restaurant serves French toast, pancakes, tofu scrambles, hot cereals, sandwiches, salads, tofu burger, lasagna. **Open daily for breakfast, lunch, and dinner. Counter service, vegan options, fresh juices, catering, $**

• Evergreen
4166 Main St., Vancouver, B.C. V5V 3P7   **(604) 879-3380**
Vegetarian/Chinese. The menu is completely vegetarian, and all foods are prepared without preservatives. Choose from Sweet Tofu Cake, Lo-Hon Mixed Vegetables, and other dishes. **Open daily. Vegan options, take-out, $**

• Greens and Gourmet
2681 W. Broadway, Vancouver, B.C. V6K 2G2   **(604) 737-7373**
Vegetarian/macrobiotic/natural foods. Items included on the extensive vegetarian menu are cooked with purified water, which is also served for drinking. At the self-service hot and cold buffet, food is sold by weight. **Open daily. Full service, macrobiotic, vegan options, fruit juices, take-out, catering, VISA/MC, $–$$**

• Miu Jay Garden Vegetarian Restaurant
363 E. Hastings St., Vancouver, B.C. V6A 1P3   **(604) 687-5231**
Vegetarian/Chinese. Bean curd, vegetarian (all-simulated) gluten meats, and deluxe clear vegetarian soups are the types of food you will find at this authentic Chinese vegetarian restaurant. **Open daily. Full service, vegan options, take-out, VISA, $$**

• The Naam Restaurant ❧
2724 W. 4th Ave., Vancouver, B.C. V6K 1R1   **(604) 738-7151**
Vegetarian/ethnic. A completely vegetarian menu offers a wide assortment of dishes, from Mexican to East Indian. All foods are made on the premises. Live music is provided at lunch and dinner. **Open daily. Full service, vegan/macrobiotic options, fruit juices, wine/beer, take-out, VISA/MC, $–$$**

The Noodle Maker Restaurant
122 Powell St., Vancouver, B.C. V6A 1G1   **(604) 683-9196**
Chinese. This gourmet Chinese restaurant offers nine vegetarian entrees. Appetiz-

ers and soup are also available. **Open Monday through Friday. Full service, vegan options, wine/beer/alcohol, VISA /MC/AMX, $$$**

Noor-Mahal Restaurant
4354 Fraser St., Vancouver, B.C. V5V 4G3 **(604) 873-9263**
South Indian. A choice of dosas and other vegetable dishes as well as several vegetarian appetizers. **Open daily. Full service, take-out, VISA/MC, $–$$**

Nyala African Restaurant
2930 W. 4th Ave., Vancouver, B.C. V6K 1R2 **(604) 731-7899**
Ethiopian. Choose from six vegan options including Shuro Watt and Yeshebera Asa. Nyala also offers a couple of salads. **Open daily. Full service, vegan options, wine/beer/alcohol, catering, take-out, VISA/MC/AMX, $$**

• Surat Sweets
6665 Fraser St., Vancouver, B.C. V5X 3T6 **(604) 322-9544**
Vegetarian/Indian. Serves a variety of pure vegetarian Gujarati foods. **Open daily. Limited service, vegan options, take-out, $$**

• Woodlands Restaurant ❧
2582 W. Broadway, Vancouver, B.C. V6J 2V1 **(604) 733-5411**
Vegetarian/North American. The menu contains numerous vegetarian dishes. None of the food contains meat, fish, fowl or eggs. Desserts are prepared in Woodlands' own bakery. **Open daily. Full service and buffet style, vegan options, fruit juices, wine/beer, catering, take-out, VISA/MC, $$**

VERNON

• Sunseed Vegetarian Cafe
2919 30th Ave., Vernon, B.C. V1T 2B8 **(604) 542-7892**
Vegetarian. In addition to two soups daily, including one special vegan soup, Sunseed offers Vegetable Lasagna, Shepherd's Pie, and international dishes. **Open morning and afternoon. Closed Sunday. Cafeteria style, vegan options, fresh juice, espresso/non-dairy cappuccino, non-alc. beer, take-out, MC/VISA, $**

VICTORIA

• Chili Non Carne at Viteway
1019 Blanshard St., Victoria, BC V8W 2H4 **(604) 384-5677**
Vegetarian. This primarily vegan restaurant offers daily specials in addition to its regular menu of curries, lasagna, pasta, and Mexican dishes. Each month, the work of a local young artist is featured. Live music is provided in a smoke-free environment. **Open Monday through Saturday for lunch and dinner. Limited service, vegan options, fresh juices, VISA/MC, $–$$**

Eugene's Greek Restaurant
1280 Broad St., Victoria, B.C. V8W 2A5 **(604) 381-5456**
Greek. Eugene's specializes in traditional Greek food. The menu includes Vegetarian Soullaki. **Open Monday through Saturday. Self-service, $**

•• Green Cuisine
560 Johnson, Victoria, B.C. V8W 3C6 **(604) 385-1809**
Vegan. In the Market Square area, this totally vegan restaurant offers a hot buffet and a salad buffet that changes daily. Desserts made without white sugar are available as are bean and grain dishes. Organic items are used whenever possible. **Open daily. Self service, vegan options, fresh juices, espresso/cappuccino, non-alc. beer, catering, take-out, VISA/MC, $**

India Curry House
506 Fort St., Victoria, B.C. V8T 4P6 **(604) 384-5622**
Indian. No MSG or preservatives are used in the preparation of ten vegetarian main courses. Free parking is available. **Open daily for lunch and dinner. Full service, reservations recommended, formal, non-alc. beer, wine/beer/alcohol, take-out, VISA/MC/AMX/DISC, $$–$$$**

Jack Lee's Chinese Village
755 Finlayson St., Victoria, B.C. V8T 4W4 **(604) 384-8151**
Chinese. Jack Lee's offers vegetarian options, and meals can be prepared to satisfy any dietary preferences. **Open daily. Full service, wine/beer/alcohol, catering, take-out, VISA/MC/AMX, $$**

Re-Bar
50 Bastian Sq., Victoria, B.C. V8W 1J2 **(604) 361-9223**
Natural foods. Re-Bar is mostly vegetarian, with fish served once a week. All baked goods are made in Re-Bar's kitchen daily, with minimum use of refined sugars and flours. Organic produce is used when available in the summer. Soups are made with 100-percent vegetable stock, and the tortillas do not contain animal fats. Re-Bar uses filtered water. Typical breakfasts include bagels, cinnamon raisin toast, scrambled eggs, and muffins. Lunch options include Miso Soup, Szechuan Noodle Salad, Almond Burger, and Enchilada. **Open daily for breakfast, lunch, and dinner. Full service, fresh juices, non-alc. beer, wine/beer, take-out, VISA/MC, $–$$**

Taj Mahal Restaurant
679 Herald St., Victoria, B.C. V8W 1S8 **(604) 383-4662**
Indian. Taj Mahal serves vegetarian dishes from all regions of India and also has various kinds of leavened and unleavened breads. All foods are prepared without MSG or preservatives. **Open Monday through Saturday for lunch and dinner, Sunday for dinner only. Full service, wine/beer/alcohol, catering, take-out, VISA/MC/AMX, $$**

• Viteway
1019 Blanshard St., Victoria, B.C. V8W 2H4 **(604) 384-5677**
Vegetarian/natural foods. Enjoy terrific chili, a large bakery selection, and music in a relaxing environment. **Open daily. Limited service, take-out, VISA/MC, $**

Capers
2496 Marine Dr., West Vancouver, B.C. V7V 1L1   **(604) 925-3316**
Natural foods/health-food store. A wide variety of vegetarian foods such as Caper's Falafel, assorted salads, and an organic stir-fry are offered. **Open daily. Full service, fruit juices, wine/beer, catering, take-out (deli only), VISA/MC, $$**

MANITOBA

WINNIPEG

Desserts Plus
1595 Main St., Winnipeg, MB R2V 1Y2   **(204) 339-1957**
Dairy. All food in this smoke-free restaurant is homemade without additives. Pastries, vegetable soups, blintzes, knishes of all types, and vegetarian egg rolls are typical vegetarian selections. Catering is the main business. **Open Monday through Friday for lunch and Thursday for dinner. Full service, reservations recommended, catering, take-out, VISA/MC, $$**

Falafel Place and Deli
612 Academy Road, Winnipeg, MB R3N 0E6   **(204) 489-5811**
Middle Eastern. The owner claims that customers say his is the best apple strudel and baklava in town. You can also try the Hummus, Veggie Burgers, Couscous, Potato Pancakes, meatless soups, and foul (fava beans). **Open daily. Counter service, vegan options, fresh juices, non-alc. beer/wine, catering, take-out, $**

Moti-Mahal Curry Place
998 St. Mary's Road, Winnipeg, MB R2M 3S3   **(204) 257-8218**
Indian. Large selection of vegetarian curries. **Open daily for dinner. Full service, reservations recommended, vegan options, Indian beer/wine/alcohol, VISA/ MC, $$**

Mrs. Lipton's
Ardjuna
962 Westminster Ave., Winnipeg, MB R3G 1B8   **(204) 775-6743**
Natural foods/Indonesian/international. At the same location, using the same tables, are two different restaurants, run by totally different owners who share space. In the daytime, Mrs. Lipton's serves lunch items such as veggie burgers, Falafel, curries, salads, and vegetarian soups. Table service is provided. In the evening, the restaurant is Ardjuna, which serves Indonesian dishes. Vegetarian selections include Steamed Vegetables with Peanut Sauce and Tofu, Bean Cake in Hot Tomato Sauce, and Peanut Wafers. **Mrs. Lipton's is open Tuesday through Saturday for lunch. Full service, alcohol, VISA, $. Ardjuna is open Tuesday through Sunday for dinner. Full service, reservations recommended on weekends. Vegan options, beer/wine, catering, take-out, VISA/MC/AMX, $$**

- ## Wheat Song Cafe and Bakery
  578 Broadway (at Balmoral), Winnipeg, MB R3C 0W5   (204) 775-0031
  Vegetarian/natural foods. The bakery uses 100-percent stone-ground flour in its whole-wheat, multi-grain, and sandwich buns. It also offers cinnamon buns, cookies, date squares, muffins, cakes, logs, and apple pie slices prepared without white sugar. The cafe serves homemade soups, sandwiches such as Sunflower Lentil Burger, spinach pie, and vegetarian pizza. **Open Tuesday through Saturday. Counter service, take-out, limited catering, $**

NOVA SCOTIA

ANTIGONISH

Sunshine Cafe
194 Main St., Antigonish, N.S. B2G 2R6   (902) 863-1194
Natural foods. Located in the Sunflower Natural Foods Store, Sunshine Cafe offers simple breakfasts such as coffee and bran muffins. For lunch, the cafe features hearty whole-wheat sandwiches and Chili as well as salads—including Tabouleh. Desserts in this smoke-free cafe are made with local maple syrup. **Open Monday through Saturday. Full service, catering, take-out, VISA/MC, $$**

HALIFAX

- ## Satisfaction Feast Vegetarian Restaurant
  1581 Grafton St., Halifax, N.S. B3J 2C3   (902) 422-3540
  Vegetarian. The menu includes a large selection of appetizers, soups, sandwiches, salads, and entrees that are all vegetarian. **Open daily. Full service, vegan options, fruit juices, catering, take-out, VISA/MC/AMX, $–$$**

ONTARIO

CONCORD

East Moon Restaurant
2150 Steeles Ave. W., Concord, ON L4K 2T5   (905) 738-1428
Chinese. The menu lists approximately ten vegetarian entrees plus vegetarian egg and spring rolls. **Open daily. Full service, catering, take-out, wine/beer/alcohol, VISA/MC/AMX, $$**

🍴 Reviewers' choice   • Vegetarian restaurant   •• Vegan restaurant
$ less than $6 $$ $6–$12 $$$ more than $12
VISA/AMX/MC/DISC/DC—credit cards accepted
Non-alc.—Non-alcoholic   Fresh juices—freshly squeezed

•• Health Haven

5555 Elington Ave. W., Etobicoke, ON M9C 5M1   **(416) 621-3636**

Vegan/Chinese. Dine on Spring Rolls, tofu dishes, stir-fried veggies, soups, noodle dishes, and more. **Open daily for lunch and dinner. Full service, completely vegan, fresh juices, take-out, VISA/MC, $$**

Darbar Restaurant

479 Princess St., Kingston, ON K7L 1C3   **(613) 548-7053**

Indian. Darbar offers more than ten vegetarian dishes. **Open daily. Darbar Coffee, lassi, $**

• Sunflower Restaurant ⭐

20 Montreal St., Kingston, ON K7L 3G6   **(613) 542-4566**

Vegetarian. The all-vegetarian international menu includes vegan entrees, soups, salads, a soy burger, and wheat-free items. There are daily specials, and organic produce is used when possible. **Open Tuesday through Saturday. Full service, vegan options, fresh juice, natural beer/wine, MC/VISA, $$**

Champion House Restaurant

25 Watline Ave., 2nd Fl., Mississauga, ON L4Z 2Z1   **(905) 890-8988**

Chinese. The menu has a vegetarian section with vegetable and tofu dishes. **Open daily. Full service, vegan options, wine/beer, take-out, VISA/MC/AMX/DC, $$**

Haifa Restaurant

3022-3024 Bathurst St., North York, ON M6B 3B6   **(416) 783-6406**

Ethnic. This restaurant offers BBQ Eggplant, Stuffed Grape Leaves, Fried Chick Peas, and more. **Open daily. Full service, wine/beer/alcohol, catering, VISA, $**

La Mexicana Restaurant

3337 Bathurst St., North York, ON M6A 2B7   **(416) 783-9452**

Mexican. This Mexican restaurant features authentic Mexican cuisine, Latin American music, and an open outdoor patio. Choose from several vegetarian dishes including Vegetable Enchiladas, Chilaquiles (Mexican lasagna), Chili Rellenos, and an eggplant casserole. **Open daily. Full service, wine/beer/alcohol, catering, take-out, VISA/MC/AMX, $$**

Domus Cafe

269 Dalhousie St., Ottawa, ON K1N 7E3   **(613) 241-6410**

Natural foods. Eclectic gourmet foods are prepared with fresh produce from local farmers. There's a daily change in the menu. The restaurant is connected to a kitchen/housewares store. **Open daily for breakfast and lunch. Full service, wine/beer, take-out, VISA/MC/AMX, $$**

The Green Door
198 Main St., Ottawa, ON K1S 1C6   **(613) 234-9597**
Vegetarian/natural foods. Open the door and find organic grains, beans, salads, and sea vegetables. Organic flours are used in sourdough baking, yeast-free baked goods, wheat-free breads, and sugar-free baked goods (no honey is used.) The Green Door specializes in macrobiotic foods and organic foods; very few dairy products or eggs are used, and food is sold by the pound. **Open daily except Monday. Self service, vegan/macrobiotic options, fresh juices, wine/beer, catering, take-out, VISA/MC, $**

• Peace Garden Cafe
47 Clarence St., Ottawa, ON K1N 9K1   **(613) 562-2434**
Vegetarian. This small cafe offers vegetarian dishes such as Lasagna, baked potatoes, soy burgers, and more. **Open daily for three meals. Counter service, espresso/cappuccino, smoothies, catering, vegan options, take-out, $$**

Rosie Lee Cafe
167 Laurier Ave. E, Ottawa, ON K1N 6N8   **(613) 234-7299**
French. Enjoy French-style quiches, sandwiches, entrees, and soups. **Open daily. Full service, wine/beer/alcohol, take-out, $$**

Silk Roads Restaurant
300 Sparks St., Mall, Ottawa ON K2C 2E9   **(613) 236-4340**
Afghan. The Afghan cuisine includes vegetarian options. **Open daily. Full service, wine/beer/alcohol, VISA/MC/AMX, $$–$$$**

SCARBOROUGH

• Chowpatty
1541 Victoria Park, Scarborough, ON M1L 2T5   **(416) 750-7854**
Vegetarian/Indian. Enjoy a wide variety of Indian vegetarian dishes in a comfortable environment at Chowpatty restaurant. **Open for lunch and dinner Wednesday through Monday. Closed Tuesday. Counter service, vegan options, catering, take-out, $**

THORNHILL

Sonny Langer's Vegetarian Dairy Restaurant
180 Steeles Ave. W., Thornhill, ON L4J 2L1   **(905) 881-4356**
Kosher. Sonny Langer's is vegetarian except for fish and is famous for pierogies. Everything is made from scratch with no preservatives or food colorings. **Open daily. Full service, vegan options, take-out, catering, VISA/MC, $$**

(For additional restaurants in the surrounding area, see Thornhill.)

• Annapurna
1085 Bathurst St., Toronto, ON M5R 3G8   (416) 537-8513
Macrobiotic/Indian. Macrobiotic foods and southern Indian cuisine are served. **Open daily. Full service, macrobiotic/vegan options, catering, take-out, $**

•• Bo De Duyen Restaurant
254 Spadina Ave., 2nd Floor, Toronto, ON M5T 2E2   (416) 601-1247
Vegan/Chinese. Bo De Duyen Restaurant serves more than forty different Chinese vegetarian dishes. **Open daily for lunch and dinner. Full service, completely vegan, take-out, $$**

• Cafe Verité
686 Bloor St. West, Toronto, ON M6G 1L2   (416) 537-0579
Vegetarian. Enjoy Lasagna, Cabbage Rolls, salads, Spanakopita, soup, samosas, and more at Cafe Verité. Don't forget to ask about the special vegan desserts! **Open daily for lunch and dinner. Full service, vegan options, take-out, $**

Champion House Restaurant
480 Dundas St. W., Toronto, ON M5T 1G9   (416) 977-8282
Chinese. Enjoy Northern Chinese cuisine, a separate vegetarian menu, and a full Chinese tea menu. **Open daily. Full service, vegan options, wine/beer/alcohol, take-out, catering, $$**

Charmers Cafe
1384 Bathurst St., Toronto, ON M5R 3J1   (416) 657-1225
Tex-Mex. Charmers offers vegetarian tostadas, burritos, enchiladas, sauces, Baba Ghanouj, soups, salads, and desserts. **Open daily. Limited service, wine/beer, take-out, catering, VISA/MC, $$**

• Chinese Vegetarian House 🍃
39 Baldwin St., Toronto, ON M5T 1L1   (416) 599-6855
Vegetarian/Chinese. The Chinese vegetarian cuisine is based on contemporary and 1000-year-old recipes. Some wheat-gluten dishes are available. No MSG is used. **Closed Monday. Full service, vegan options, organic wine/beer, catering, take-out, $$**

• Earth Tones Whole Food Emporium and Vegetarian Restaurant
357 Queen St. W., Toronto, ON M5V 2A4   (416) 599-9054
Vegetarian. Enjoy the restaurant's wide selection of vegetarian foods, and visit the health food store and deli at the same location. **Open daily. Cafeteria style, wine/beer, take-out, catering, VISA/MC, $**

Epicure Cafe

512 Queen St. W., Toronto, ON M5V 2B2   **(416) 363-8942**

Natural foods. Enjoy items from the traditional Italian and French bistro black-board menu, which changes daily and is seasonal. **Open daily. Full service, wine/beer/alcohol, take-out, catering, VISA/MC/AMX, $$**

Grainfield's Bakery

1464 Kingston Rd., Toronto, ON M1N 1R6   **(416) 691-6061**

Natural foods. This alternative bakery specializes in sourdough and yeast-free breads and pasteries. Organic flours are used, and most products are dairy- and egg-free. **Open 9 A.M. to 5 P.M. Tuesday through Friday, to 4:30 P.M. Saturday. Take-out only.**

The Groaning Board

287 King St. West, Toronto, ON M5V 1JS   **(416) 595-7232**

North American style/natural foods. The Groaning Board appropriately features a self-serve soup, salad, and make-your-own-sundae bar. There is also waiter service for such items as Vegetarian Lasagna, Spanakopita, Brown Rice Pilaf, and Mush-room-Spinach Quiche. **Open daily. Limited service, wine/beer, take-out, VISA/MC/AMX/DISC, $$**

• Hare Krishna Center

243 Avenue Rd., Dupont, Toronto, ON M5R 2J6   **(416) 922-5415**

Vegetarian. In downtown Toronto, you'll find this all-you-can-eat buffet. Foods are egg-free, and different dishes are featured daily—usually rice, dahl, and soups. **Open Monday through Saturday, Sunday evening feast. Cafeteria style, limited catering, take-out, $**

• Hey Good Cooking

238 Dupont St., Toronto, ON M5R 1V7   **(416) 929-9140**

Vegetarian. Daily specials include Chickpea and Vegetable Curry, Texan Chili, Mush-room Nut Loaf, and Southern Spiced Tofu, as well as homemade veggie burgers, soups, and salads. **Open daily. Cafeteria style, vegan options, take-out, $**

•• Juice for Life

238 Queen St. W., Toronto, ON M5V 1Z1   **(416) 408-3581**

Vegan. You'll find vegan dishes and an extensive juice bar. **Open daily. Cafeteria style, vegan options, fresh juices, take-out, catering.**

• Kensington Natural Bakery, Inc.

460 Bloor St. West, Toronto, ON M5S 1X8   **(416) 534-1294**

Vegetarian. This smoke-free bakery offers vegetarian baked goods, entrees, and fresh juices. **Open daily for three meals. Full service, vegan/macrobiotic options, catering, take-out, $**

Le Kashmire
605 Bloor St. W., Toronto, ON M6G 1K5 (416) 533-5955
Indian/Pakistani. Indian/Pakistani cusine here includes a special luncheon buffet and Saturday and Sunday brunch. **Closed Monday. Buffet lunch, full service dinner, vegan options, wine/beer/alcohol, take-out, catering, $$**

La Mexicana Restaurant
229 Carlton St., Toronto, ON M5A 2L2 (416) 929-6284
Mexican. This Mexican restaurant features authentic Mexican cuisine, Latin American music, and an open outdoor patio. Choose from several vegetarian dishes including Vegetable Enchiladas, Chilaquiles (Mexican lasagna), Chili Rellenos, and an eggplant casserole. **Open daily. Full service, wine/beer/alcohol, catering, take-out, VISA/MC/AMX, $$**

Le Papillon
16 Church St., Toronto, ON M5E 1M1 (416) 363-0838
French. Savor the crêpes in a comfortable French atmosphere. Children are welcome. **Closed Monday. Full service, wine/beer/alcohol, take-out, catering, VISA/MC/AMX, $$**

Motimahal Restaurant
1422 Gerrard St. East, Toronto, ON M4L 1Z6 (416) 461-3111
Indian. This Northern Indian restaurant offers a wide variety of curries. **Closed Tuesday. Cafeteria style and full service, wine/beer/alcohol, take-out, catering, VISA/MC/AMX, $**

Queen Mother Café
208 Queen St. W., Toronto, ON M5V 1Z2 (416) 598-4719
Laotian/Thai. Queen Mother has been serving Lao-Thai food and vegetarian burgers since 1978. In spring and summer, you can eat on the garden patio. **Closed Sunday. Full service, wine/beer/alcohol, take-out, catering, VISA/MC/AMX, $$**

The Queen of Sheba
1198 Bloor St. W., Toronto, ON M6H 1N2 (416) 536-4162
Ethiopian. Some vegetarian dishes are featured and are served with injera, Ethiopian bread. There's also a six-dish vegetarian sampler. **Open daily. Full service, wine/beer/alcohol, take-out, catering, VISA/MC, $$**

• Renaissance Cafe
509 Bloor St. W., Toronto, ON M5S 1Y2 (416) 968-6639
Vegetarian. West Indian and Indonesian dishes are just a sample of the type of vegetarian food served here. Renaissance Cafe is open late into the evening every day. Outdoor patio. **Open daily for lunch and dinner. Full service, vegan options, catering, take-out, VISA/MC/AMX, $$**

The Rivoli
332 Queen St. W., Toronto, ON M5V 2A2   **(416) 596-1908**
Oriental. In the summertime, a sidewalk cafe affords additional seating. Live entertainment is sometimes offered. **Open daily. Full service, wine/beer/alcohol, catering, take-out, VISA/MC, $$**

United Bakers Dairy Restaurant
506 Lawrence Ave. W., Toronto, ON M6A 1A1   **(416) 789-0519**
Ethnic/Jewish dairy. Toronto's oldest dairy restaurant features European-style dishes including blintzes, kreplach, quiche, Cabbage Rolls, Stuffed Green Peppers, Vegetarian Lasagna, Vegetarian Chopped Liver, bagels, soups, and salads. **Open daily. Full service, vegan options, take-out, catering, VISA/MC, $$**

• The Vegetarian Restaurant
4 Dundonald St., Toronto, ON M4Y 1K2   **(416) 961-9522**
Vegetarian/natural foods. This restaurant avoids frying and uses filtered water. Organic food is used when possible, and the menu lists ingredients for all items—an international selection, salad bar, prepared salads, burritos, Lasagna, bean dishes, Nut Loaf, and vegan desserts. Live music is featured on Wednesday. **Open daily, Sunday for dinner only. Cafeteria style, vegan options, fresh juices, non-alc. beer/wine, take-out, VISA/MC/DC**

• The West End Vegetarian Restaurant
2849 Dundas St. W., Toronto, ON M6P 1Y6   **(416) 762-1204**
Vegetarian/natural foods. This vegetarian restaurant has been open for more than eighteen years. Dishes, which vary seasonally, are listed on a chalkboard menu. Organic products are used when available. **Open daily. Cafeteria style, vegan options, take-out, VISA/MC, $$**

Willow Restaurant
193 Danforth Ave., Toronto, ON M4K 1N2   **(416) 469-5315**
Mexican. The Mexican fare includes vegetarian burritos, chimichangas, enchilladas, quesadillas, and fajitas. **Open daily. Full service, wine/beer/alcohol, take-out, VISA/MC/AMX, $$**

Yofi's Restaurant and Patio
19 Baldwin St., Toronto, ON M5T 1L1   **(416) 977-1145**
Primarily vegetarian/ethnic. This restaurant is vegetarian with the exception of one tuna entree. A wide variety of different ethnic dishes includes Middle Eastern Hummus, Baba Ghanouj, and Tabouli; Mexican Nachos; Greek Salad; and many different vegetarian burgers. **Patio dining. Closed Sunday. Full service, vegan options, take-out, catering, VISA/MC, $–$$**

🐾 Reviewers' choice   • Vegetarian restaurant   •• Vegan restaurant
$ less than $6 $$ $6–$12 $$$ more than $12
VISA/AMX/MC/DISC/DC—credit cards accepted
Non-alc.—Non-alcoholic   Fresh juices—freshly squeezed

Yonge Garden Restaurant and Tavern
5186 Yonge St., Willowdale, ON M2N 5P6   **(416) 225-2383**
Chinese. This Chinese restaurant offers more than a dozen different vegetarian dishes including Mixed Greens and Tofu, Vegetable Balls (made out of wheat gluten), Chow Mein, Vegetable Fried Rice, and Mixed Vegetables. **Open daily. Full service, wine/beer/alcohol, take-out, catering, VISA/MC/AMX, $$**

QUEBEC

LAFEBVRE
• Vegies Story Land
169 St. Jean D'Arc, Lafebvre, P.Q. J0H 2C0   **(514) 733-6299**
Vegetarian. Visit this vegetarian restaurant by appointment—mostly during the summertime. Vegies also has a bed-and-breakfast arrangement. **Open weekends during summer. Cafeteria style, $**

MONTREAL
• Le Commensal
2115 St-Denis, Montreal, P.Q. H2X 3K8   **(514) 845-0248**

1204 McGill College Ave., Montreal, P.Q. H3B 4J8   **(514) 871-1480**

5122 Coteneiges, Montreal, P.Q. H3T 1X8   **(514) 733-9755**
Vegetarian. Voted best vegetarian restaurant by the *Montreal Monitor* in 1992, Le Commensal has been in business for more than fifteen years and offers various ethnic dishes. **Open daily. Buffet, take-out, catering, VISA/MC/AMX, $$**

Cuillere D'or (Golden Spoon)
5217 De Carie, Montreal, P.Q. H3W 3C2   **(514) 481-3431**
Kosher. Vegetarian with the exception of a few dishes, this kosher dairy restaurant serves Stuffed Grape Leaves, blintzes, vegetarian burgers, Lasagna, pizza, and Middle Eastern platters. **Full service, vegan options, take-out, catering, VISA, $$**

Foxy's Kosher Pizza
5987 Victoria, Montreal, P.Q. H3W 2R9   **(514) 739-8777**
Kosher/natural foods. Foxy's features kosher pizza. **Closed Saturday. Cafeteria style, beer, take-out, $**

Pizza Pita
5710 Victoria Ave., Montreal, P.Q. H3W 2X5   **(514) 731-7482**
Natural foods/kosher. Vegetarians can dine on a wide variety of pizzas, Falafel, Hummus, and much more. **Open Sunday through Thursday for three meals. Open Friday for breakfast and lunch. Open for late dinner Saturday. Limited service, vegan options, take-out, $–$$**

- ## Pushap Restaurant and Sweets
5195 Pare, Montreal, P.Q. H4P 1P4   **(514) 737-4527**

11999 Boul. Goulin W., Pierrefonds, P.Q. H8Z 1V8   **(514) 683-0556**
Vegetarian/Indian. Pushap is a family-run restaurant offering Indian vegetarian food. **Open daily. Full service, Indian spice tea, $$**

Bouquinerie-Café Mille Feuille
32 Rue Ste.-Angele, Quebec City, Quebec G1R 4G4   **(418) 692-2147**

1405 Chemin Ste.-Foy, Quebec, G1S 2N7   **(418) 681-4520**
Natural foods. Situated in an historic house with a fireplace, the café offers outdoor dining in the summer. In addition to dining, you can also enjoy an art exhibition. The primarily vegetarian menu features Chili (without meat), Cauliflower with Mushroom and Cheese in Tomato Sauce, Millet Pie, quiche, bread with cheese, salads, and Spanakopita. **Open daily for breakfast, lunch, and dinner in the summer. Closed October 3rd to May 1st of each year. Full service, reservations recommended, espresso/cappuccino, non-alc. beer and wine, beer/ wine/alcohol, catering, take-out, VISA/MC, $$**

SASKATCHEWAN

Alfredo's
1801 Scarth St., Regina, Saskatchewan S4P 2G9   **(306) 522-3366**
Italian. Appealing to vegetarians are Baked Zucchini Parmesan, Spinach Tortelini, and Eggplant Parmesan. Homemade pasta (with eggs) is prepared fresh daily. **Open Monday through Saturday. Full service and cafeteria options, reservations recommended, espresso/cappuccino, beer/wine/alcohol, catering, take-out, VISA/MC/AMX/DC, $–$$$**

Vegetarian
Vacation Spots

"From Atlantic to Pacific, gee, the traffic is terrific!"—it must be vacation time. Whether you choose to vacation on one of the coasts or any place in between, you'll find that vegetarians now have a multitude of options. Choose one of the following spots and combine rafting, yoga, or what have you with tastes galore.

ALABAMA

Yuchi Pines Institute
Route 1, Box 443, Seale, AL 36875　　　　　　　**(205) 855-4781**

A health-conditioning center for ambulatory people who have health problems, the institute operates within the framework of Seventh-day Adventist beliefs and is supervised by two M.D.'s. All meals are vegan.

ARIZONA

Canyon Ranch Health & Fitness Resort
8600 E. Rockcliff Rd. Tucson, AZ 85715　　　　　**(602) 749-9000**

Each lunch and dinner menu includes the option of a vegan soup and/or appetizer and entree.

Healing Center of Arizona
25 Wilson Canyon Rd., Sedona, AZ 86336　　　　　**(602) 282-7710**

Recycling, composting, and use of earth-friendly products are characteristic of this smoke-free center, which offers vegetarian meals. Enjoy the sauna, hot tub, massages, and more.

ARKANSAS

The Garden of Eve Health Spa
1 Washington Street, Eureka Springs, AR 72632　　　**(501) 253-7777**

Located in the Ozarks, this spa serves vegetarian cuisine from a variety of ethnic cultures.

The Oasis
HC 33, Box 10, Tilly, AR 72679   **(501) 496-2364**
A health retreat located in the Boston Range of the Ozark Mountains, The Oasis specializes in organically grown foods as a mainstay of its vegetarian meals. Nearby is Buffalo River National Park.

CALIFORNIA

Ananda
14618 Tyler Foote Road, Nevada City, CA 95959   **(800) 346-5350**
The beauty of the Sierra Nevadas has been the setting of Ananda's meditative and yoga retreats for more than twenty-five years. It is a strictly vegetarian establishment, and almost always serves a vegan option.

EarthSave
706 Frederick Street, Santa Cruz, CA 95062   **(408) 423-4069**
Wilderness retreats and river-rafting trips are conducted in California, and there are environmental youth camps nationwide. All are "pure vegetarian."

La Maida House and Bungalows
11159 La Maida Street, North Hollywood, CA 91601   **(818) 769-3857**
For ethical reasons, this "romantic city-hideaway executive retreat" no longer serves animal products.

Land of Medicine Buddha
5800 Prescott Road, Soquel, CA 95073   **(408) 462-8383**
Health retreats here include organic, vegetarian meals.

Mendocino Summer Retreat
21109 Costanso St., Woodland Hills, CA 91364   **(818) 716-6332**
Programs here integrate macrobiotic living and Waldorf education. The retreat is vegan.

Mount Madonna Center
445 Summit Road, Watsonville, CA 95076   **(408) 847-0406**
The center is a community for the creative arts and health sciences within a context of spiritual growth. Campgrounds in redwood groves are located on the site. The center is strictly lacto-vegetarian but can accommodate vegans.

The Oaks at Ojai
122 E. Ojai Ave., Ojai, CA 93023   **(805) 646-5573**
This resident health spa located in the Ojai Valley serves vegetarian meals on an "alternative" basis, but is looking into a more extensive veggie cuisine.

The Palms
572 North Indian Canyon Drive, Palm Springs, CA 92262   **(619) 325-1111**
The Palms calls itself one of the top ten health spas in the country. It offers vegetarian options at every meal.

Rancho La Puerta
P.O. Box 2548, Escondido, CA 92033   **(619) 744-6677**
The ranch prides itself on being the world's first fitness spa. Largely vegetarian since its opening fifty years ago, it does serve fish.

Royal Gorge Cross Country Ski Resort
P.O. Box 1100, Soda Springs, CA 95728   **(800) 634-3086**
The resort serves vegetarian food to its guests.

Sivananda Yoga Vedanta Center
Sivananda Ashram Yoga Farm,
14651 Ballantree Lane, Grass Valley, CA 95949   **(916) 272-9322**
The center offers a lacto-vegetarian menu at all of its yoga retreats. It also conducts weekend workshops on vegetarian lifestyles.

Stony Brook Inn
309 W. Colombero, P.O. Box 1860   **(916) 964-2300**
McCloud, CA 96057-1860   **or (800) 369-6118**
This Shasta Mountain bed-and-breakfast retreat offers "diverse international vegetarian cuisine with vegan alternatives."

Vega Study Center's Summer Camp
1511 Robinson Street, Oroville, CA 95965   **(916) 533-7702**
An annual affair in Tahoe National Forest, the program centers around macrobiotic living.

We Care Health Center
18000 Long Canyon Rd.   **(619) 251-2261**
Desert Hot Springs, CA, 92240   **or (800) 888-2523**
The center is run by a wholistic health group devoted to physical and mental wellness. It offers a wide variety of raw vegetable juices as part of its vegetarian regimen.

Weimar Institute
P.O. Box 486, 20601 W. Paoli Lane
Weimar, CA 95736-0486   **(916) 637-4111**
A strictly vegan health resort, Weimar also offers a variety of health-related seminars.

Zosa Ranch Bed and Breakfast
9381 West Lilac Rd., Escondido, CA 92026   **(619) 723-9093**
This bed and breakfast offers primarily vegan meals. The ranch, located on twenty-two acres of Monserate Mountain, offers eight fully furnished bedrooms, tennis, basketball, volleyball, and more.

Mind and Body River Adventures

P.O. Box 863, Hotchkiss, CO 81419 (303) 527-3365

This organization specializes in "river adventures to self-awareness." Yoga and tai chi are part of its program. The adventures are primarily organically vegan, but other diets will be catered to upon request.

Butterbrooke Bed and Breakfast

78 Barry Road, Oxford, CT 06483 (203) 888-2000

This restored 1711 colonial house is located on a small organic farm, and serves a vegetarian breakfast.

Savannah Inn

330 Savannah Road, Lewes, DE 19958 (302) 645-5592

Located near the Atlantic Ocean, this vegetarian bed-and-breakfast serves food only in the summer months.

Abundant Health Lifestyle Center

Rt. 2 Box 451A, Webster, FL 33597 (904) 568-1119

A Christian health resort specializing in a vegan diet, the center offers twenty-six-day lifestyle sessions.

Club Hygiene

105 Bruce Court, Marathon, FL 33050-2915 (305) 743-3168

Located in the Keyes area, Club Hygiene offers "comprehensive hygienic vacations" including 100-percent raw, vegan meals.

Crystal Springs Wilderness Retreat

1932 Deer Lane, Zephyrhills, FL 33540 (813) 782-4226

Various outdoor activities are available on the retreat's grounds, and it is close to many Florida resorts. Management told us that many dietary preferences can be accommodated.

The Great Outdoors Inn

65 N. Main Street, P.O. Box 387, High Springs, FL 32643 (904) 454-2900

This bed-and-breakfast inn is located on forty acres near a state park, and serves vegetarian food. The inn can accommodate up to twenty-four people for conferences. Nearby is the Great Outdoors Cafe offering vegetarian entrees.

Hippocrates Health Institute

1443 Palmdale Court, West Palm Beach, FL 33411 (407) 471-8876

A strictly vegan health resort, the institute now offers a singles program.

Hygeia Center
P.O. Box 845, Estero, FL 33928 **(813) 489-3337**

This is a wholistic preventive health-care retreat serving gourmet vegetarian cuisine. A vegan option is offered. Vegetarian trips to places such as Paros, Greece, are sometimes offered.

Indigo Inn
Drayton Island, Box 5, Georgetown, FL 32139 **(904) 467-2446**

A bed-and-breakfast open all year, the inn is located on a twelve-acre working farm on an island. The proprietor, a vegetarian/vegan cook for eighteen years, completed macrobiotic studies at the Kushi Institute.

Palm-Aire Spa Resort
2601 Palm-Aire Drive North, Pompano Beach, FL 33069 **(305) 968-2750**

Vegetarian options are offered every day.

Regency Health Resort and Spa
2000 S. Ocean Drive, Hallandale, FL 33009 **(305) 454-2220**

This is a luxury-class beach resort offering gourmet vegetarian cuisine.

Royal Atlantic Health Spa
1460 S. Ocean Blvd., Pompano Beach, FL 33062 **(800) 583-3500**

Enjoy gourmet vegetarian cuisine and attend health seminars at this beach health spa.

Russell House of Key West
611 Truman Avenue, Key West, FL 33040 **(305) 294-8787**

Russell House, which bills itself as a tropical wellness retreat, serves a vegetarian diet with a vegan option.

Safety Harbor Spa and Fitness
105 N. Bayshore Dr., Safety Harbor, FL 34695 **(800) 237-0155**

Calling itself the "ultimate spa vacation," Safety Harbor offers a few vegetarian/vegan options on its regular menu.

HAWAII

Hana Plantation Houses
P.O. Box 489, Hana Maui, HI 96713 **(808) 248-7248**

This beach resort is operated by a vegetarian who was a founder of the Ecologically Conscious Host Network and operates two Environmental Information Centers.

Hawaiian Fitness Holiday
P.O. Box 279, Koloa, Kauai, HI 96756 **(808) 332-9244**

Focus on total health and fitness in a tropical paradise. Vegetarian cuisine (fish is also served) with a vegan option is offered.

Kalani Honua
RR2 Box 4500, Pahoa, HI 96778   **(808) 965-7828**

This conference and retreat center specializes in vegetarian cuisine although fish and fowl entrees are offered. The center also conducts a wide variety of workshops and festivals.

The Plantation Spa
51-550 Kam Hwy., Ka'a'awa, Oahu, HI 96730   **(800) 422-0307**

This Swedish Polynesian retreat bills itself as a "spa resort for body and mind," and offers lacto-vegetarian cuisine with a vegan option.

IDAHO
Idaho Afloat
P.O. Box 542, Grangeville, ID 83530   **(208) 983-2414**

A white-water rafting organization in the Pacific Northwest, Idaho Afloat can accommodate vegetarians, and would be happy to bring in a local vegan cook for a group of more than twelve.

ILLINOIS
The Heartland
20 E. Jackson Blvd., Chicago, IL 60604   **(312) 427-6465**

Located eighty miles south of Chicago, this health and fitness retreat is situated on thirty-one acres of woods and farmland. The cuisine is "basically vegetarian supplemented with fish."

MAINE
Bouldaire
Blue Hill Falls, ME 04615   **(207) 359-4692**

Located on the shorefront, Bouldaire is a newly renovated older home. It is close to Acadia National Park, and offers yoga and cooking classes. The cuisine is macrobiotic.

Kingsbury House
35 Northport Avenue, Belfast, ME 04915   **(207) 338-2419**

A macrobiotic bed-and-breakfast, Kingsbury House regularly serves miso soup and tofu French toast.

Northern Pines
559 Rt. 85, Raymond, ME 04071- 6248   **(207) 655-7624**

A lakeside resort in southern Maine, Northern Pines is largely vegetarian, serving fish once a week and offering soy substitutes for dairy. The resort can provide kosher foods, and accommodate diabetics and vegans.

Poland Spring Health Institute
Summit Spring Road, RFD 1, Box 4300
Poland Spring, ME 04274   **(207) 998-2894**
This institute offers a lifestyle improvement program including a vegan regimen.

The Roaring Lion
995 Main Street, P.O. Box 756, Waldoboro, ME 04572   (207) 832-4038
Open all year, this bed-and-breakfast caters to vegetarian and macrobiotic diets.

West of Eden
Rt. 102 and Kelleytown Rd., P.O. Box 114
Seal Cove, ME 04674   **(207) 244-9695**
You'll find this small bed-and-breakfast on Mt. Desert Island, just outside of Acadia National Park. It is macrobiotic with a very strong vegan emphasis.

MARYLAND

Gramercy Bed & Breakfast
1440 Greenspring Valley Rd., Box 119
Stevenson, MD 21153   **(410) 486-2405**
Located outside of Baltimore on fifty-four acres of forest, organic flower and herb gardens, Gramercy's facilities include a pool, tennis court, and hiking trails. Breakfast items include omelettes, French toast, pancakes, cereals, and fresh fruit.

MASSACHUSETTS

Canyon Ranch in the Berkshires
165 Kemble St., Lenox, MA 01240   **(413) 637-4100**
Each lunch and dinner menu includes the option of a vegan soup and/or appetizer and entree.

Insight Meditation Society
1230 Pleasant St., Barre, MA 01005   **(508) 355-4378**
Eighty wooded acres is the perfect setting for vipassana (insight meditation). Meals are vegetarian.

The Kushi Institute
P.O. Box 7, Becket, MA 01223   **(413) 623-5741**
The Institute is a nonprofit educational resort located in the Berkshire Mountains. It is macrobiotic with a vegan emphasis.

Rowe Camp and Conference Center
Kings Highway Rd., Box 273, Rowe, MA 01367   **(413) 339-4216**
The center offers all types of programs to aid in the revitalization of mind and body for all ages. It is surrounded by 1,400 acres of protected forest, and the cuisine is "gourmet vegetarian."

The Turning Point Inn

RD2 Box 140, Great Barrington, MA 01230   **(413) 528-4777**

A year-round bed-and-breakfast, The Turning Point is a 200-year-old inn in the heart of the Berkshires. The inn serves lacto-ovo vegetarian meals and can accommodate vegans.

Whispering Maples

P.O. Box 382, Surriner Road, Becket, MA 01223   **(413) 623-2392**

This bed-and-breakfast specializes in natural and macrobiotic foods.

MICHIGAN

Circle Center Pines

8650 Mullen Road, Delton, MI 49046   **(616) 623-5555**

This cooperative recreation and education center provides vegetarian meals in a campground setting.

MONTANA

Feathered Pipe Foundation

Box 1682, Helena, MT 59624   **(406) 442-8196**

Located in the Rockies, the foundation offers programs for those seeking a healthier mind and body. It also organizes international tours. The cuisine is primarily vegetarian, but fish and chicken are occasionally served.

NEW HAMPSHIRE

Star Island Corporation

110 Arlington St., Boston, MA 02116   **(617) 426-7988**

Summer conferences covering a wide-range of topics are offered on Star Island off the coast of New Hampshire. Meals are vegetarian.

The Tuc'Me Inn

68 North Main St., Box 657, Wolfeboro, NH 03894   **(603) 569-5702**

Located in a quaint New England town on the Eastern Shore of Lake Winnipe-saukee, this bed and breakfast serves vegetarian breakfasts. Enjoy swimming, boating, hiking, mountain-climbing, or skiing nearby.

NEW JERSEY

Appel Farms

P.O. Box 770, Elmer, NJ 08318-2472   **(609) 358-2472**

This dormitory-style conference center specializes in home-style vegetarian and kosher vegetarian cuisine. Some of the produce is organically grown on the grounds.

Mayer's Manor

57 Dupont Avenue, P.O. Box 85
Seaside Heights, NJ 08751 **(908) 793-6606**
Located close to many places of interest in New Jersey, Mayer's bills itself as a vegetarian guest house.

Serendipity Bed and Brunch

712 9th Street, Ocean City, NJ 08226-3554 **(609) 399-1554**
Vegetarian and macrobiotic entrees are served buffet style.

NEW YORK

Farm Sanctuary

P.O. Box 150, Watkins Glen, NY 14891 **(607) 583-2225**
This shelter for abused farm animals also has a bed-and-breakfast serving a continental vegetarian breakfast. The shelter is open year round.

Highland House

Airport Road, Yulan, NY 12792 **(914) 557-8391**
Located on the Delaware River in the Shawangunk Mountains, this hotel follows a philosophy of "Supernutrition." It is strictly lacto-vegetarian, buffet style, and caters to vegans and those with food allergies. Camping inquiries are welcome.

Living Springs Lifestyle Center

136 Bryant Lifestyle Center, Putnam Valley, NY 10579 **(800) SAY-WELL**
In cooperation with Seventh-day Adventists, the center offers seminars on health issues. Vegan meals are a mainstay of the program.

New Age Health Spa

Neversink, NY 12765 **(800) 682-4348**
This spa is located on 155 acres in the Catskill Mountains. It offers three types of dietary regimens: non-vegetarian with a vegetarian option; vegan; and juice fast.

Omega Institute

RD 2, Box 377, Rhinebeck, NY 12572 **(914) 266-4301**
This conference and workshop resort "exists to encourage and promote a hopeful response to personal and cultural challenges . . . based on the belief that a sane world starts with healthy people." The institute also offers outdoor journeys and kids' camps. It is primarily lacto-ovo vegetarian but serves fish.

The Open Space

HCR 1 Box 171, Livingston Manor, NY 12758 **(914) 439-3119**
Located in the Catskill Mountains, this conference center is committed to Zen practice and offers vegetarian meals.

VATRA Vegetarian Lodge
P.O. Box F, Rte. 214, Hunter, NY 12442   **(518) 263-4919**
The name says it all.

The Woodstock Center for Healing and Renewal
PO Box 127, Woodstock, NY 12498   **(800) 398-2630**
Enjoy kosher vegetarian cuisine at this healing center located on thirty-five acres.
Take classes, swim in the pool, play tennis, go hiking, learn yoga, enjoy the indoor
jacuzzi, plus much more.

NORTH CAROLINA

Mountain Mist
420 Country Club Dr., Hazelwood, NC 28738   **(704) 452-1550**
This vegetarian retreat is located in the mountains of North Carolina. It offers a
health program, cooking classes, an exercise program, and more.

North Carolina Macrobiotic Oceanside Retreat
P.O. Box 262, Corolla, NC 27927   **(919) 453-3553**
The retreat is located one block from the ocean.

OHIO

Sans Souci
3745 Rte. 725, Bellbrook, OH 45305   **(513) 848-4851**
A spa resort located on an eighty-acre private estate, Sans Souci offers a highly
individualized program including vegetarian meals. The spa grows its own vegetables.

PENNSYLVANIA

Himalayan Institute
RR 1, Box 400, Honesdale, PA 18431   **(717) 253-5551**
The institute, devoted to teaching yoga and meditation, serves vegetarian meals
and offers workshops on vegetarianism.

The Peetham: A Center for Well-Being
RD 8, Box 8116, Stroudsburg, PA 18360   **(717) 629-0481**
This retreat nestled in the heart of the Poconos has conference facilities and serves
vegetarian meals.

Quest Center
RR 1, Box 1366, Hop Bottom, PA 18824   **(717) 289-4021**
At a rustic log cabin in the Pocono Mountains, you'll find three dormitory-style
bedrooms, vegetarian meals, and yoga and meditation workshops.

White Cloud
RD 1, Box 215, Newfoundland, PA 18445   **(717) 676-3162**
Meals at this country inn located in the Poconos are strictly lacto-ovo vegetarian, and vegans can be accommodated.

PUERTO RICO

Grateful Bed & Breakfast
Box 568 - VJ, Luquillo, PR 00773   **(809) 889-4919**
Enjoy vegetarian meals and the nearby rainforest, as well as snorkeling and scuba diving.

SOUTH DAKOTA

Black Hills Health and Education Center
Box 19, Hermosa, SD 57744   **(605) 255-4101**
This strictly vegan health resort is situated in the famous Black Hills.

TEXAS

Church of the White Eagle Lodge
P.O. Box 930, Montgomery, TX 77356   **(409) 597-5757**
This spiritual retreat center is dedicated to following and teaching White Eagle's philosophy. It is strictly lacto-ovo vegetarian and will accommodate vegans.

UTAH

Capitol Reef Inn
360 West Main St., Torrey, UT 84775   **(801) 425-3271**
This Inn also offers a natural foods restaurant. Located in southern Utah a few miles from Capitol Reef National Park, it has ten motel units.

Snowbird Ski and Summer Resort
Snowbird, UT 84092   **(801) 742-2222**
The resort offers 11,000-foot peaks for your enjoyment all year round, and is also a conference facility. The menu contains a few vegetarian entrees.

VERMONT

Greenhope Farm
RFD, Box 2260, E. Harwick, VT 05836   **(802) 533-7772**
At this women-only vacation farm in a tiny hamlet in northeast Vermont, the cooking is vegetarian/vegan.

VIRGIN ISLANDS

Majo Bay Camps, Inc.
Cruz Bay, St. John USVI 00830   **(809) 776-6240**
Majo Bay Camps is strongly committed to environmental preservation. It consists of a community of tent-cottages within a national park. Every cottage has a

propane stove and an ice cooler for food storage. A restaurant offers one vegetarian option at each meal.

VIRGINIA

Hartland Health Center
P.O. Box 1, Rapiden, VA 22733   **(703) 672-3100**
Located on 500 acres of gently rolling hills, Hartland is just two hours from Washington, D.C. With a Seventh-day Adventist orientation, the Center is determinedly vegetarian.

Satchidananda Ashram-Yogaville
Buckingham, VA 23921   **(804) 969-3121**
This spiritual center offers a strictly lacto-vegetarian menu and has an annual summer camp.

WASHINGTON

Annapurna Inn
538 Adams at Clay Street, Port Townsend, WA 98368   **(206) 385-2909**
A relatively new vegetarian bed-and-breakfast, the Inn is smoke-free and located in an historic district.

Towerhouse Bed and Breakfast
San Juan Island, 1230 Little Road
Friday Harbor, WA 98250   **(206) 378-5464**
Located on ten acres, Towerhouse offers vegetarian (vegan upon request) breakfasts.

WEST VIRGINIA

The Woods
P.O. Box 5, Hedgeville, WV 25427   **(800) 248-2222**
This 18,000-acre resort and conference center, located close to the Baltimore-Washington area, offers a few vegetarian entrees.

WISCONSIN

Ralph and Jan's Roadside Attraction
703 Railroad Street, Blanchardville, WI 53516   **(608) 523-2001**
Ralph and Jan run a vegetarian bed-and-breakfast.

CANADA

• Golden Dreams B and B
6412 Easy St., Whistler, BC, Canada V0N 1B6 **(604) 932-2667**
At this vegetarian bed-and-breakfast, rooms are tastefully decorated in Victorian, Oriental, and Aztec themes and feature sherry decanters, moccasins, and duvets. Relax in the private jacuzzi bath and awake to a nutritious, hearty breakfast including homemade jams and fresh herbs served in a country kitchen.

Hollyhock Farm
Box 127, Manson's Landing
Cortes Island, BC Canada V0P IKO **(604) 935-6465**
Wholistic-living workshops and retreats are offered, and camping is available. There is also a "Journeys Program." Fresh vegetarian and seafood fare is served buffet-style.

Strathcona Park Lodge
Box 2160S, Campbell River
British Columbia, Canada V9W 5C9 **(604) 286-2008**
Located in the center of Vancouver Island in a wilderness area, the lodge offers outdoor expeditions that are mostly vegetarian. Special trips are offered for young students.

Nada Hermitage
Box 119, Crestone, CO 81131 **(719) 256-4778**
The Hermitage is a monastic spiritual institute in the wilderness of the Sangre de Cristo mountains. People may eat as they choose, but the institute is primarily vegetarian. A sister institute, **Nova Nada**, is in Kemptville, Nova Scotia, Canada B0W 1Y0.

Forest Edge Bed & Breakfast
RR#3, Durham, Ontario, Canada N0G 1R0 **(519) 369-5661**
Enjoy a vegetarian breakfast at this bed and breakfast.

Hidden Valley Farm
RR 2, Chatsworth, Ontario, Canada, N0H 1G0 **(519) 794-3727**
Most of the food served on this farm is home-cooked and home-grown on 120 acres of organic farmland located close to many points of interest. Meals are vegan but dairy and eggs are available for those in transition.

Oats 'n' Honey Bed & Breakfast
General Delivery, Camden East
Ontario, Canada K0K 1J0   **(613) 378-0174**
Enjoy vegetarian breakfasts at this vegetarian bed and breakfast.

Philoxia
P.O. Box 56, Marlbank
Toronto, Ontario, Canada K0K 2L0   **(613) 478-6070**
This vacation resort serves macrobiotic and vegetarian foods with an international flavor.

QUEBEC

Vegetarian Story Village
Box 136, S. Durham, P.Q. Canada, J0H 2C0   **(514) 738-9062**
The strictly vegan village bills itself as a "vegetarian mini-resort for nature's lovers and for relaxation."

AMERICAN VEGETARIAN TRAVEL TOURS & SERVICES

When you're smitten by wanderlust, peruse this alphabetical listing of organizations; you're sure to find an American expedition that will satisfy your needs.

Always Travel
4701 Sangamore Road, Bethesda, MD 20816   **(800) 783-8990**
Ask for or write to Donna Zeigfinger who specializes in arranging travel plans for vegetarians.

Ancient Forest Adventures
800 NW 6th Avenue, Suite 201, Portland, OR 97209   **(503) 248-0492**
Interpretive tours of the Pacific Northwest are conducted on foot, snowshoe, or cross-country skis. Vegetarian meals are served; on some tours, vegan is standard. The organization donates 5 percent of the proceeds to conservation efforts.

AZI Guide Service
CVSR Box 2207, Moab, UT 84532   **(801) 259-7620**
This service wants to assist those wishing to approach zero impact on an outdoor expedition in the Southwest. The service offers an organic vegetarian menu.

The Biking Expedition
Box 547V, Henniker, NH 03242   **(800) 245-4649**
Bike tours in New Hampshire feature vegetarian meals as an option at every meal; vegan meals are available upon request. Vegetarian dishes include Pasta Primavera, Chili, Lentil Stew, and Curried Rice and Vegetables. The emphasis is on healthy meals.

Celebrity Cruises
5200 Blue Lagoon Drive, Miami, FL 33126   **(800) 437-6111**
With twenty-four hours' notice, vegetarian or vegan meals will be arranged on cruises.

Country Walkers, Inc.

P.O. Box 180, Waterbury, VT 05676-0180   **(802) 244-1387**

Specializing in fine walking and hiking vacations around the country with an emphasis on natural history, Country Walkers donates some of its proceeds to conservation groups. The inns and hotels used by the group usually offer a vegetarian option. Upon request, vegans will be accommodated gladly.

The Crash Network

519 Castro St., #7, San Francisco, CA 94114

Billing itself as "the new guide to traveling through the underground," the network publishes a directory of folks to home-exchange with as you travel.

Desert Journeys

P.O. Box 241, Bodega, CA 94922   **(707) 874-3342**

Small groups are organized for trips into the deserts of California and Arizona. Journeys take place four times a year, one every season. Lacto-vegetarian food is offered (the dairy products are kept separate and vegans can be accommodated).

Environmental Travel

P.O. Box 253, Kew Gardens, NY 11415   **(800) 929-3005**

This is a new travel service run by vegetarians.

Figaro Cruises

P.O. Box 1336, Camden, ME 04843   **(800) 473-6169**

Figaro offers sailing cruises along the Maine coast for health-minded folks. The menu is lacto-ovo vegetarian although macrobiotic and vegan preferences can be accommodated. Figaro makes most of the foods from scratch, and offers a seafood side option.

Hatch River Expeditions

P.O. Box 1150, Vernal, UT 84078   **(800) 342-8243**

You can take a white-water rafting trip down the Colorado River; request vegetarian/vegan meals in advance.

Hawk, I'm Your Sister

P.O. Box 9109, Santa Fe, NM 87504-2268   **(505) 984-2268**

Women's wilderness canoe trips feature primarily vegetarian meals. A few co-ed trips are also offered.

Her Wild Song

P.O. Box 6793, Portland, ME 04101   **(207) 773-4969**

Specializing in wilderness journeys for women, Her Wild Song serves vegetarian fare.

Kaibab Mountain Bike Tours

37 S. First West, Moab, UT 84532   **(800) 451-1133**

Kaibab easily outfits vegetarians and vegans for tours in Utah.

Laughing Heart Adventures
P.O. Box 669, Willow Creek, CA 95573 **(916) 629-3516**
Laughing Heart specializes in "consciousness-raising canoe outings on wild and scenic rivers throughout the West and Mexico." The meals are mostly vegetarian, and vegans can be accommodated. All staff members are vegetarian.

Michigan Bicycle Touring
3512 Red School Road, Kingsley, MI 49649 **(616) 263-5885**
"Glen Lake Veggie Amble" tours feature food prepared by a chef who "creates magic with her non-dairy, international cuisine."

Mind Body River Adventures
P.O. Box 863, Hotchkiss, CO 81419 **(303) 527-4466**
This service specializes in wilderness river-retreats in Colorado and Utah. Vegetarian meals are served.

Resources
Box 1067 Harvard Square Station
Cambridge, MA 02238 **(617) 825-8895**
This is a directory of more than 12,000 alternative groups and organizations. A travel guide is also available.

River Travel Center
Box 6, Pt. Arena, CA 95468 **(800) 882-RAFT**
River Travel specializes in rafting and kayaking in the American West. Most of its outfitters can accommodate vegetarians.

Sierra Club
730 Polk Street, San Francisco, CA 94109 **(415) 776-2211**
The club offers a wide range of outdoor expeditions. A trip to New Mexico features vegetarian food.

Uncle John's Foods
500 Hathaway, P.O. Box 489, Fairplay, CO 80440 **(719) 836-2710**
or (800) 530-8733
Supplies nutritious, air-dried, vegan food suitable for camping and backpacking.

Vermont Bicycle Touring
Box 711, Bristol, VT 05443 **(802) 453-4811**
On biking tours in Vermont as well as elsewhere, this group serves vegetarian meals upon request.

Woodswomen Adventure Travel for Women of All Ages
25 West Diamond Lake Road, Minneapolis, MN 55419 **(800) 279-0555**
Woodswomen's trips are primarily vegetarian.

Working Assets Travel Service

701 Montgomery Street #400, San Francisco, CA 94111   (415) 788-0777

This service donates 2 percent of the proceeds from travel purchases to some nonprofit organizations working for peace, human rights, economic justice, or the environment.

INTERNATIONAL VEGETARIAN TRAVEL TOURS & VACATION SPOTS

The many ethnic foods described in this book may well give you a taste for a foreign adventure. If so, contact one of the following groups for assistance in finding just the right trip.

Adventure Associates
P.O. Box 16304, Seattle, WA 98116   **(206) 932-8352**
Offers co-ed and women-only expeditions around the world. The Associates serve primarily vegetarian meals in the field; they can accommodate special requests but may ask the guest to supply some food.

Amazonia Expeditions
163 Russell Street, Brooklyn, NY 11222   **(212) 642-5405**
Amazonia offers trips to the South American rain forests. All meals are vegan, with eggs and canned milk an option. Much of the fruit is native to the area.

Animal Amnesty
Galleria Passarella 1, 20122 Milano, Italy   **02-4224620 or 02- 4224506**
Vegetarian holidays are available to members.

Carnival Cruise Lines
327 E. 49th Street, Hialeah, FL 33013   **(800) 232-4666**
A vegetarian menu is offered to guests.

Crackington Manor
Crackington Haven
North Cornwall, England EX23 OJG   **(08403) 397 or 536**
A beach hotel owned by vegetarians, Crackington was voted "Vegetarian Restaurant of the Year" by *Vegetarian Living* magazine. Token meat and fish dishes are offered, but the manor is primarily ovo-vegetarian.

D'Astros Le Pin
82 340 Auvillar, France   **63-95-95-20**
This bed-and-breakfast offers vegetarian meals.

Forum Travel International
91 Gregory Lane, #21, Pleasant Hill, CA 94523   **(510) 671-2900**
Specializing in "classic and unusual travel" all over the world, Forum employees told us that most of its European biking trips can accommodate vegetarians very easily.

Greg Johnson Associates
60 E. 42nd Street, Ste. 1111, NY, NY 10165   **(212) 599-0300**
This organization arranges trips throughout the world. The service accommodates vegetarians and can easily arrange a tour for a large group of vegetarians.

Hi-Lo Travel
459 Route 79, PO Box 27, Morganville, NJ 07751   **(908) 591-9292**
Worldwide travelers themselves, staff members have had experience arranging trips for both diabetics and vegetarians. Ask for or write to Tema.

Hippocrates Health Center
Elaine Avenue, Mudgeeraba 4213, Gold Coast
Queensland, Australia   **(075) 302860**
A guest described the center as a national park with luxuries. It offers raw vegan foods on Ann Wigmore's Wheatgrass Program.

The Invented City
41 Sutter Street, #1090, San Francisco, CA 94104   **(415) 673- 0347**
                                                         or (800) 788-CITY

This international home-exchange service offers travelers a way to swap lodgings. The service does not designate kitchens as vegetarian or not, although we were told that many members are vegetarians.

Inverdene
11 Bridge Square, Ballater, Scotland AB35 5QJ   **(03397) 55759**
This vegan guest house is nestled in the mountains near the river Dee.

Kesher Worldwide Jewish Home Link
75 Solvent Road, West Hampstead,
London, England NW6 1TY   **071-794-0073**
An exchange and rental organization servicing the world, Kesher works only with vegetarian, kosher, and other Jewish families.

Miranda's Veranda
Umaran 122, San Miguel de Allende
Guanajuato 37700, Mexico   **011-52-465-22659**
Miranda's is a smoke-free, vegetarian bed-and-breakfast that has a water treatment system.

Moshav Amirim
Bikat Beit Hakarem, Carmel, Israel 20115   **06-980946**
Billing itself as a vegetarian/naturalist village, Moshav Amirim is located in the beautiful upper Galilee overlooking the Kinnert. Most of the foods and herbs are organically grown on the premises.

O'Reilly's Guest House
Via Canungra, QLD 4275, Australia   **(075) 440-644**
Located in Lamington National Park, O'Reilly's offers lacto-ovo vegetarian meals.

Rio Caliente
c/o Barbara Dane Associates, 480 California Terrace
Pasadena, CA 91105   **(818) 796-5577**
This spa and mineral hot springs resort in Guadalajara, Mexico, is lacto-ovo vegetarian.

Royal Caribbean Cruise Line
1890 Park Marina Drive, #107, Redding, CA 96001   **(800) 852-3268**
The cruise line now offers vegetarian cruises to the Caribbean.

The Safari Connection
245 E. 35th Street, Ste. 5G, NY, NY 10016   **(800) 245-9234**
Arranges safaris to Africa . . . and beyond. The organization will cater to vegetarians upon request, and can easily arrange a tour for a large group of vegetarians.

Sea Quest Expeditions
Zoetic Research, P.O. Box 2424
Friday Harbor, WA 98250   **(206) 378-5767**
Experts in the field lead whale-watching trips. Kayaking expeditions in Washington and Mexico, some of which are parts of research projects, are also offered. All meals are vegetarian; much of the food is organically grown.

Sivanda Yoga Vedanta Center
243 W. 24th Street, NY, NY 10011
The center will connect you with ashrams around the world. Accommodations are strictly lacto-vegetarian. Camping is available.

Southwind Adventures
P.O. Box 621057, Littleton, CO 80162   **(303) 972-0701**
Vegetarian and vegan diets are accommodated on trips to the Andes and Amazon.

Tigh-Na-Mara
The Shore, Ardindrean, Loch broom
Wester Ross, Scotland IV23 2SE   **0854 85 282**
This guest house is close to many Scottish attractions and serves principally vegetarian meals. Some vegan and seafood entrees are offered.

Tivoli Ltd.
Merkazim Building, P.O. Box 2045, Maskit Street 5, Industrial Area
Herzliya, Israel 46120   **052-557108**
This organization books hotels and tours that cater to vegetarians.

Transitions Abroad Magazine
18 Hulst Road, Box 344, Amherst, MA 01004   **(413) 256-0373**
This is an international resource guide for educational and socially responsible travel.

Wildland Adventures
3516 NE 155th St., Seattle, WA   **(800) 345-4453**
Wildland specializes in "authentic, worldwide expeditions." Some of the proceeds go to local conservation groups. The organization is always able to provide alternatives to meat-based diets; 60 percent of the clientele request alternatives.

Local Contacts for More Information

When traveling, you may want to contact the following groups for the latest information about restaurants in their areas. Our thanks to many of these contacts for helping us locate information for this guide and apologies to any group that we may have accidentally failed to acknowledge.

For updated information about local groups or to ask questions about vegetarianism, contact The Vegetarian Resource Group, P.O. Box 1463, Baltimore, MD 21203, or call (410) 366-VEGE.

United States

ARIZONA

Jewish Vegetarians of Arizona
P.O. Box 32842, Phoenix, AZ 85064   (602) 840-7142

CALIFORNIA

Bay Area Jewish Vegetarians
46 Southwind Circle, Richmond, CA 94804-7404   (415) 465-0403

EarthSave
706 Frederick St., Santa Cruz, CA 95062   (408) 423-4069

Los Angeles Vegetarian Association
505 S. Beverly Dr., Suite 690, Beverly Hills, CA 90212   (213) 964-4FUN

Peninsula Vegetarians
284 Margarita Ave., Palo Alto, CA. 94306   (415) 493-0211

Sacramento Vegetarian Society
P.O. Box 163583, Sacramento, CA 95816   (916) 446-9334

San Francisco Vegetarian Society
1450 Broadway #4, San Francisco, CA 94109   (415) 775-6874

COLORADO

Vegetarian Society of Colorado
P.O. Box 6773, Denver, CO 80206   (303) 777-4828

CONNECTICUT

ARIES (Animal Rights Information and Education Service)
P.O. Box 332, Rowayton, CT 06853

Friends of Animals
P.O. Box 1244, Norwalk, CT 06856   (203) 866-5223

DISTRICT OF COLUMBIA

Vegetarian Society of D.C.
P.O. Box 4921, Washington, DC 20008   (301) 589-0722

FLORIDA

I CARE
P.O. Box 279, Osprey, FL 34229

Vegetarian Gourmet Society
P.O. Box 8060, Hollywood, FL 33084   (305) 791-1562

Vegetarian Society of Southern Florida Environmental Center
11011 SW 104th St., Miami, FL 33176-3393   (305) 347-2600

GEORGIA

Vegetarian Society of Georgia
P.O. Box 2164, Norcross, GA 30091   (404) 447-5561

HAWAII

Vegetarian Society of Honolulu
P.O. Box 25233, Honolulu, HI 96825   (808) 395-1499

ILLINOIS

Chicago Vegetarian Society
P.O. Box 6154, Evanston, IL 60204 (312) 764-VEGY

Vegetarians in Motion
P.O. Box 6943, Rockford, IL 61125 (815) 397-5579

IOWA

Heartland Products
P.O. Box 218, Dakota City, IA 50529 (515) 332-3087

MAINE

Maine Vegetarian Resource Group
RFD 2 Box 194, Belfast, ME 04915

MARYLAND

Bowie Area Vegetarian Society
P.O. Box 1478, Bowie, Maryland 20717 (301) 249-7926

Jewish Vegetarians of North America
6938 Reliance Road, Federalsburg, MD 21632 (410) 754-5550

The Vegetarian Resource Group
P.O. Box 1463, Baltimore, MD 21203 (410) 366-8343

MASSACHUSETTS

Boston Vegetarian Society
P.O. Box 38-1071, Cambridge, MA 02238 (617) 424-8846

Cape Cod Vegetarians
P.O. Box 243, Sagamore Beach, MA 02562 (508) 888-2106

New England Anti-Vivisection Society
333 Washington St., Suite. 850, Boston, MA 02108

MICHIGAN

Michigan Vegetarian Society
P.O. Box 258, Clawson, MI 48017 (810) 435-3514

MINNESOTA

Vegetarian Information Service
5049 Thomas Ave., S., Minneapolis, MN 55410 (612) 920-6412

Vegetarian Society of Southern Minnesota
P.O. Box 3532, Mankato, MN 56002   (507) 625-4448

NEBRASKA

Nebraska Vegetarian Society
P.O. Box 30631, Lincoln, NE 68503-0631   (402) 476-7252

NEVADA

Sierra Vegetarian Society
15425 Fawn Lane, Reno, NV 89511-9068

NEW JERSEY

American Vegan Society
501 Old Harding Hwy., Malaga, NJ 08328   (609) 694-2887

New Jersey Animal Rights Alliance (NJARA)
P.O. Box 174, Elizabethtown, NJ 07726-0174   (908) 855-9092

Vegetarian Society of South Jersey
P.O. Box 272, Marlton, NJ 08053   (609) 983-3964

NEW MEXICO

Sangre de Cristo Animal Protection, Inc.
P.O. Box 5179, Albuquerque, NM 87185   (505) 983-2200

NEW YORK

Binghamton Area Vegetarian Society
P.O. Box 614, Vestal, NY 13850-0614   (607) 757-9463

Long Island Vegetarians
P.O. Box 1146, Huntington, NY 11743-0656   (516) 349-8639

North American Vegetarian Society (NAVS)
P.O. Box 72, Dolgeville, NY 13329   (518) 568-7970

Rochester Area Vegetarian Society
P.O. Box 20185, Rochester, NY 14602-0185   (716) 381-2208

Vegetarian Society of New York
128 E. 83rd Street, New York, NY 10028   (212) 535-9385

NORTH CAROLINA

Mecklenburg Vegetarian Society
7302 Lancashire Dr., Charlotte, NC 28227   (704) 545-3796

Triangle Vegetarian Society
P.O. Box 61069, Durham, NC 27705-1069   (919) 471-4453

Vegetarian Society of the Lower Cape Fear
P.O. Box 3411, Wilmington, NC 28406   (919) 791-4907

Very Vegetarian Society
620 Bellview St., Winston-Salem, NC 27103-3502   (919) 765-2614

OHIO

Vegetarian Club of Canton
P.O. Box 9079, Canton, OH 44711   (216) 497-2859

The Vegetarian Society of Greater Dayton Area
P.O. Box 404, Englewood, OH 45322   (513) 429-9163

Vegetarian Society of Toledo and Northwest Ohio
2655 Calverton Rd., Toledo, OH 43607   (419) 536-4073

OREGON

Portland Vegetarians
P.O. Box 19521, Portland, OR 97219   (503) 223-5596

Salem Vegetarians
P.O. Box 13932, Salem, OR 97309-1932   (503) 585-1829

PENNSYLVANIA

Lehigh Valley Vegetarians
1035 Flexer Ave., Allentown, PA 18103   (215) 437-3278

Mobilization for Animals, PA, Inc.
P.O. Box 99762, Pittsburgh, PA 15233   (412) 232-5106

Vegetarian Education Network
P.O. Box 3347, West Chester, PA 19380   (215) 696-VNET

Vegetarian Society of Central Pennsylvania
P.O. Box 11066, State College, PA 16805-1066   (814) 238-2239

The Vegetarians of Philadelphia
P.O. Box 24353, Philadelphia, PA 19120   **(215) 276-3198**

RHODE ISLAND

Rhode Island Vegetarians
P.O. Box 716, N. Satuate, RI 02857

SOUTH CAROLINA

South Carolina Vegetarian Society
P.O. Box 1093, Lexington, SC 29072   **(803) 957-8155**

TENNESSEE

East Tennessee Vegetarian Society
P.O. Box 1974, Knoxville, TN 37901   **(615) 522-5555**

Tennessee Vegetarian Society
P.O. Box 854, Knoxville, TN 37901   **(800) 280-8343**

TEXAS

Austin Vegetarian Society
P.O. Box 2335, Cedar Park, TX 78613   **(512) 331-5287**

Denton Area Vegetarian Organization
2040 West Oak, Denton, TX 76201   **(817) 383-3858**

San Antonio Vegetarian Society
P.O. Box 23127, San Antonio, TX 78233-0127   **(210) 658-6557**

Vegetarian Society of Houston
P.O. Box 980093, Houston, TX 77008

VERMONT

Vermont Vegetarian Society
RR1 Box 1797, N. Ferrisburg, VT 05473   **(802) 453-3945**

VIRGINIA

Virginia Vegetarian Society
6451 Cotton Hill Rd., Roanoke, VA 24018   **(703) 772-3316**

(See also D.C. Vegetarian Society)

WASHINGTON

Animal Advocates of the Inland Northwest
P.O. Box 4262, Spokane, WA 99202   (509) 459-8502

CANADA

Canadian Vegans for Animal Rights
620 Jarvis St.,Ste. 2504, Toronto, Ontario
M4Y 2R8   (416) 924-1377

Ottawa Vegetarian Society
P.O. Box 4477, Station E, Ottawa, Ontario K1R 6P9   (613) 230-1798

Toronto Vegetarian Association
736 Bathurst St., Toronto, Ontario, M5S 2R4   (416) 533-3897

Vancouver Island Vegetarian Association
529 Stornoway Dr., Victoria, British Columbia
V9C 3G8   (604) 478-8477

Vegetarians of Alberta
9211 72nd St., Edmonton, Alberta T6B 146   (403) 469-1448

CAMPS OFFERING VEGETARIAN MEALS

When the cry of "School's out for the summer" echoes across North America, legions of youngsters trade their school jackets for camp tee-shirts. Happily, vegetarian youngsters can find a variety of camps that will cater to their diets.

The Vegetarian Resource Group conducted a mail survey of more than 2,000 camps throughout the United States and parts of Canada. In addition to completing the survey, many camps ordered recipe packets and subscriptions to *Vegetarian Journal*–a sign of their commitment to the vegetarian lifestyle. The survey asked each camp whether it offered vegetarian meals, either upon request or as an option at every meal. The same question was asked with respect to vegan meals and kosher meals. We also asked camps to list some of the vegetarian dishes they prepare and to note whether they will cater to special dietary needs.

The following is a summary of the responses we received from this survey. Since we intend to keep this list updated, we'd like to hear about your experiences obtaining vegetarian meals at the camps listed. We'd also like information about any other camps that serve vegetarian and/or vegan meals.

VEGETARIAN CAMPS OR CAMPS WITH A LARGE VEGETARIAN CLIENTELE

NEW YORK

CAMP TE' YEHUDA located in New York City offers vegetarian/vegan/kosher meals as options at every meal. Regular vegetarian food service is available for those campers who register as vegetarians. For further information write to Camp Te' Yehuda, 50 West 58th Street, New York, NY 10019, or call (212) 246-9215.

VERMONT

CRAFTSBURY SPORTS CENTER offers programs in running, sculling (rowing), weight loss, walking, bird watching, swimming, guided nature walks, etc. (Beware that fly-fishing is also taught.) All ages and abilities are welcome.

Vegetarian meals are always offered as an option. Dishes served include Mushroom-Tofu Stroganoff, Spinach Casserole, Ground Nut Stew, Lasagna, Pizza, Chili, Hummus, Mushroom Pâté, seitan, and homemade breads, salads, and soups. The camp frequently accommodates those who eat fat-free or yeast- and gluten-free diets, diabetics, and vegans. For information write to Craftsbury Sports Center, P.O. Box 31, Craftsbury Common, VT 05827, or call (802) 586-7767.

KILLOOLEET says that 20 percent of its campers sign up for vegetarian dinners and that all other meals are vegetarian. Some of the dishes served include Vegetable Lasagna, Chili, Stuffed Peppers, Quiche, Pita with Hummus, and Zucchini Fritata. Killoolet will cater to campers who are allergic to milk, milk products, and/or wheat. Write to Killooleet, Hancock, VT 05748, or call (802) 767-3152 for further information.

VIRGINIA

LEGACY INTERNATIONAL is a nonprofit, educational organization, affiliated with the United Nations Department of Public Information as a non-governmental organization. The camp offers vegetarian meals primarily, but will occasionally serve meat dishes, too. Many international vegetarian dishes are served, prepared with foods such as whole grains, legumes, breads, a variety of vegetables, some dairy products and eggs, fruits, and nuts. The camp is happy to accommodate non-dairy or non-wheat diets.

Campers aged eleven through eighteen come from around the world and have ample time to enjoy Legacy's various workshops, including "Intrigued by International Affairs? — Leadership and Global Issues"; "Motivated to Help the Environment?"; "Concerned about Resolving Conflicts?"; "Inspired to Promote Global Thinking through Theater Arts?"; and "Attracted to Serving Others?" For information write to Legacy International, c/o Mary Helmig, Route 4, Box 265, Bedford, VA 24523, or call (703) 297-5982.

CANADA

AU GRAND BOIS is a nonprofit camp and resource center located on 565 acres of rolling hills, woods, fields, streams, and ponds in Quebec, Canada. The camp serves vegetarian meals including grains, beans, vegetables, nuts and seeds, fruits and a few dairy products. No eggs are used. Campers may also choose non-dairy and macrobiotic meals. An organic garden supplies the camp with fresh greens and some vegetables.

Au Grand Bois accommodates children and teens between the ages of eight and sixteen. Since it is a small camp with approximately fifty children per session, everyone gets to know one another and some nice friendships are made. Activities reflect the camp's desire to encourage respect for others and an understanding of our natural environment. For further information write to Lenny and Arleen Prost, Au Grand Bois, Ladysmith, Quebec J0X 2A0, Canada, or call (819) 647-3522.

CAMPS OFFERING VEGETARIAN MEALS AS AN OPTION AT EACH MEAL

CALIFORNIA

BOYS AND GIRLS CLUB OF HOLLYWOOD CAMP offers vegetarian meals as options at each meal and vegan meals are available upon request. For information write to Boys and Girls Club of Hollywood Camp, 2103 Wilderness Road, P.O. Box 751, Running Springs, CA 92382, or call (714) 867-2155.

MONTECITO-SEQUOIA FAMILY VACATION CAMP offers vegetarian meals as options at each meal and vegan meals upon request. Dinners are served buffet-style, and a salad bar is available. Write to Montecito-Sequoia Family Vacation Camp, Box 858 Grant Grove, Kings Canyon, CA 93633, or call (209) 565-3388 for information.

COLORADO

TROJAN SUMMER CAMP has vegetarian meals as options at every meal. Write to Trojan Summer Camp, P.O. Box 711, Boulder, CO 80306, or call (303) 442-4557 for details.

CONNECTICUT

CAMP HORIZONS, a camp for people who are mentally handicapped, offers vegetarian meals as options at every meal. Mexican dishes and other homemade vegetarian dishes are prepared. Meals are served family-style. For more information, write to Camp Horizons, P.O. Box 323, South Windham, CT 06266, or call (203) 456-1032.

INDIANA

CAMP ALEXANDER MACK offers both vegetarian and vegan meals as options at every meal. Diabetic campers or those needing low-cholesterol, or low-sodium diets can be accommodated. Write to Camp Alexander Mack, P.O. Box 158, Milford, IN 46542, or call (219) 658-4831 for information.

MAINE

CAMP MATOAKA FOR GIRLS offers both vegetarian and vegan meals as options at every meal. The camp will cater to campers who are lactose intolerant and to dieters. For details, write to Camp Matoaka for Girls, RFD 2, East Lake, Oakland, ME 04963, or call (407) 488-6363.

KINGSLEY PINES CAMP offers both vegetarian and vegan meals as options at each meal. Italian and Chinese dishes are sometimes available. Write to Kingsley Pines Camp, 113 Plains Road, Raymond, ME 04071, or call (207) 773-4621 for further information.

MASSACHUSETTS

ROWE CAMP for adults, young people, and families is located in Rowe, Massachusetts. It offers vegetarian meals as options at every meal and vegan meals upon request. The camp uses as many regional and local foods as possible and fresh baked goods are offered at most meals. The camp will try to accommodate all dietary needs. For information, write to Rowe Camp, Kings Highway Road, Rowe, MA 01367, or call (413) 339-4954.

MICHIGAN

CIRCLE PINES CENTER offers vegetarian meals as options at every meal and vegan meals upon request. Meals are served family-style, and locally grown organic produce is used as much as possible. For information, write to Circle Pines Center, 8650 Mullen Road, Delton, MI 49046, or call (616) 623-5555.

NEW HAMPSHIRE

INTERLOCKEN INTERNATIONAL SUMMER CAMP offers vegetarian meals as options at every meal and vegan meals upon request. Meals include meatless pizza, chili, and lasagna. A salad bar is available along with fresh breads. Campers can choose what they wish as they go through the meal lines. For information, write to Interlocken International Summer Camp, RR 2, Box 165, Hillsboro, NH 03244, or call (603) 478-3166.

NEW JERSEY

CAMP DARK WATERS offers both vegetarian and vegan meals as options at every meal. Write to Camp Dark Waters, P.O. Box 263, Medford, NJ 08055-0263, or call (609) 654-8846 for further information.

NEW YORK

CAMP KINDERLAND is located in New York City. Vegetarian meals are offered as options at every meal. For details write to Camp Kinderland, 1 Union Square West, New York, NY 10003, or call (212) 255-6283.

CAMP REGIS-APPLEJACK, located in White Plains, New York, offers vegetarian meals as options at every meal. For information write to Camp Regis-Applejack, 107 Robinhood Road, White Plains, NY 10605, or call (914) 997-7039.

CAMP SOMERHILL is situated in the Adirondack Mountains near Lake George, New York. The camp offers both vegetarian and vegan meals as options at every meal. A salad bar is available and cafeteria-style service is provided. For information write to Camp Somerhill, 20 Huntley Road, Box 295, Eastchester, NY 10709, or call (914) 793-1303.

NORTH CAROLINA

CAMP JUDAEA offers kosher vegetarian meals as options at every meal. Vegan meals are available upon request. Vegetarian dishes include falafel, vegetarian hot dogs, and lasagna. For details, write to Camp Judaea, Rt. 9, Box 395, Hendersonville, NC 28739, or call (404) 634-7883.

PENNSYLVANIA

KEN CREST offers vegetarian meals as options at every meal and vegan meals upon request. Different combinations of pasta and quiches, plus much more are offered. Write to Ken Crest, Rt. 29, Mont Clare, PA 19453, or call (215) 935-1581.

VIRGINIA

CAMP HANOVER offers vegetarian meals as options at many meals and upon request. Dishes served include lasagna, chili, and squash/zucchini casserole. A sandwich and salad bar is also available. Freshly baked bread is offered. For further information write to Camp Hanover, Rt. 1, Box 492, Mechanicsville, VA 23111, or call (804) 779-2811.

WEST VIRGINIA

CAMP ALLEGHANY offers both vegetarian and vegan meals as options at every meal. Camp cooks bake their own bread. Write to Camp Alleghany, Greenbrier County, Lewisburg, WV 24901-0086, or call (304) 645-1316.

WISCONSIN

CAMP INTERLAKEN offers kosher vegetarian meals as options at each meal and vegan meals upon request. Write to Camp Interlaken, 6255 North Santa Monica Blvd., Milwaukee, WI 53217, or call (414) 964-4444.

MENOMINEE SPORTS CAMP FOR BOYS offers vegetarian and vegan meals as options at every meal. For information, write to Menominee Sports Camp for Boys, 4985 Highway D, Eagle River, WI 54521, or call (715) 479-CAMP.

CAMPS OFFERING VEGETARIAN MEALS UPON REQUEST

CALIFORNIA

CAMP A-LOT
5384 Linda Vista Road #100, San Diego, CA 92110   (619) 574-7575

PILGRIM PINES
39566 Clearwater, Yucaipa, CA 92399   (714) 797-1821

SKY MOUNTAIN CHRISTIAN CAMP
P.O. Box 79, Emigrant Gap, CA 95715   (916) 389-2118

COLORADO

CHELEY COLORADO CAMPS, INC.
P.O. Box 6525, Denver, CO 80206

COLORADO LIONS CAMP
FOR THE HANDICAPPED
P.O. Box 90434, Woodland Park, CO 80866   (219) 687-2087

PRESBYTERIAN HIGHLANDS CAMP
P.O. Box 446, Allenspark, CO 80510   (303) 747-2888

GEORGIA

CAMP PINE ACRES
100 Edgewood Avenue, Suite 1100, Atlanta, GA 30303   (404) 527-7500

ILLINOIS

CAMP MEDILL McCORMICK
P.O. Box 1616, Rockford, IL 61110   (815) 962-5591

WOODLAND FOR GIRLS
AND TOWERING PINES FOR BOYS
242 Bristol Street, Northfield, IL 60093   (708) 446-7311

MASSACHUSETTS

CAMP YAVNEH
43 Hawes Street , Brookline, MA 02146   (617) 739-0363

MICHIGAN

JUDSON COLLINS CAMP
1000 Hane Highway, Onsted, MI 49265   (517) 467-7711

PRESBYTERIAN CAMPS
631 Perryman Street, Saugatuck, MI 49453   (616) 857-2531

MISSOURI

SALVATION ARMY CAMP MO-KAN
16200 East 40 Highway, Kansas City, MO 64136   (816) 373-4153

NEW HAMPSHIRE

WAUKEELA CAMP
Rt. 153, Eatoo Center, NH 03832   (603) 447-2260

NEW JERSEY

CAMP TECUMSEH
4 Gary Road, P.O. Box 3170, Union, NJ 07083   (908) 851-9300

NEW YORK

BACO/CHE-NA-WAH
80 Neptune Avenue, Woodmere, NY 11598   (516) 374-7757

CAMP MONROE
P.O. Box 475, Monroe, NY 10950   (914) 782-8695

NORTH CAROLINA

CAMP ELLIOTT
601 Camp Elliott Road, Black Mountain, NC 28711   (704) 669-8639

CAMP NEW HOPE
4805 Highway 86, Chapel Hill, NC 27516   (919) 942-4716

OHIO

CAMP ALLYN
1414 Lake Allyn Road, Batavia, OH 45103

OREGON

TILIKUM RETREAT CENTER
15321 NE North Valley, Newberg, OR 97132   (503) 538-2763

PENNSYLVANIA

CAMP BLUE DIAMOND
Box 240, Petersburg, PA 16669-0240   (814) 667-2355

CAMP EDER
914 Mt. Hope Road, Fairfield, PA 17320   (717) 642-8256

WASHINGTON

BUCK CREEK CAMP
67404 S.R. 410 East, Enumclaw, WA 98022   (206) 663-2201

RESTAURANT SURVEY FORM

Restaurants continually change locations, new ones open, and others close. Please help us to update the next edition of this book by returning this survey with any new information we should have. Feel free to make copies of this form. Your help and support are greatly appreciated.

Return to Restaurant Survey, The Vegetarian Resource Group, P.O. Box 1463, Baltimore, MD 21203. Please include a menu. Call (410) 366-VEGE.

RESTAURANT NAME: _____

STREET ADDRESS:_____

CITY:_____

STATE OR PROVINCE: _____ ZIP:_____

TELEPHONE NUMBER: (_____) _____

Please circle choice(s):

TYPE OF RESTAURANT: Vegetarian (no meat, fish, fowl); Vegan (no meat, fish, fowl, dairy, eggs); Natural Foods; Macrobiotic; California style; American; Juice Bar; Juice Bar in Natural Foods Store; Take-Out Only; Italian; Chinese; Indian; Thai; Middle Eastern; Mexican; Other: _____

DESCRIPTION/SPECIAL FEATURES (examples of dishes, special foods, decor, music, view; what makes this place special?):

_____

_____

_____

Formal restaurant (you need to dress up); Typical, informal; Suitable for business entertaining; Earthy; Totally non-smoking

HOURS:_____

MEALS SERVED: Breakfast   Lunch   Dinner
Late evening service   Sunday brunch   Open 24 hours

TYPE OF SERVICE: Full service (regular table service); Cafeteria; Take-out; Take-out only; Limited service (order at counter, but food taken to table); Counter service (eat at counter); Catering

RESERVATIONS: Required; Recommended; Not needed; Not taken

OPTIONS: Vegan (no meat, fish, fowl, dairy, eggs); Macrobiotic; Vegetarian

BEVERAGES: Juices made in the store (e.g. carrot juice); Espresso; Cappuccino; Non-alcoholic beer or wine; Smoothies; Soy milk; Special drinks; Beer; Wine; Alcohol

CREDIT CARDS: Visa   Mastercard   American Express
Discover   Diners Club

COST: $–less than $6 ; $$–$6–$12; $$$–more than $12

Should this restaurant be given a four-carrot rating? _____

NAME OF READER:_____

ADDRESS:_____

CITY: _____

STATE OR PROVINCE: _____ **ZIP:**_____

TELEPHONE NUMBER: (_____)_____

Attach to this questionnaire any additional comments you may have.

VEGETARIAN JOURNAL

The practical magazine for those interested in health, ecology, and ethics.

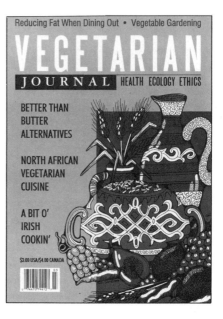

Each issue features:
- **Nutrition Hotline** -- answers your questions about vegetarian diets.
- **Low-fat Vegetarian Recipes** -- quick and easy dishes, international cuisine, and gourmet meals.
- **Natural Food Product Reviews**
- **Scientific Updates** -- a look at recent scientific papers relating to vegetarianism.
- **Vegetarian Action** -- projects by individuals and groups.

VEGETARIAN Journal ISSN 0885-7636 is published bi-monthly by the independent Vegetarian Resource Group.

To receive a one year subscription, send a check for $20.00 to The Vegetarian Resource Group, PO Box 1463, Baltimore, MD 21203. Canadian and Mexican subscriptions are $30.00 per year and must be paid in U.S. funds. All other foreign countries subscriptions are $40.00 per year and must be paid in U.S. funds.

Name:_____

Address: _____

_____Zip: _____